SELECTED PAPERS ON ELECTROCARDIOGRAPHY OF WILLEM EINTHOVEN

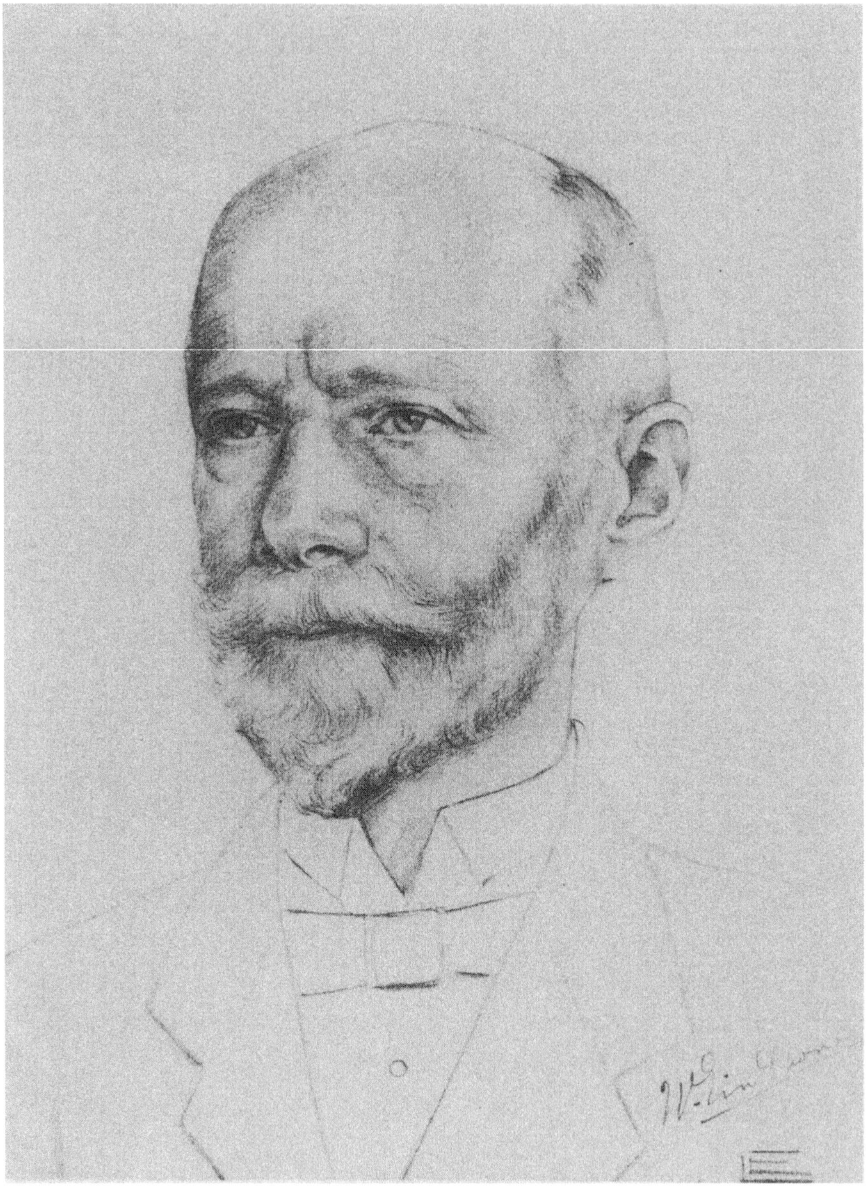

WILLEM EINTHOVEN

SELECTED PAPERS ON ELECTROCARDIOGRAPHY OF WILLEM EINTHOVEN

WITH A BIBLIOGRAPHY,
BIOGRAPHICAL NOTES AND COMMENTS
BY

H. A. SNELLEN

LEIDEN UNIVERSITY PRESS
1977

ISBN-13: 978-94-010-1303-1 e-ISBN-13: 978-94-010-1301-7
DOI: 10.1007/ 978-94-010-1301-7

Softcover reprint of the hardcover 1st edition 1977

ACKNOWLEDGEMENTS

The helpful cooperation of the Museum Boerhaave, the department of Physiology and the University Library of Leiden is gratefully acknowledged.

Financial assistance was given by the «Leids Universiteits-Fonds» and by the Herman Snellen Fund from the cardiological department of Leiden University.

TABLE OF CONTENTS

INTRODUCTION

It is not difficult to explain why it was decided to reproduce some of Einthoven's papers with photographic fidelity. The immense amount of information provided by electrocardiography, which in spite of its natural limitations has become one of the main diagnostic procedures in cardiology and at the same time a cornerstone of scientific research, is universally acknowledged. On the other hand, we have also come to realize how important it is not only to know the historical perspective of cardiology, or any other field of medicine, but also to study the original sources from which our knowledge stems, without the contamination of later opinions or traditional interpretation, however well founded they may seem.*

There is also a reason for the timing of this publication of facsimile reprints: Einthoven died 50 years ago; about 75 years ago the string galvanometer was invented and used for electrocardiography (first publication on the instrument in 1901, first publication of electrocardiograms taken with it in 1903). The papers, which are reproduced here, constitute a selection, necessarily limited and arbitrarily chosen. I should like to add, that the selection was made from several points of view.

In the first place, only those articles were selected which had a definite and direct relation with cardiology, in particular electrocardiography. Although it is obvious from Einthoven's bibliography (chapter 2) that several of his papers deal with other subjects, the prominent place which electrocardiography occupies in Einthoven's work, justifies this choice. Only one paper from this selection is concerned with the string galvanometer itself. It describes the new instrument for the first time in its essential features. Later papers about it often have a strictly mathematical and/or technical character.

Secondly, Einthoven published in several languages: Dutch, German, French and English. It was felt that, as this book is intended for an international public, it was desirable to omit all Dutch papers (although included in the bibliography of chapter 2), and to shift the emphasis from German (the language in which most of Einthoven's publications were

* Footnote. Of course the advantage of photographic reproduction is still more evident, if the publication is older (c.f. the papers on angina pectoris and cardiac infarction, republished earlier). However, even during Einthoven's lifetime and shortly after, misunderstandings and misrepresentations of his writings were already frequent; they became more so when Frank Wilson, who was probably his best interpreter, also died.

N.B. For references see ch. I.

written) to English. Some important articles in French have also been included.

Thirdly, given these priorities and the necessary limitation in number of papers, the first publications (including the lesser known) of any particular aspect were preferred. In chapter 3 more detailed information about the selected papers is given.

It should be added, that this kind of selection was possible, and at the same time necessary, because Einthoven repeatedly published some papers without any substantial changes in two or even three different languages. Moreover, he occasionally published a second article on the same subject in more detail and in another language.

A comprehensive review of Einthoven's work on electrocardiography was given by himself in one of his last publications: his acceptance speech at the Nobel Prize ceremony (134, A, 13 E). This lecture, read in German, was published as such by the Nobel Foundation in 1926 and again in 1965 in English. The latter version was chosen; it is a fitting conclusion to this series of reprints, which, as I hope, illustrates clearly the fundamental but also very practical, and far-seeing but always rectilinear character of Einthoven's work. A more comprehensive and general review of electrocardiography was completed by Einthoven at the end of his life and published posthumously in Bethe's Handbuch der normalen und pathologischen Physiologie. It contains interesting indications about the final stage of development of Einthoven's ideas and is therefore quoted several times in chapter I, which contains an introduction to Einthoven's work. This chapter gives only limited information about the general history of electrocardiography; for a complete review the reader can be referred to Burch and DePasquale (b).

CHAPTER 1

LIFE AND WORK OF WILLEM EINTHOVEN (1860-1927)*

Einthoven's life was outwardly uneventful; his personality made it rich. The latter is so interwoven with his work, that there is little to be gained from a separate discussion of both. After a very brief review of the course of his life I shall therefore try to describe Einthoven's personality and his work together, often quoting his friends and contemporary colleagues. What they wrote about Einthoven, is largely contained in obituaries or later commemorative tributes and perhaps may appear biased. On the other hand, a statement of this kind may reveal deeply felt and well considered thoughts, which were not and perhaps could not be expressed during Einthoven's lifetime.

As far as his work is concerned, this chapter leads the way to the complete bibliography in chapter 2 and to the selected papers in chapter 3.

Willem Einthoven's father was an army doctor and later a public health officer in the (then) Dutch East Indies. He died in 1866, when his son Willem was only 6 years old, leaving a widow with six children, among whom Willem was the eldest son with two older sisters. Mrs. Einthoven left for Holland four years later, together with her unmarried brother, who stayed with her when she settled in Utrecht. It was there that Einthoven was educated and where he studied medicine, accepting a government grant which committed him to a career in the Dutch colonial army. Early in his studies he made his first scientific contribution when he broke his wrist during gymnastics (Einthoven was a keen and allround sportsman in his youth). As a result of this accident his attention was drawn to the articulation of the elbow, which he studied thoroughly (42). Equally characteristic, he overcame the handicap in his movements by rigorous and successful training in fencing.

As a young assistant to the ophthalmologist H. Snellen, and wishing to specialize in this field, he came into closer contact with Donders, the famous physiologist and pioneer in ophthalmology. This led to Einthoven's thesis in 1885 on stereoscopy by difference in colour. Soon after this, the chair of physiology in Leiden became vacant and Einthoven was

* N.B. References, indicated with numbers, are listed in the bibliography of chapter 2; those indicated with letters will be found at the end of this chapter. An asterix is added to the number, if that specific paper has been reprinted in full in chapter 3.

appointed in spite of his youth. He soon obtained his medical license, was released from his army engagements – at great financial sacrifice – and went to Leiden where he remained for his entire life.

His first publication from Leiden concerned subjects which he had encountered in Donders' laboratory. One of these was a very original, until lately insufficiently recognized, experimental research into bronchial function, by which he identified bronchial spasm as the cause of asthma. (10,13,14). An interesting opportunity for another study offered itself when the professor of surgery van Iterson showed him a patient, whose left upper jaw and orbita had been resected so extensively for carcinoma, that the movements of the soft palate could be viewed and photographed. This led to the writing of a chapter on the physiology of the pharynx in Heymann's Handbuch der Laryngologie (42) and some other papers (40,417). Soon however, his main interest shifted to electrophysiology, in particular that of the heart, after Waller (c,d,e) had shown that electrical currents accompanying the heart-beat could be recorded from the human body. The appeal of electrophysiology to Einthoven was probably however, not only founded on the new and unexplored character of this field but also on the opportunity for exact registration and measurement of organic activity, which it provided. For, as Samojloff, his Russian colleague and long time friend, later wrote (f) "His mind was like an instrument of precision. He worked only on what could be measured and his measurements reached the limit of precision possible under the circumstances."

Einthoven's first step was to study the best available instrument for measuring small and rapid changes in potential: the capillary electrometer, introduced by Lippmann (a glass capillary, filled with mercury and sulphuric acid, the boundary between these two moving with change of potential). As Wiggers pointed out in 1960 (g): "It is at this point, that we gain a good insight into Einthoven's genius – a human trait, that Carlisle has defined as 'the ability to take infinite pains' ". Einthoven like several other physiologists, was naturally impelled to repeat Waller's significant observations. Instead of merely using such capillary electrometers as were available in his laboratory, he first tested their physical characteristics and found that their performance could be materially improved by attention to minor expedients, including the resistance of the external circuits. "Through technical improvements of the instrument and of the recording system he was able to obtain tracings, which Wiggers called "immeasurably superior to those recorded by Waller."

The first two human electrocardiograms taken in Leiden (the third and fourth in history after those of Waller and of Bayliss and Starling) were published in the thesis of Einthoven's assistant de Vogel (1893 h). The curves showed two small deflections for each heart-beat: a rapid, followed by a slow, respectively called p and q and presumably corresponding to our present R and T waves. In 1894 Einthoven and Geluk (20*) were able to present a method for registration of heart sounds, by which frequencies could be recorded beyond those of the human voice. Their main object was to use the time interval between the heart sounds for measuring the length of the systole, which at that time was a point of controversy, ranging from the whole to less than half of the plateau in the apex cardiogram (estimations by Marey and Landois respectively, as quoted by Einthoven in an address to a Dutch medical audience in 1893. This address is interesting because Einthoven introduced therein the brand-new electrocardiogram as a method of clinical examination and also stressed the necessity for standardizing the units of potential and time to allow comparison of different electrocardiograms). The time relations of the heart sounds with the carotid pulse and apex beat were also studied by Einthoven and Geluk. This first publication in the literature of a detailed registration of the heart sounds was completed by an abnormal phonocardiogram i.e. that of experimental aortic insufficiency in the dog. It showed the typical crescendo-decrescendo contour of the diastolic murmur, which was compared to a pulse wave. The sound waves were not further analysed.

In the same year 1894, however, Einthoven published a paper on the registration of rapidly changing potentials (18,19). He showed that, although the capillary electrometer was the most suitable instrument then available for this purpose, the friction of the mercury and sulphuric acid when moving in a capillary caused a deformation of the registered curve, which had to be corrected mathematically. For this purpose he used a method (44,46) which was different to and developed independently from that of Burch (i). In 1895 Einthoven applied this method of correction to the electrocardiogram and showed its true form (26). While in the recorded curve 4 peaks were visible indicated as A,B,C,D, the corrected curve now showed 5 peaks, which Einthoven called P,Q,R,S,T. From these R,S, and T were recognized as belonging to ventricular activity, while P and Q were tentatively ascribed to atrial contraction. Standardization regarding potential differences (at this time still in Millidaniell) and speed of registration was also introduced. Further studies to investigate the importance of different leads (at this period both hands were always used, i.e. lead I), of the body position, and of heart frequency, were planned as well as comparisons between different individuals and between patients and normal subjects.

This ambitious programme, which was to occupy electrocardiography for many years, had already been carried out to a certain extent, when a later publication (with the Lint) (48) on the electrocardiogram appeared in 1900. A series of normal electrocardiograms in their original and corrected form was studied with relation to the leads used (divided, as Waller did, in favorable and infavorable, i.e. of high and low voltage). Potential differences were now expressed in Millivolts. The essential similarity of different normal electrocardiograms was emphasized and the time lag between electrocardiogram and the apex beat cardiogram was measured. In connection with the latter, the relation between electrical and mechanical activity was discussed explicitly for the first time. Einthoven returned to this subject more than once, finally summarising his view on the invariably linked and simultaneous appearance of these two functions in his lecture for the Harvey Society of New York (132*). It is important to note that the (corrected) electrocardiograms of 2 patients with aortic insufficiency were also shown; they displayed in lead I a flat and a negative T wave respectively.

At this stage it becomes obvious, how logically and consistently Einthoven proceeded in his investigations. After having obtained the "true" (corrected) electrocardiogram, he realized that the mathematical correction would have to be replaced by a directly registered, but equally reliable tracing, if the electrocardiogram was to be used more generally, as he hoped and believed it would. In this he was greatly helped by his mathematical and physical capabilities. As expressed by the physiologist A.V. Hill (j): "Einthoven, in spite of his medical training and his office was essentially a physicist, and the extraordinary value of his contributions to physiology, and therewith indirectly to medicine, emphasises the way in which an aptitude – in Einthoven's case a genius – for physical methods can aid in the solution of physiological problems". There will be another opportunity to comment on Einthoven's relationship to medicine at the end of this chapter. With regard to mathematics (and physics) it is interesting to quote from a letter which Einthoven wrote to Frank Wilson, after his visit to Ann Arbor during his 1924 tour of the United States: "May I send you the excellent book of Lorentz 'Differential- und Integralrechnung.' I have learnt my mathematics from it after my nomination a a professor in this University, and I hope you will have as much pleasure and profit by it as I have had myself."

The considerations which led Einthoven to construct the string galvanometer were based on calculations designed to improve sensitivity and speed simultaneously, starting from the most rapid instrument available i.e. the mirror galvanometer of Deprez-d'Arsonval. Its mirror was attached to a coil with many turns of conducting wire and suspended between the poles of a magnet. Einthoven calculated that sensivity could be enhanced by reducing the number of turns as far as possible (i.e. to a straight wire) and by minimising dimensions and weight, therefore omitting the mirror, but increasing the range of recordable deflections by observation through a microscope and intensifying the magnetic field. During the subsequent investigations, which continued for several years, Einthoven was confronted with many technical and physical problems which he studied exhaustively. This resulted in publications in the "Annalen der Physik" and the "Proceedings of the Kon. Akademie voor Wetenschappen" on such subjects as damping (electrical and mechanical), isolation against vibrations in the environment, mass and tension of the string, visibility of thin threads etc. Finally, in 1909 (95) he published all details of the construction of his galvanometer, which was of course tantamount to waiving any inventors's rights.

The first publication of the string galvanometer was in 1901 (52*), while more detailed papers with reproduction of electrocardiograms (58,59* and a technical discussion of the instrument (60)) were published in 1903. The same man whose corrected electrocardiogram had been published in 1900, was then re-examined and the identity of both tracings established. In substance all the technical research described above, was foreseen and prepared in these first publications. In a sense therefore Wenckebach (k) was justified in saying "Dieses wunderbare Instrument kam, wie Pallas Athene aus dem Kopf von Zeus, vollendet aus einem Haupte zur Welt."

It was pointed out by Einthoven (52) that a publication by Ader from 1897 dealing with a string instrument for use in telegraphy had come to his attention in the meantime. In accordance with Ader's purpose, speed of deflection was the chief requirement; its sensitivity was about 100.000 times less than the string galvanometer, as Einthoven later estimated (95).

In the publication of 1903 the definitive standardization of voltage and recording speed, now still in use, was introduced, but not yet that of leads, although the necessity for consistently using the same leads was mentioned. An observation, already made in 1895, was confirmed, i.e. of the occurrence of small vibrations in the electrocardiogram, independent of the heart-beat. It was now concluded that they must originate inside the body, but their muscular origin was not yet established.

A very important step forward was taken in 1906. In "Le Télécardiogramme" (77) Einthoven described his arrangements for examining patients in the hospital through a long distance connection (a specially stabilised telephone cable) to the string galvanometer in his laboratory, thereby initiating its use as a diagnostic tool. The three leads were taken, which became customary from then on. Although they were defined in words rather numbered, the principle of what was later called Einthoven's law (we shall return later to this unjustified term), i.e. lead I = lead II - lead III, was mentioned. Various electrocardiograms of patients were shown, which were pathological both in terms of hypertrophy (auricular in cases of mitral stenosis, but also left ventricular in aortic insufficiency) of arrhythmia. The latter included several examples of ventricular extrasystoles, which enabled Einthoven to warn the clinician by telephone, that an intermission of the pulse was imminent. It appears that this and perhaps even more his occasional electrocardiographic arguments against a clinical diagnosis displeased the clinicians so much, that in due course the latter severed the connection (Hoogewerf (1)). Other types of arrhythmia e.g. atrial flutter and fibrillation[1], were also observed, but not or incompletely understood. A case of clinical heart block was presented together with some tracings of experimental heart block from vagal stimulation in the dog. The occurrence of a U wave was also shown for the first time.[2]

In this same period Einthoven again published registrations of heart sounds, together with Flohil and Battaerd (79,82,87*). (The latter wrote subsequently in more detail on this subject in Heart (m)). The lack of corrected tracings in the publication of 1894 was now compensated by a new and much improved technique. Several new examples of pathological phonocardiograms were shown, in particular from a patient with mitral stenosis and insufficiency, with a presystolic, systolic and diastolic murmur. These phonocardiograms were taken with the long distance connection described in "Le Télécardiogramme" and were meant to demonstrate their usefulness for clinical diagnosis. It should be noted that for this phonocardiographic study no mechanical reference tracings could be used. One could add, however, that the carotid pulse and apex beat tracings from the earlier publication (20*) were definitely less informative than those published much earlier by Marey (n). There was in fact a certain lack of interest on Einthoven's part in findings that could be interpreted haemodynamically and clinically, but not measured quantitatively. Wit regard to the apex cardiogram, he complained about its

[1] For atrial flutter this was pointed out by Einthoven himself in his last and comprehensive publication on the electrocardiogram (137), in which he again showed the same tracing. Atrial fibrillation was discussed by him in a publication of 1911 (98).

[2] This article in French has twice been translated in part into English and published in the American Heart Journal (77A and 77B).

inconstancy and inexactitude as opposed to the electrocardiogram (90*). At this time (1907) Einthoven did not yet possess a combined set of 2 galvanometers, and therefore could not add an electrocardiogram as reference tracing to the "cardiophonogram" as he called his sound registration. Later he recorded from two or even three string galvanometers simultaneously (107,108,111) and Battaerd was able to use this method in his paper, cited above (m). Before doing so Einthoven sometimes combined phonocardiogram and electrocardiogram in one single curve, to identify simultaneous points of the ECG in different leads, as published by Fahr in Heart (15).

A separate publication (83,84,85,86) was devoted to his discovery of the third heart sound which turned out to be a confirmation of an auscultatory observation by Gibson. In this case mechanical tracings were used for identification of this sound and its possible cause. Einthoven sought the latter in aftervibration of the aortic valves, because the third sound occurred immediately after the second aortic sound. He found this third heart sound originally in a healthy young man, but later in several other subjects in whom it was weaker and less certain.

From his electrophysiological studies of nerves and sense organs I can mention the demonstration of two sets of centripetal impulses in the vagus nerve, simultaneous with respiration and heart beat respectively (91,92* 94). In other studies Einthoven examined the effect of vagus stimulation upon the heart (97,100,103), especially in the occurrence of heart block (already observed and described in 78* and 90*) and of changes in the shape of P and T waves.

Perhaps the most influential and certainly the best known conception of Einthoven was his scheme of the equilateral triangle, combined with the rule of lead I = lead II - lead III. It was pointed out by Einthoven that the latter was a self-evident truth (he would certainly have been surprised to hear it called Einthoven's law). Self-evident, because the potential difference between two points must always be the same, irrespective of the way chosen for proceeding from one to the other. Einthoven was aware, however, that this truth is not always obvious if you compare R waves etc. from different leads, because these waves, although bearing the same name, are not always completely synchronous. The scheme of the equilateral triangle was evolved in order to explain both the difference between the electrocardiographic complexes in the three leads and the change brought about in one lead (in particular lead III) by variations in the position of the heart. The latter are usually caused either by respiration or by shifting the position of the body.

Einthoven gave a lecture to the Chelsea Clinical Society in London on the different forms of the human electrocardiogram and their significance, which was published in the Lancet (99*). In this lecture he reviewed several of his earlier findings and at the same time introduced his equilateral triangle and the rule of the link between the three leads, mentioned above. Einthoven himself was not quite satisfied with the way in which his paper was published (typographical errors such as Wilhelm for his first name, reduction in size of the figures etc.). Perhaps he also said too little about the schematic, but for practical purposes sufficiently accurate character of his concept. A year later he published with Fahr and de Waart his famous, more elaborate article on the triangle (102). As this has been translated into English and published in the American Heart Journal (102 A), it seemed more interesting to reprint the earlier paper from the Lancet, because, concise as it may be, it contains every really important aspect. This choice was the more attractive as it proved possible to add some elucidation by Einthoven himself in answer to questions from Lewis (in 1915) and Frank Wilson (in 1921).[3] It is interesting to note that in his Lancet article (99*) Einthoven stressed the fact that he was concerned with the momentary magnitude (and direction) of the combined potential differences in the heart and that it is irrelevant in this connection, whether one thinks of an integration of the electrical activity of the base and the apex of the heart, or of the left and right heart, or even of two different strata of heart muscle. This thought was repeatedly expressed by Einthoven during the following years, up to his last and posthumously published review of action currents of the heart (137).

However, in this last review he made an exception to a certain extent for Lewis's concept of the electrocardiogram as the result of interference of the electrical waves from the right and left heart (dextrogram and laevogram). Einthoven wrote in that chapter p. 832 (137): Die erst genannte Vorstellung, die von Selenius und Buchanan erörtert und namentlich von Lewis ausführlich begründet worden ist, hat den groszen Vorzug vor allen anderen, dass sie eine anatomische und physiologische Grundlage hat. Die beiden Schenkel functionieren nicht immer gleich. Wenn der rechte seine Leitfähigkeit verloren hat, oder wenn ein Reiz autonom im linken Schenkel entsteht, zieht sich der linke Ventrikel früher als der rechte zusammen. Es kommen dann im Anfang der Systole die Folgen der Systole des linken Herzens allein zum Ausdruck".

[3] Permission was granted by the Museum Boerhaave of Leiden to select and reproduce this correspondence. A survey of all Einthoven's documents, preserved in this Museum, will be published before long.

Einthoven was impressed by the synthesis, made by Lewis, of laevogram and dextrogram to a curve, which very much resembled the normal electrocardiogram. He was presumably also impressed by the seemingly overwhelming evidence from experimental bundle branch block in the dog and from the few human cases with electrocardiographic evidence, in which the histology of the conduction system was verified (e.g. Eppinger and Stoerk (p)). We know now, of course, that the histological examination was not so complete as it should have been, that human bundle branch block lesions are often partial and bilateral, and that infarction patterns may have interfered.[4] Moreover, the conclusions from experimental bundle branch block in the dog (in situ) were for several reasons not or only partly applicable to human cases. All of this resulted in an universally accepted, but mistaken notion about the pattern of right and left bundle branch block in man, which had to be reversed after the paper of Wilson and his co-workers in 1932 (q).

This is one of the rare occasions on which Einthoven – although guardedly – favoured a hypothesis on a subject about which he himself had no exact data. However, as previously stated, his main concern was the summated electrical response of the heart and here his ideas proved very fruitful. His schematic concept of the manifest potential difference in the heart, which possesses – as he pointed out in his first article (99) – not only a definite magnitude but also a definite direction, in other words the characteristics of a vector, laid the foundation for vectorcardiography.[5]

In 1912 Einthoven reviewed in another paper critically (101) the various attempts at explaining the electrocardiogram and added his own, in which he again stressed the global, integrated nature of the electrocardiogram as the sum of all simultaneous potential differences in the heart at successive instants. He also mentioned in this context – and this was repeated in his last review (137) – that whichever of the existing theories one accepted for the electrical events at the local level, the fact had to be faced that the part of the muscle which is being activated, becomes negative (or less positive) compared with other parts. But in contrast to his papers from 1912, in later publications (122,129,134,137) he viewed the microscopical cardiac muscle segments (i.e. cells) as electrical units, which make the cardiac syncytial muscle different from the skeletal muscle with its long fibres. Einthoven refrained from a more detailed and

[4] From the history and the electrocardiogram it appears likely that this occurred in the case described by Kauf (r).

[5] Vectorcardiography was introduced in 1920 by Mann (s) as "a method of analysing the electrocardiogram". It was called monocardiogram by him.

speculative discussion, presumably because he saw no possibility of quantitative measurements at the cellular level.

The explanation of the electrocardiogram given in 1912, included the P wave as representing atrial activity, the QRS complex as ventricular activity with the T wave as its final phase of retreat. The U wave was regarded as a continuation of the same process. The difference in level between the PR-interval and the diastolic period, sometimes found in normals, was noticed and here tentatively ascribed to similar processes as those underlying the U wave. In the last review (137) the Ta wave was mentioned as an influence on the PR segment.

One of the non-electrocardiographic papers by Einthoven, but still of cardiological interest, concerned the height of the pulse of the unequal and irregular type, by then recognized to be caused by atrial fibrillation. Einthoven, together with Korteweg (109), pointed out that even though there is often some correlation with the length of the proceeding diastolic period[6] (and therefore with ventricular filling) this cannot be the only determinant. He showed that there was also an inverse correlation with the height of the preceding pulse and explained this on the basis of increased or diminished filling of the aorta with resultant change in the resistance to ventricular ejection. In other words, he stressed the significance of still earlier events than the diastole preceding the pulse, but did not envisage the heart rate as a determinant of contraction force as Kruta did in 1937 (t) and Rothberger and Sachs in 1938 (u).

In the early twenties an important technical gap could, at least in part, be overcome. This was best demonstrated on the two subsequent occasions in which Einthoven at the request of others, that is Byrnes and Karplus with Kreidl respectively, studied the action currents of the sympathic nerve.

Einthoven's string galvanometer and especially the instruments made in his own laboratory had proved a great advance in electrophysiology. The commercial types were divergent in quality, but in general less reliable. Yet, while the instrument could meet all requirements concerning action currents produced by cardiac and skeletal muscle, neural electrophysiology demanded much more speed and sensitivity in recording technique. Einthoven was therefore not satisfied with the results of the first investigation, although informative with respect to timing. (126). In accordance with his plans, announced in this paper, he experimented with further amplification through thermionic valves but was not satisfied thereby either. Only when he had completed – together with his son

[6] Mentioned earlier in a review from 1911 (98).

W. F. Einthoven, an engineer – the construction of a galvanometer with a much shorter and very thin string, placed in a vacuum, where even Brownian molecular movement could be a disturbing factor (134), he undertook to study the sympathic action currents again. Even so, the records show in retrospect that timing and appearance after stimulation of other centres – in this case the hypothalamus – could very well be examined, but that the finest details were not discernible (135). It is now obvious that improvement of amplification together with registration by inertia free electronic oscilloscopes have provided the only practicable road to rapid progress in this field.

It should be noted that the main use for the vacuum string galvanometer, indeed the object of its construction, was to establish wireless communication with the Dutch East Indies. The string functioned in this case as an electrically reverberating instrument which could be tuned to the incoming high frequency oscillations. It received the signals directly without rectification, which had not proved successful in earlier attempts. In 1932 the Einthovens were able to register Morse signals from Bandung as well as from stations in other countries (W. F. Einthoven (v)).

A similar short and very thin string placed in a funnel, was used as a resounding appliance for direct registration of sound (string phonograph of Einthoven and Hoogerwerf (127,128,129,135). With this very sensitive instrument it was possible to register the sound of a Galton whistle and to analyse the harmonics of vowels from human speech and song. It was concluded that the instrument would be useful in studying the physiology of voice and hearing, but here again, amplifying techniques soon offered an easier method.

At the end of this chapter some remarks of a general nature can be made. It appears that the most productive years of Einthoven's work were those before World War I culminating in his scheme of the equilateral triangle and the determination of the manifest potential. Neither the limitations, because of their schematic character, nor their significance were always fully appreciated. This will be discussed in connection with the letters to Lewis and Wilson in chapter 3.

On the other hand, it is also clear that foundations for new and important work were laid in the subsequent period. Although this work remained unfinished, it shaped his ideas as laid down in his last review and influenced others.

One of the fundamental issues concerned his segmental theory, already mentioned. It was probably formulated for the first time clearly in Einthoven's letter to Wilson in 1921 (chapter 3) and published succinctly a few years later (122,129,137). In 1922 Lewis wrote what was his last important contribution to cardiac electrophysiology (because he then turned to the study of the peripheral circulation). This paper contained his Mellon Lecture, entitled "Interpretations of the initial phases of the electrocardiogram with special reference to the theory of 'limited potential differences'" (w). The latter was similar to Einthoven's segmental theory, which was, however, founded on a histological basis and in that respect closer to present conceptions.

In his notes, preserved in the Museum Boerhaave for the history of sciences and medicine at Leiden, Einthoven wrote down, that he agreed fully with the theory of Lewis, adding that it was an inducement to perform the experiments which Lewis proposed but did not carry out and to write a paper on this subject himself. Although he did not mention it specifically, it is also very likely, that he concurred completely with the following introductory remark by Lewis in that paper: "In studying the electrocardiogram we attempt to explain its general deflections in rational terms, yet the terms which we are forced to employ are terms which refer to intimate and intangible effects of cellular physics and chemistry" ... . Understanding was deepened by the work of Craib and Wilson towards the end of Einthoven's lifetime and still more thereafter, but it appears likely in retrospect, that Einthoven to a certain extent kept aloof for want of a quantitative method, which was available only much later, i.e. when the intracellular and transmembrane potentials could be measured (see also X b). Einthoven was certainly not always aware of the clinical implications of electrocardiography. This is evident for instance from Sam Levine's story (x) about the electrocardiographic diagnosis of cardiac infarction made by a technician from his hospital, when Einthoven visited him in 1924. This astonished Einthoven very much (as it probably would have most European clinicians at that time). However, it gave him deep satisfaction. It may be true, that Einthoven was essentially a physicist, as A.V. Hill (j) and others for example Wenckebach (k), maintained, but his wish to help the patient was sincere and the clinical application of his work was in his mind from the beginning. When the connection of the string galvanometer with the hospital was broken, he placed his instrument at the disposition of doctors who wanted their patients to be examined. Several of his collaborators have testified about his thoughtful and obliging attitude towards these patients. From the records made at these occasions it is obvious that he wanted them as perfect as he did for his research. If necessary, the examination was repeated for that purpose.

I conclude by quoting Wiggers again (g): ... " It may here be noted that when Einthoven reached the zenith of his career, he had many characteristics in common with Donders. Both were intent on constantly improving apparatus for living processes. Both attempted as far as possible to reduce functional processes to physical and mathematical terms. Both were not merely concerned with the orderly solution of problems for the sake of science, but were anxious to apply them to practical clinical problems..." And this about Einthoven's visit to Wiggers' laboratory: "We mutually agreed that our evidence pointed toward different conclusions. Einthoven then made a significant statement, that I have never forgotten: When evidence is at variance, the respective investigators should spend more time in attempting to harmonize differences, rather than to direct their energies toward procurement of more data for a favored hypothesis. The truth is all that matters, what you or I think is inconsequential."

a) H. A. SNELLEN: A Disorder of the Breast, *Collection of original texts on ischaemic heart disease*. Rotterdam 1976.
b) G. E. BURCH and N. P. DEPASQUALE: *A History of Electrocardiography*. Chicago 1964.
c) A. D. WALLER: A demonstration on man of electromotive changes accompanying the heart's beat. *J. Physiol.* **8**: 17, 1887.
d) A. D. WALLER: The electromotive properties of the human heart. *Brit. Med. J.*: Oct. 6, 731, 1888.
e) A. D. WALLER: On the electromotive changes with the Beat of the Mammalian Heart, and of the Human Heart in particular. *Phil. Transact. Royal Soc. London.* **180**: 169, 1890.
f) A. SAMOJLOFF: Reminiscences of the late Professor Willem Einthoven. *Am. Heart J.* **5**: 545, 1930.
g) C. J. WIGGERS: Willem Einthoven (1860-1927). Some facets of His Life and Work. *Circulation Research.* **9**: 225, 1961.
h) W. T. DE VOGEL: *Thesis.* Leiden 1893.
i) G. J. BURCH: On the Time-relations of the Excursions of the Capillary Electrometer, with a Description of the Method of Using it for the Investigation of Electrical Changes of Short duration. *Phil. Transact. Royal Soc. London.* **183**: 81, 1893.
j) A. V. HILL: Obituary. Prof. W. Einthoven For. Mem. R.S. *Nature.* **120**: 591, 1927.

k) K.F. WENCKEBACH: W. Einthoven †. *D. med. Wschr.* **53**, II: 2176, 1927.

l) S. HOOGERWERF: Willem Einthoven. In: *Nederlandse Helden der Wetenschap.* Amsterdam 1946.

m) P.J.T.A. BATTAERD: Further graphic researches on the acoustic phenomena of the heart in normal and pathological conditions. *Heart.* **6**: 121, 1915-'17.

n) E.J. MAREY: *La circulation du sang à l'état physiologique et dans les maladies.* Paris 1881.

o) G. FAHR: On simultaneous records of the heart sounds and the electrocardiogram. *Heart.* **4**: 147, 1912-'13.

p) H. EPPINGER and O. STOERK: Zur Klinik des Elektrokardiogramms. *Zschr. f. klin. Med.* **71**: 157, 1910.

q) F.N. WILSON, A.G. MACLEOD and P.S. BARKER: The order of ventricular excitation in human bundle-branch block. *Am. Heart J.* **7**: 305, 1932.

r) E. KAUF: Zur Diagnose des Schenkelblocks beim menschlichen Herzen. *Zschr. f. klin. Med.* **98**: 126, 1924.

s) H. MANN: A method of analyzing the electrocardiogram. *Arch. Int. Med.* **25**: 283, 1920.

t) V. KRUTA: Sur l'activité rythmique du muscle cardiaque. I. Variations de la réponse mécanique en fonction du rythme. *Arch. Internat. Physiol.* **45**: 332, 1937.

u) C.J. ROTHBERGER and A. SACHS: Über den Zusammenhang zwischen Schlagfrequenz und Zuckungshöhe am Vorhofstreifen des Warmblüterherzens. *Pflügers Arch. ges. Physiol.* **240**: 60, 1938.

v) W.F. EINTHOVEN: The string galvanometer in wireless telegraphy. *Proc. Kon. Akad. Wet.* **26**: 635, 1923.

w) TH. LEWIS: Interpretations of the initial phases of the electrocardiogram with special reference to the theory of "limited potential differences." *Arch. Int. Med.* **30**: 269, 1922.

CHAPTER 2

BIBLIOGRAPHY

The following bibliography of Einthoven's writings is based on that in De Waart's biography of Einthoven (A. de Waart: Einthoven; Haarlem, 1957. Written in Dutch with an English summary) and on a list which was largely made under Einthoven's supervision and corrected in part by himself. However, a few additions and corrections proved necessary after careful scrutiny by Mrs. M. Blaauw-Koch.

The papers reproduced in chapter 3, have been marked with an asterisk.

1882

1 Mededeling in gewone vergadering van 30 sept. 1882 (gedaan door prof. Koster).
Proces verbaal Natuurk. Kon. Akad. Wet. 3:4-6, 1882/83

2 Quelques remarques sur le mécanisme de l'articulation du coude.
Arch. néerl. des Sciences Exact. Nat. 17:289-298

1885

3 Stereoscopie door kleurverschil.
Proefschrift, Utrecht, 4 juli 1885

4 Stereoscopie durch Farbendifferenz.
Albr. v. Graefes Arch. Ophthalm. 31 III:211-238

1886

5 Stéréoscopie dépendant d'une différence de couleur.
Arch. néerl. des Sciences Exact. Nat. 20:361-387

6 De leer der specifieke energieën. Redevoering 24 februari 1886 bij de aanvaarding van het hoogleraarsambt aan de R.U. te Leiden.
Leiden, S.C. van Doesburgh

1888

7 Donders' intrathoracale drukking en de gasspanningen in de pleuraholte. In: Feestbundel van Natuur- en Geneeskundige Onderzoekingen ter gelegenheid van den 70sten verjaardag van Franciscus Cornelis Donders.
Amsterdam, F. van Rossen
(Onderzoekingen Physiologisch Laboratorium Leiden* 2e reeks 1:1-27, 1894)

8 Der Donders'sche Druck und die Gasspannungen in der Pleurahöhle.
Pflügers Arch. ges. Physiol. 44:152-174

1889

9 Het eerste Internationale Physiologen-congres te Bazel (10-12 September 1889).
Ned. T. Geneesk. 25 II:457-462; 496-503

1891

10 De werking der bronchiaalspieren, naar een nieuwe methode onderzocht.
Handelingen van het Derde Ned. Natuur- en Geneesk. Congres (3, 4 April 1891) pp. 153-155.
Utrecht, J. van Boekhoven, 1891

11 In memoriam Dr. Adriaan Isebree Moens.
Ned. T. Geneesk. 27 II:1-2

1892

12 Verslag der werkzaamheden verricht in het zoölogisch station van

* Collection of selected reprints and doctoral theses from Einthoven's laboratory, many of them in Dutch.

dr. A. Dohrn te Napels, gedurende de maanden Juli-September 1892.
Staatscrt. 247 (20 October 1892)

13 Über die Wirkung der Bronchialmuskeln, nach einer neuen Methode untersucht, und über Asthma nervosum.
Pflügers Arch. ges. Physiol. 51:367-444
(Onderzoekingen Physiologisch Laboratorium Leiden 2e reeks 1:28-122, 1894)

1893

14 Sur l'action des muscles bronchiques, étudiée suivant une nouvelle méthode, et sur l'asthme nerveux.
Arch. néerl. des Sciences Exact. Nat. 26:1-90

15 On the production of shadow and perspective effects by difference of colour.
Brain J. Neurol. 16:191-202

16 Over asthma nervosum.
Ned. T. Geneesk. 29 II:469-495

17. Nieuwe methoden voor clinisch onderzoek. (Voordracht 44ste Alg. Verg. der Ned. Maatschappij ter bev. der Geneeskunst)
Ned. T. Geneesk. 29 II:263-286

18 Het meten van snel wisselende potentiaalverschillen met behulp van Lippmann's capillair-electrometer.
Mndbl. Nat. Wet. 18:109-120
(Onderzoekingen Physiologisch Laboratorium Leiden 2e reeks 1 : 199-216, 1894)

1894

19. Lippmann's Capillar-Electrometer zur Messung schnell wechselnder Potentialunterschiede.
Pflügers Arch. ges. Physiol. 56:528-541

*20 Die Registrirung der Herztöne.
(mit M.A.J. Geluk)
Pflügers Arch. ges. Physiol. 57:617-639

21 In memoriam Hermann von Helmholtz.
Ned. T. Geneesk. 30 II:490-492

22 Demonstratie van een methode van kleurmenging.
Ned. T. Geneesk. 30 II:186-187

23 De vorming van schaduw en perspectief door kleurverschil.
Onderzoekingen Physiologisch Laboratorium Leiden 2e reeks 1:185-198

1895

24 Over den invloed, dien de geleidingsweerstand uitoefent op de bewegingssnelheid van den meniscus in Lippmann's capillair-electrometer.
Mndbl. Nat. Wet. 19:61-69
(Onderzoekingen Physiologisch Laboratorium Leiden 2e reeks 2:30-42, 1896)

25 Über den Einfluss des Leitungswiderstandes auf die Geschwindigkeit der Quecksilberbewegung in Lippmann's Capillarelectrometer.
Pflügers Arch. ges. Physiol. 60:91-100

26 Über die Form des menschlichen Electrocardiogramms.
Pflügers Arch. ges. Physiol. 60:101-123

27 In memoriam J.W.F.J. van Eecke.
Ned. T. Geneesk. 31 I:933-934

28 Particuliere correspondentie. Het derde «Internationale Physiologen-congres» te Bern 9-13 September 1895.
Ned. T. Geneesk. 31 II:645-652

29 Een isolatie-inrichting tegen trillingen der omgeving.
Verslagen Natuurk. Kon. Akad. Wet. Amsterdam 4:38-41, 1895/96
(Onderzoekingen Physiologisch Laboratorium Leiden 2e reeks 2:85-101. 1896)

30 Vertheidigung gegen J. Burdon Sanderson.
Centralbl. Physiol. 9:277-278
(Onderzoekingen Physiologisch Laboratorium Leiden 2e reeks 2:102-104, 1896)

31 Eine Isolationsvorrichtung gegen Erschütterungen der Umgebung.
Ann. Physik. Chem. 56:161-166

32 Die Cardinalpunkte des Auges für verschiedenfarbiges Licht.
Pflügers Arch. ges. Physiol. 62:166-171

1896

33 Sur les points cardinaux de l'œil pour les lumières de couleur différente.
Arch. néerl. des Sciences Exact. Nat. 29:346-351

34 Het registreeren der hartstonen.
(met M. A. J. Geluk)
Onderzoekingen Physiologisch Laboratorium Leiden 2e reeks 2:1-29

35 Over den vorm van het menschelijk electrocardiogram.
Onderzoekingen Physiologisch Laboratorium Leiden 2e reeks 2:43-76

36 De cardinale punten van het oog voor verschillend gekleurd licht.
Onderzoekingen Physiologisch Laboratorium Leiden 2e reeks 2:169-176

1897

37 In memoriam Emil du Bois-Reymond.
Ned. T. Geneesk. 33 I:10-12

38 Over eenige optische illusies.
Handelingen zesde Ned. Natuur- en Geneesk. Congres Delft, 23 en 24 April 1897. pp. 271-274
Haarlem, J. L. E. I. Kleynenberg, 1897

1898

39 Eine einfache physiologische Erklärung für verschiedene geometrisch-optische Täuschungen.
Pflügers Arch. ges. Physiol. 71:1-43
(Onderzoekingen Physiologisch Laboratorium Leiden 2e reeks 3:133-188, 1898)

40 Über die Bewegungen des Pharynx. Bemerkungen zu einigen stereoskopischen Momentaufnahmen.
Internat. Photograph. Monatschr. Med. 5:17-19
(Onderzoekingen Physiologisch Laboratorium Leiden 2e reeks 3:189-194, 1898)

41 Over de bewegingen van den pharynx. Aanteekeningen bij eenige stereoscopische momentphotographieën.
Ned. T. Geneesk. 34 II:1053-1056

1899

42 Physiologie des Rachens. In: Handbuch der Laryngologie und Rhinologie. II. Band : Der Rachen, pp. 46-64.
Wien, Alfred Hölder, 1899

43 Explication physiologique simple de diverses illusions optiques-géométriques.
Arch. néerl. des Sciences Exact. Nat. série 2, 2:103-143

44 Bijdrage tot de theorie van Lippmann's capillair-electrometer.
Verslagen Natuurk. Kon. Akad. Wet. Amsterdam 8:177-191, 1899/1900

45 On the theory of Lippmann's capillary electrometer.
Proceed. Section of Sciences, Kon. Akad. Wet. Amsterdam 2:108-120, 1899/1900

1900

46 Beitrag zur Theorie des Capillar-Elektrometers.
Pflügers Arch. ges. Physiol. 79:1-25
(Onderzoekingen Physiologisch Laboratorium Leiden 2e reeks 4:1-32, 1900)

47 Eine Vorrichtung zum Registriren der Ausschläge des Lippmann'schen Capillar-Elektrometers.
Pflügers Arch. ges. Physiol. 79:26-38
(Onderzoekingen Physiologisch Laboratorium Leiden 2e reeks 4:33-49, 1900)

*48 Über das normale menschliche Elektrokardiogramm und über die capillar-elektrometrische Untersuchung einiger Herzkranken.
(mit K. de Lint)
Pflügers Arch. ges. Physiol. 80:139-160

49 Onderzoek van eenige lijders aan hartziekten met den capillair-electrometer.
(m.m.v. M.A.J. Geluk en H.W. Blöte)
Ned. T. Geneesk. 36 I:1031-1035
(Onderzoekingen Physiologisch Laboratorium Leiden 2e reeks 4:152-158, 1900)

50 Über Nervenreizung durch frequente Wechselströme.
Pflügers Arch. ges. Physiol. 82:101-133
(Onderzoekingen Physiologisch Laboratorium Leiden 2e reeks 4:159-202, 1900)

1901

51 Over den invloed van het bedrag der demping op het prikkelend effect van een frequenten wisselstroom. In: Feestbundel Dr. Sape Talma bij gelegenheid van zijn 25-jarig hoogleeraarschap, den 6en October 1901, pp. 169-187.
Haarlem, Erven F. Bohn

*52 Un nouveau galvanomètre.
Arch. néerl. des Sciences Exact. Nat. série 2, 6:625-633

53 Demonstraties op het physiologisch laboratorium bij gelegenheid van de 52ste Alg. Verg. der Ned. Maatschappij tot bev. der Geneesk. te Leiden.
Ned. T. Geneesk. 37 II:69-75

1902

54 Weitere Untersuchungen über Nervenreizung durch frequente Wechselströme.

II. Mittheilung. Über den Einfluss der Dämpfung auf die erregende Wirkung einer sinusoïdal oscillirenden Elektricitätsbewegung.
Pflügers Arch. ges. Physiol. 89:547-591
(Onderzoekingen Physiologisch Laboratorium Leiden 2e reeks 5:91-150, 1904)

55 Die Accommodation des menschlichen Auges.
Ergebn. Physiol. 1 II:680-694

56 Galvanometrische registratie van het menschelijk electrocardiogram. In: Herinneringsbundel prof. S.S. Rosenstein, pp. 101-106. Leiden, Eduard IJdo, 1902

1903

57 De snaargalvanometer en het menschelijk electrocardiogram.
Verslagen Natuurk. Kon. Akad. Wet. Amsterdam 12:122-131, 1903/04

58 Die galvanometrische Registrirung des menschlichen Elektrokardiogramms, zugleich eine Beurtheilung der Anwendung des Capillar-Elektrometers in der Physiologie.
Pflügers Arch. ges. Physiol. 99:472-480
(Onderzoekingen Physiologisch Laboratorium Leiden 2e reeks 6:106-117, 1907)

*59 The string-galvanometer and the human electrocardiogram.
Proceed. Section of Sciences, Kon. Akad. Wet. Amsterdam 6:107-115, 1903/04

60 Ein neues Galvanometer.
Ann. Physik 12:1059-1071
(Onderzoekingen Physiologisch Laboratorium Leiden 2e reeks 5:168-184, 1904)

1904

61 Sur le galvanomètre à corde (deuxième communication).
Arch. néerl. des Sciences Exact. Nat. série 2, 9:186-201

62 Enregistrement galvanométrique de l'électrocardiogramme humain et contrôle des résultats obtenus par l'emploi de l'électromètre capillaire en physiologie.
Arch. néerl. des Sciences Exact. Nat. série 2, 9:202-209

63 Eenige toepassingen van den snaargalvanometer.
Verslagen Natuurk. Kon. Akad. Wet. Amsterdam 12:876-884, 1903/04

64 On some applications of the string-galvanometer.
Proceed. Section of Sciences, Kon. Akad. Wet. Amsterdam 6:707-714, 1903/04

65 Über einige Anwendungen des Saitengalvanometers.
Ann. Physik 14:182-192
(Onderzoekingen Physiologisch Laboratorium Leiden 2e reeks 6:118-130, 1907)

66 Sur la précision et la sûreté des mouvements de la main.
Arch. Internat. Physiol. 1:72-77
(Onderzoekingen Physiologisch Laboratorium Leiden 2e reeks 6:131-139, 1907)

67 In memoriam E.J. Marey.
Ned. T. Geneesk. 40 I:1109-1113

68 Een nieuwe methode om oscilleerende galvanometeruitslagen te dempen.
Verslagen Natuurk. Kon. Akad. Wet. Amsterdam 13:284-293, 1904/05

69 On a new method of damping oscillatory deflections of a galvanometer.
Proceed. Section of Sciences, Kon. Akad. Wet. Amsterdam 7:315-323, 1904/05

1905

70 Über eine neue Methode zur Dämpfung oszillierender Galvanometerausschläge.
Ann. Physik 16:20-31
(Onderzoekingen Physiologisch Laboratorium Leiden 2e reeks 6:140-154, 1907)

71 Une nouvelle méthode d'amortissement des oscillations dans les indications galvanométriques.
Arch. néerl. des Sciences Exact. Nat. série 2, 10:137-147

72 Analyse der snaargalvanometrische krommen. Massa en spanning van den kwartsdraad en weerstand der draadbeweging.
Verslagen Natuurk. Kon. Akad. Wet. Amsterdam 13:824-886, 1904/05

73 Analysis of the curves obtained with the string-galvanometer. Mass

and tension of the quartz wire and resistance to the motion of the string.
Proceed. Section of Sciences, Kon. Akad. Wet. Amsterdam 8:210-268, 1905/06

74 Sur le galvanomètre à corde (3ème communication) (Analyse des courbes galvanométriques. Masse et tension du fil de quartz et résistance au mouvement du fil).
Arch. néerl. des Sciences Exact. Nat. série 2, 10:414-482

1906

75 Over de beteekenis der electro-physiologie als een onderdeel van de leer der levensverrichtingen. Rede uitgesproken op den 331sten verjaardag der Universiteit te Leiden, 8 februari 1906.
Leiden, Brill

76 Le télécardiogramme.
Arch. néerl. des Sciences Exact. Nat. série 2, 11:239-272

*77 Le télécardiogramme.
Arch. Internat. Physiol. 4:132-164
(Onderzoekingen Physiologisch Laboratorium Leiden 2e reeks 7:1-44, 1908)

77A The telecardiogram.
Partial translation
by Mathewson FAL and Jackh H. Amer. Heart J. 49:77-82, 1955
by Blackburn HW. Amer. Heart J. 53:602-615, 1957

78 Het tele-cardiogram.
Ned. T. Geneesk. 50 II:1517-1547

79 Het registreeren van menschelijke hartstonen met den snaargalvanometer.
(m.m.v. A. Flohil en P.J.T.A. Battaerd)
Ned. T. Geneesk. 50 II:818-826

80 Weitere Mitteilungen über das Saitengalvanometer. Analyse der saitengalvanometrischen Kurven. Masse und Spannung des Quarzfadens und Widerstand gegen die Fadenbewegung.
Ann. Physik 21:483-514; 665-700
(Onderzoekingen Physiologisch Laboratorium Leiden 2e reeks 6:155-244, 1907)

81 Verslag van de lotgevallen der Universiteit, 17 September 1906. Jaarboek der Rijksuniversiteit te Leiden 1905-1906, pp. 35-67. Leiden, Brill, 1906

1907

82 Die Registrirung der menschlichen Herztöne mittels des Saitengalvanometers.
(Mitwirkung von A. Flohil und P. J. T. A. Battaerd)
Pflügers Arch. ges. Physiol. 117:461-472
(Onderzoekingen Physiologisch Laboratorium Leiden 2e reeks 7:45-60, 1908)

83 Over een derden hartstoon.
(m.m.v. J. H. Wieringa en E. P. Snijders)
Verslagen Natuurk. Kon. Akad. Wet. Amsterdam 16:108-110, 1907/08

84 Een derde hartstoon.
(m.m.v. J. H. Wieringa en E. P. Snijders)
Ned. T. Geneesk. 51 II:470-480

85 On a third heart sound.
(in collab. with J. H. Wieringa and E. P. Snijders)
Proceed. Section of Sciences, Kon. Akad. Wet. Amsterdam 10:93-95, 1907/08

86 Ein dritter Herzton.
(Mitwirkung von J. H. Wieringa und E. P. Snijders)
Pflügers Arch. ges. Physiol. 120:31-43
(Onderzoekingen Physiologisch Laboratorium Leiden 2e reeks 7:61-78, 1908)

*87 L'enregistrement des bruits du cœur de l'homme à l'aide du galvanomètre à corde.
(avec collab. de A. Flohil et P. J. T. A. Battaerd)
Arch. néerl. des Sciences Exact. Nat. série 2, 12:401-411

1908

88 Over de electrische reactie van het oog op lichtprikkels van verschillende intensiteit.
(met W. A. Jolly)
Verslagen Natuurk. Kon. Akad. Wet. Amsterdam 16:693-699, 1907/08

89 The electric response of the eye to stimulation by light at various intensities.
(with W. A. Jolly)
Proceed. Section of Sciences, Kon. Akad. Wet. Amsterdam 10:698-703, 1907/08

*90 Weiteres über das Elektrokardiogramm. Nach gemeinschaftlich mit Dr. B. Vaandrager angestellten Versuchen mitgeteilt.
Pflügers Arch. ges. Physiol. 122:517-584

91 Über Vagusströme. Nach gemeinschaftlich mit A. Flohil und P. J. T. A. Battaerd angestellten Versuchen mitgeteilt.
Pflügers Arch. ges. Physiol. 124:246-270
(Onderzoekingen Physiologisch Laboratorium Leiden 2e reeks 7:177-210, 1908)

*92 On vagus currents examined with the string galvanometer.
(in collab. with A. Flohil and P. J. T. A. Battaerd)
Quart. J. Exp. Physiol. 1:243-245

93 The form and magnitude of the electrical response of the eye to stimulation by light at various intensities.
(with W. A. Jolly)
Quart. J. Exp. Physiol. 1:373-416
(Onderzoekingen Physiologisch Laboratorium Leiden 2e reeks 8:1-72, 1912)

1909

94 Sur les courants du nerf vague.
(avec le concours de A. Flohil et P. J. T. A. Battaerd)
Arch. néerl. des Sciences Exact. Nat. série 2, 14:157-179

95 Die Konstruktion des Saitengalvanometers.
Pflügers Arch. ges. Physiol. 130:287-321
(Onderzoekingen Physiologisch Laboratorium Leiden 2e reeks 8:98-145, 1912)

1911

96 Ongelijksoortige vaguswerkingen op het hart, electrocardiographisch onderzocht.
(met J. H. Wieringa)
Verslagen Natuurk. Kon. Akad. Wet. Amsterdam 20:99-100, 1911/12

97 On different vagus effects upon the heart investigated by means of electrocardiography.
(with J. H. Wieringa)
Proceed. Section of Sciences, Kon. Akad. Wet. Amsterdam 14:165-166, 1911/12

98 Neuere Ergebnisse auf dem Gebiete der tierischen Elektrizität.
Verh. Ges. dtsch. Naturf. Aerzte, pp. 80-113

1912

*99 The different forms of the human electrocardiogram and their signification. (Paper read before the Chelsea Clinical Society on March 19th, 1912)
Lancet I:853-861

100 Ungleichartige Vaguswirkungen auf das Herz, elektrokardiographisch untersucht.
(mit J. H. Wieringa)
Pflügers Arch. ges. Physiol. 149:48-64
(Onderzoekingen Physiologisch Laboratorium Leiden 2e reeks 9:1-22, 1916)

101 Über die Deutung des Elektrokardiogramms.
Pflügers Arch. ges. Physiol. 149:65-86
(Onderzoekingen Physiologisch Laboratorium Leiden 2e reeks 9:23-51, 1916)

1913

102 Über die Richtung und die manifeste Grösse der Potentialschwankungen im menschlichen Herzen und über den Einfluss der Herzlage auf die Form des Elektrokardiogramms.
(mit G. Fahr und A. de Waart)
Pflügers Arch. ges. Physiol. 150:275-315
(Onderzoekingen Physiologisch Laboratorium Leiden 2e reeks 9:96-149, 1916)

102A On the direction and manifest size of the variations of potential in the human heart and on the influence of the position of the heart on the form of the electrocardiogram.
(Translated by Hoff H E, Sekelj P)
Amer. Heart J. 40:163-211, 1950

1914

103 Etude électrocardiographique des diverses actions des nerfs vagues sur le cœur.
(avec J. H. Wieringa)
Arch. néerl. des Sciences Exact. Nat. série 3B 2:91-108

104 Sur l'explication de l'électrocardiogramme.
Arch. néerl. des Sciences Exact. Nat. série 3B 2:109-129

105 Over verschillende soorten van hartcontracties.
Ned. T. Geneesk. 58 II:2113-2131

1915

106 In memoriam K. F. L. van der Woerd
Jaarboekje voor Gesch. en Oudheidk. Leiden en Rijnland.
Leiden, Théonville, 1915

107 Over het gelijktijdig registreeren van electrische verschijnselen met behulp van twee of meer galvanometers en over de toepassing daarvan op de electro-cardiographie.
(met F. L. Bergansius en J. Bijtel)
Verslagen Natuurk. Kon. Akad. Wet. Amsterdam 24:29-33, 1915/16

108 Upon the simultaneous registration of electric phenomena by means of two or more galvanometers, and upon its application to electrocardiography.
(with F. L. Bergansius and J. Bijtel)
Proceed. Section of Sciences Kon. Akad. Wet. Amsterdam 18:242-246, 1915/16

109 On the variability of the size of the pulse in cases of auricular fibrillation.
(with A. J. Korteweg)
Heart 6:107-120
(Onderzoekingen Physiologisch Laboratorium Leiden 2e reeks 10:1-20, 1922)

110 Eine Vorrichtung zur photographischen Registrierung der Zeit.
Z. biol. Techn. Methodik 3:1-6, 1915
(Onderzoekingen Physiologisch Laboratorium Leiden 2e reeks 9:88-95, 1916)

1916

111 Die gleichzeitige Registrierung elektrischer Erscheinungen mittels zwei oder mehr Galvanometer und ihre Anwendung auf die Elektrokardiographie.
(mit F. L. Bergansius und J. Bijtel)
Pflügers Arch. ges. Physiol. 164:167-197
(Onderzoekingen Physiologisch Laboratorium Leiden 2e reeks 10:31-66, 1922)

112 Über Bindeelektroden nebst einigen Bemerkungen über das Kinder-E.-K.-G.
Nach Untersuchungen von P. Meerburg und J. Endtz mitgeteilt.
Wiener Mediz. Wschr. 66:507-511
(Onderzoekingen Physiologisch Laboratorium Leiden 2e reeks 10:67-75, 1922)

113 Über die angebliche positive Stromschwankung in der Schildkrötenvorkammer bei Vagusreizung nebst Bemerkungen über den Zusammenhang zwischen Kontraktion und Aktionsstrom.
(mit A. C. A. Rademaker)
Pflügers Arch. ges. Physiol. 166:109-143
(Onderzoekingen Physiologisch Laboratorium Leiden 2e reeks 10:76-117, 1922)

1918

114 Sur les phénomènes électriques du tonus musculaire.
Arch. néerl. Physiol.* 2:489-499
(Onderzoekingen Physiologisch Laboratorium Leiden 2e reeks 10:185-197, 1922)

1919

115 Over het electrocardiogram bij het uitblijven van elke zichtbare samentrekking van het hart.
(met F. W. N. Hugenholtz)
Ned. T. Geneesk. 63 I:310-319

* This journal forms a continuation of the Arch. néerl. des Sciences Exact. Nat.

1920

116 Über den Zusammenhang zwischen Elektro- und Mechanokardiogramm.
Ber. ges. Physiol. 2:178

117 Over de waarneming en afbeelding van dunne draden.
Verslagen Natuurk. Kon. Akad. Wet. Amsterdam 29:388-389, 1920/21

118 On the observation and representation of thin threads.
Proceed. Section of Sciences, Kon. Akad. Wet. Amsterdam 23:705-706, 1920/21

1921

119 L'électrocardiogramme tracé dans le cas où il n'y a pas de contraction visible du cœur.
(avec F. W. N. Hugenholtz)
Arch. néerl. Physiol. 5:174-184

120 Über Widerstand und Potentialdifferenz bei dem psychogalvanischen Reflex.
(mit J. Roos)
Pflügers Arch. ges. Physiol. 189:126-136

121 Über die Beobachtung und Abbildung dünner Fäden.
Pflügers Arch. ges. Physiol. 191:60-98

1922

122 De weg, die door de contractiegolf in de hartspier wordt afgelegd, en de vorm van het electrocardiogram.
Ned. T. Geneesk. 66 I:2313-2315

123 Stroomgeleiding door het menschelijk lichaam.
(met J. Bijtel)
Verslagen Natuurk. Kon. Akad. Wet. Amsterdam 31:9-11

124 Conduction du courant électrique par le corps humain.
(avec J. Bijtel)
Arch. néerl. Physiol. 7:407-410

1923

125 Über Stromleitung durch den menschlichen Körper.
(mit J. Bijtel)
Pflügers Arch. ges. Physiol. 198:439-482

126 Functions of the cervical sympathetic as manifested by its action currents.
(with J. Byrne)
Amer. J. Physiol. 65:350-362

127 De snaarphonograaf.
(met S. Hoogerwerf)
Verslagen Natuurk. Kon. Akad. Wet. Amsterdam 32:656-659

1924

128 Le phonographe à corde.
(avec S. Hoogerwerf)
Arch. néerl. Physiol. 9:100-104

129 La voie, suivie par l'onde de contraction dans le muscle cardiaque et la forme de l'électrocardiogramme.
Arch. néerl. Physiol. 9:406-408

130 Der Saitenphonograph.
(mit S. Hoogerwerf)
Pflügers Arch. ges. Physiol. 204:275-294

1925

131 La détermination de l'axe électrique du cœur.
Acta Paediat. 4:136-140
(Vide: Gorter E: Sur la dextrocardie. ibid. 4:125-136)

132 Brownsche bewegingen van een gespannen snaar.
(met W.F. Einthoven, W. van der Horst en H. Hirschfeld)
Physica 5:358-360

1926

*133 The relation of mechanical and electrical phenomena of muscular contraction, with special reference to the cardiac muscle.
(Lecture Dec. 6, 1924)
The Harvey Society Lectures 1924-1925.
Philadelphia, London, J.B. Lippincott, 1926

134 Nobel Lecture, December 8, 1925: Das Saitengalvanometer und die Messung der Aktionsströme des Herzens.
A. Les prix Nobel en 1924-1925. Stockholm, P.A. Norstedt & Fils, 1926
B. Acta Societas Medicorum Suecanae 51:213-226, 1926
*C. The string-galvanometer and the measurement of the action currents of the heart.
Nobel Ed. Physiology or Medecine 1922-1941.
Amsterdam, New York, Barking, Elsevier, 1965

1927

135 Gehirn und Sympathicus. VI. Mitteilung von Einthoven, Hoogerwerf, Karplus und Kreidl.
A. Die Aktionsströme des Halssympathicus.
(mit S. Hoogerwerf)
Pflügers Arch. ges. Physiol. 215:443-452

136 Expériences avec le phonographe à corde.
(avec S. Hoogerwerf)
Arch. néerl. Physiol. 11:496-508

1928

137 Die Aktionsströme des Herzens (Elektrokardiogramm). In: Handbuch der normalen und pathologischen Physiologie. Ed: A. Bethe et al. pp. 785-862.
Berlin, Springer

CHAPTER 3

SELECTED PAPERS OF WILLEM EINTHOVEN

The following reproductions of papers (marked with an asterisk in the bibliography of chapter 2) and of correspondence with Lewis and Wilson about the equilateral triangle, which follow, have already been referred to in the first chapter.

They constitute together a fairly representative collection of Einthoven's published work, which covers a period of more than 30 years, although the selection was limited to electrocardiography and allied subjects of cardiological interest. Why this selection was chosen has been explained in the Introduction. Here a few comments about the contents will be added together with brief summaries, in particular of the French and German texts.

The list of titles runs as follows:

I (1894) Die Registrierung der Herztöne (nr. 20 in the bibliography of chapter 2)
II (1900) Über das normale menschliche Elektrokardiogramms und über die capillar-elektrometrische Untersuchung einiger Herzkranken (48)
III (1901) Un nouveau galvanomètre (52)
IV (1903) The string galvanometer and the human electrocardiogram (59)
V (1906) Le télécardiogramme (77)
VI (1907) L'enregistrement des bruits du cœur de l'homme à l'aide du galvanomètre à corde (87)
VII (1908) Weiteres über das Elektrokardiogramm (90)
VIII (1909) On vagus currents examined with the string galvanometer (92)
IX (1912) The different forms of the human electrocardiogram and their signification (99)
XA (1916) Correspondence with Thomas Lewis
XB (1921) Correspondence with Frank Wilson
XI (1912) The relation of mechanical and electrical phenomena of muscular contraction, with special reference to the cardiac muscle (133)
XII (1965), 1926) The string galvanometer and the measurement of the action currents of the heart (134 c).

I
Die Registrierung der Herztöne

Although there were precursors, mentioned in this paper, Einthoven and Geluk were the first to publish phonocardiograms (from dogs, rabbits and normal men). Their tracings are chiefly analysed with respect to time relations; the (apex) cardiogram and carotid pulse are used as reference tracings. It is stated that opening and closure of the aortic and pulmonary valves can be identified and that the ejection period can be differentiated from the first part of systole (i.e. the isometric period) by the time interval between the first sounds at the apex and at the aorta. Attention is also given to the difference in characteristics between first and second sound as well as to the similarity of heart sounds from successive beats. It is stated that heart sounds do not consist of regular vibrations and therefore are not sounds in the physical sense.

A diastolic murmur from experimental aortic insuffiency in a dog, is shown; its shape is compared to a pulse wave.

It is to be noted, that the records are made by means of a microphone coupled with a Lippman's capillary electrometer. Although the tracings show a much improved recording technique, they have not been corrected mathematically and it is evident that high frequency components are not registered.

In an appendix the accuracy of the time interval measurements is discussed.

(Physiologisches Laboratorium in Leyden.)

Die Registrirung der Herztöne.

Von

Professor **W. Einthoven** und **M. A. J. Geluk**, Arzt.

Mit 12 Figuren im Text.

Schon vor geraumer Zeit wurde das Bedürfniss empfunden, den Schall durch Registrirung sichtbar machen zu können.

Für stärkere Laute wurden Methoden erfunden, welche directe Registrirung ermöglichten. Insofern uns bekannt ist, gelang dies zuerst mit dem Phonautographen; im neuen Edison'schen Phonographen und den schönen phonophotographischen Untersuchungen Hermann's näherte sich diese Kunst ihrer Vollendung.

Wenn wir erwägen, dass unser Gehörorgan ein ausserordentlich empfindliches Sinneswerkzeug ist, mit welchem wir thatsächlich das Gras wachsen hören könnten[1]), — wenn nur seine chemische Energie als Schall aufträte, — und dass wir ungeachtet dieser grossen Empfindlichkeit die Herztöne in der Regel nur dann hören können, wenn wir entweder das Ohr unmittelbar gegen den Thorax halten oder specielle Werkzeuge wie das Stethoskop anwenden, so wird es uns klar sein, wie grosse praktische Schwierigkeiten mit der directen Registrirung solcher schwachen Schälle verbunden sein werden.

Der erste, welcher versucht hat, eine directe graphische Darstellung[2]) der Herztöne zu erhalten, ist Léon Fredericq[3]) in

1) Citirt nach L. Hermann's Lehrbuch der Physiol. 10. Aufl. 1892, S. 507.

2) Donders' Methode der indirekten Registirung der Herztöne datirt vom Jahre 1866. Nederl. Arch. v. Genees- en Natuurkunde, Dl. II, bl. 139.

3) Léon Fredericq, Ueber die Zeit der Oeffnung und Schliessung der Semilunarklappen. Centralbl. f. Physiol. 1892, Bd. VI, S. 260.

Lüttich, der die Schwingungen einer phonautographischen Membran photographirte, aber seine Ergebnisse unseres Wissens bis jetzt noch nicht publicirte.

Nach Fredericq ist Hürthle[1]) in Breslau zu erwähnen. Dieser wendete einen Mikrophon an, welchen er in den primären Strom eines Inductionsapparates einschaltete, dessen secundäre Rolle durch Leitungsdrähte mit dem Nerv eines Froschmuskels verbunden war; jeder Schall, auch derjenige eines Herztones, der mit genügender Intensität den Mikrophon traf, veranlasste eine Contraction des Muskels.

Hürthle bemühte sich namentlich, den richtigen Anfang der Herztöne kennen zu lernen und hiermit einige schwierige Fragen inbetreff der Bedeutung des Cardiogrammes zu lösen. Seine Methode kann nicht dazu dienen, den Charakter der Herztöne näher zu studiren, weil die Zuckungen eines Froschmuskels relativ langsam sind und schon bei einer Reizfrequenz von 20 bis 30 Reizen pro Secunde vollkommen verschmelzen; ein Ton, durch Schwingungen von derselben Frequenz verursacht, würde also nur einen Tetanus der Froschmuskeln zur Folge haben.

Die Arbeit Hürthle's brachte uns auf den Gedanken, den stromprüfenden Froschschenkel durch den Capillarelektrometer zu ersetzen. Erstens macht dieses Werkzeug die Methode empfindlicher, aber es ist namentlich wegen der sehr schnellen Bewegungen, welche der Quecksilberfaden in der Capillarröhre eines Capillarelektrometers vollbringt, dass es als ein Hülfsmittel für die Untersuchung den Vorzug verdient.

Als Mikrophon wenden wir einen einfachen, bei vielen Telephonvereinen mit Erfolg gebrauchten Apparat von Berliner an. Ein Bunsenelement liefert den elektrischen Strom, welcher durch den Mikrophon und die primäre Rolle eines du Bois-Reymond'schen Schlittenapparates geführt wird. Die Schraubklemmen der secundären Rolle sind mit den Polen des Capillarelektrometers verbunden, während der selbstwirkende Stromunterbrecher festgesetzt ist.

Ist der Rollenabstand des Inductionsapparates 0 und die Vor-

---

1) K. Hürthle, Ueber die Erklärung des Cardiogramms mit Hilfe der Herztonmarkirung und über eine Methode zur mechanischen Registrirung der Töne. Deutsche medic. Wochenschr. 1893, Nr. 4.

richtung also aufs empfindlichste gestellt, so verursachen schwache Schälle in der Nähe des Mikrophons schon ausgiebige Bewegungen des Quecksilbermeniscus.

Spricht oder ruft man mit starker Stimme — sogar in einer Entfernung des Mikrophones von einigen Metern — so tritt der Meniscus ganz aus dem Gesichtsfelde des Mikroskopes hinaus.

Ein kurz andauernder Schall wie ein Klatsch in die Hände, ein Schlag des Metronomes, gibt einen Ausschlag, der unter directer Beobachtung der Quecksilberbewegung, wegen seiner grossen Geschwindigkeit ausserordentlich schwierig beurtheilt werden kann.

Der Quecksilberfaden scheint in einem unmessbar kleinen Augenblick eine auf- und niedergehende Bewegung zu machen. wonach er seine ursprüngliche Stelle genau wieder einnimmt, Hat bei einer bestimmten Stromrichtung der Ausschlag mit einer Bewegung aufwärts angefangen, so ist bei umgekehrtem elektrischem Strom die Bewegung erst nach unten.

Wird eine Stimmgabel vor dem Mikrophone angestrichen, so dass sie einen Ton hervorbringt, so zeigt sich zwischen dem schwarzen Quecksilber und der hellen durchsichtigen Schwefelsäurelösung ein grauer Streifen, dessen obere und untere Grenze beide die gewöhnliche Form des Quecksilbermeniscus zeigen. Je intensiver der Ton, desto länger wird der Streifen.

Bei intensiven Tönen bewegt sich der Quecksilberfaden zusammen mit dem grauen Streifen schwefelsäurewärts; diese Bewegung ist unabhängig von der Stromrichtung und ist bei hohen Tönen viel bedeutender als bei tiefen.

Bei sehr hohen Tönen geht die nach der Schwefelsäure hin gerichtete Bewegung so weit, dass das zum Vorschein treten des grauen Streifens unmöglich gemacht wird, weil dieser bei einem schwachen hohen Ton unmerklich klein ist, während ein intensiver hoher Ton das Quecksilber aus der Oeffnung der Capillarröhre treibt.

Die Photographie[1]) erläutert das Wesen des erwähnten grauen Streifens und zeigt, dass er durch schnell auf- und niedergehende Quecksilberbewegungen desselben Rhythmus und derselben Frequenz wie die Stimmgabelschwingungen verursacht wird.

---

1) Eine ausführliche Beschreibung der Vorrichtung zum Photographiren des Capillarelectrometers folgt später.

Wir untersuchten nicht, welcher der höchste Ton ist, den man — auf diese Weise registrirend — noch als eine Curve sichtbar machen kann, haben uns aber vorläufig begnügt mit b''' (1920 ganze Schwingungen pro Secunde), einem Tone, der höher ist als der höchste, den die menschliche Stimme je hat hervorbringen können. In der Curve, die wir erhielten, waren die Wellengipfel zwar nicht eben so schön und scharf, wie diejenigen tieferer Töne, aber sie waren doch deutlich sichtbar und leicht zählbar.

Fig. 1.

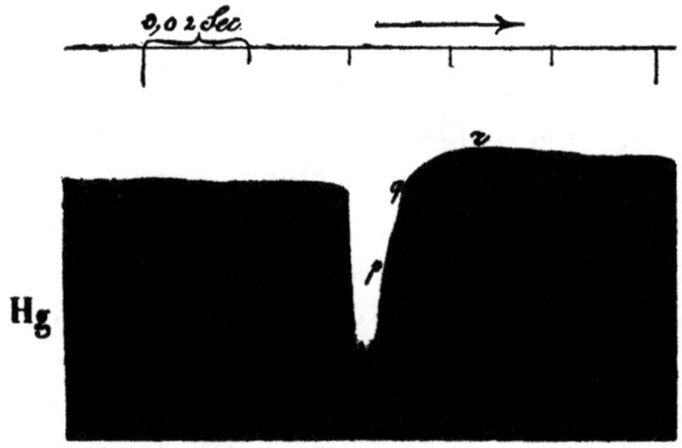

Metronomschlag. Die Bewegung des Quecksilbers ist nach dem Quecksilber hin gerichtet.

Fig. 2.

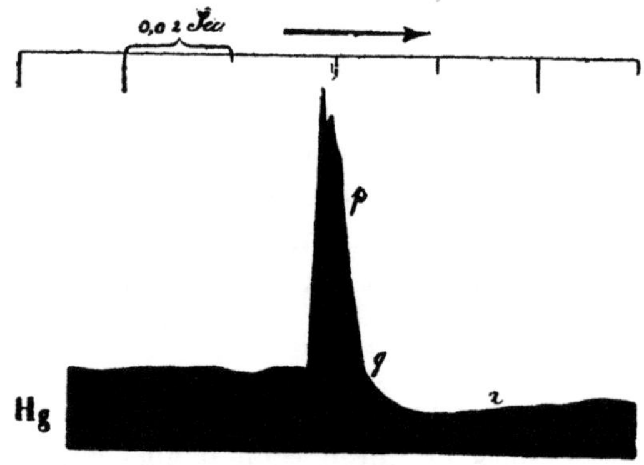

Metronomschlag. Die Bewegung des Quecksilbers ist nach der Schwefelsäure hin gerichtet.

In den Figuren 1 und 2 geben wir eine Abbildung des Klanges eines Metronomschlages. In Fig. 1 hat der elektrische Strom eine andere Richtung als in Fig. 2, daher der Unterschied der Bewegungsrichtung des Meniscus: in Fig. 1 nach dem Quecksilber, in Fig. 2 nach der Schwefelsäurelösung hin gerichtet.

Der Anfang des Klanges kann jedesmal mit sehr grosser Genauigkeit angegeben werden, weil der Meniscus sich mit grosser Anfangsgeschwindigkeit hebt und senkt. Das Ende des Klanges — also auch dessen Dauer — lässt sich jedoch nicht so scharf angeben, weil der Schall, welcher auf einmal mit voller Kraft angefangen hat, nur langsam an Intensität abnimmt. Das Ende des Klanges oder besser die Stelle, wo seine Intensität so gering ist, dass der Capillarelektrometer ihn nicht mehr anzugeben vermag, muss irgendwo auf der Curve *p q r* gefunden werden. Wollen wir diese Stelle kennen lernen, also die Stelle, wo der Wechsel der elektrischen Spannungsunterschiede zu bestehen aufhört — so müssen wir die Neigung der Curve *p q r* näher untersuchen und wir wenden hierzu die Methode an, welche von einem von uns beiden schon anderswo beschrieben ist[1]).

Wenn wir einen schwachen Nachhall vernachlässigen und annehmen, dass das Ende des Klanges da ist, wo seine Intensität bis auf nur einige wenige Procente des ursprünglichen Werthes zurückgebracht ist, so wird die Dauer des hier registrirten Metronomschlages zu 0,005 bis 0,006 Secunde berechnet.

Die nähere Analyse der Curve zeigt weiter, dass der Klang hauptsächlich aus einem einzigen Tone von 550 Schwingungen pro Secunde besteht. Durch die kurze Dauer des Klanges treten nur drei Schwingungen klar hervor, die erste Schwingung hat eine viel grössere Amplitude als die zweite und diese wieder eine viel grössere als die dritte. In Fig. 1 sind die drei Gipfel einzeln sichtbar, in Fig. 2 ist der dritte Gipfel stark abgestumpft. Die Phase *q r*, in beiden Figuren sichtbar, muss wahrscheinlich einer Nachwirkung des Mikrophones zugeschrieben werden. Die geringe Neigung, welche die Curve in dieser Phase zeigt, deutet auf einen geringen elektrischen Spannungsunterschied, der ohne grobe Fehler zu veranlassen ausser Rechnung gelassen werden darf.

Beim Registriren der Herztöne machen sich eigenthümliche Schwierigkeiten geltend.

---

1) W. Einthoven, Lippmann's Capillarelectrometer zur Messung schnell wechselnder Potentialunterschiede. Dieses Archiv. Bd. 56. S. 528.

Die Intensität des Tones ist so gering, dass man gezwungen wird, das Herz in die unmittelbare Nähe des Mikrophones zu bringen. Doch darf man sich nicht verführen lassen, den Mikrophon direkt auf die Brustwand zu setzen, weil das Werkzeug für gewöhnliche Stösse und Erschütterungen sehr empfindlich ist und man der Gefahr ausgesetzt ist, an Statt der Töne einige gröbere Herzbewegungen zu registriren, welche dem Mikrophone mitgetheilt werden könnten[1]).

Auf verschiedene Weise wurde den Beschwerden abgeholfen.

Nach einigen weniger erfolgreichen Bemühungen fertigten wir zwei Apparate an, welche den gemachten Anforderungen gänzlich entsprechen. Der erste wurde zur Registrirung der Herztöne von Hunden und Kaninchen angewendet, während der zweite zur Registrirung der menschlichen Herztöne diente.

Bei Hunden und Kaninchen wurden die Herztöne registrirt, ohne dass eine mechanische Verbindung zwischen der Brustwand des Thieres und dem Mikrophon angebracht wurde. Der Hartgummitrichter eines Schlauchstethoskopes wird mit der Hand gegen die linke Brustwand des auf einen Tisch befestigten Thieres angedrückt. Der elastische Schlauch ist mit einer kupfernen Röhre verbunden, welche an einen isolirten steinernen Pfeiler befestigt ist und sich mit ihrem freien Ende der Mikrophonröhre nähert; die letztere, welche geräumiger ist, wird sogar theils über erstere hin geschoben, ohne jedoch dieselbe zu berühren.

Der Mikrophon selbst ist an ein starkes und kurzes auf einen schweren Quaderstein festgeklemmtes Stativ befestigt. Der Quaderstein ruht — durch vier Stücke Kautschuk getragen — auf dem Pfeiler. Auf diese Weise ist ein Ueberbringen der Stösse und Erschütterungen vom Stethoskope zum Mikrophon gänzlich ausgeschlossen, und kann der letzte nur durch einen Schall in der Form von Luftschwingungen getroffen werden.

Der einschlägige Beweis wurde ausserdem noch geliefert, indem wir die Kautschukröhre oder auch eine über den Hartgummitrichter des Stethoskopes gespannte Membran auf solche Weise mit der Hand anstiessen, dass wir, ohne einen Schall hervorzubringen, den Effekt des Herzstosses vergrössert nachahmten. Diese

---

1) Siehe u. A. Ewalds Referat von Hürthle's Arbeit. Centr. f. Physiol. Bd. VII, S. 52.

Manipulationen veränderten den Stand des Meniscus nicht im Mindesten. Nicht sobald aber setzten wir den Stethoskoptrichter auf die Herzgegend des Versuchsthieres, so zeigte der Meniscus unmittelbar rhythmische, mit den Herztönen vollkommen synchronische Oscillationen.

Mit demselben Stethoskope untersucht, klingen die Herztöne des Kaninchens in der Regel stärker als diejenigen des Hundes und des Menschen und auch stärker als diejenigen grösserer Thiere wie Rinder und Pferde, was der dickeren Brustwand zugeschrieben werden muss, welche bei den letztern die Intensität der Töne bedeutend beeinträchtigt. Um bei grösseren Hunden diesen Beschwerden abzuhelfen, führten wir mit Erfolg eine grössere oder kleinere Rippenresection aus, welche Operation bei kleinern Hunden aber ganz überflüssig war.

Die Ausschläge des Capillarelektrometers waren oft so gross, dass sie bis aus dem Gesichtsfelde des Mikroskopes reichten; wir verkleinerten sie dann, indem wir den Rollenabstand des Schlittenapparates vergrösserten.

Gewöhnlich wurde bei Rollenabständen von 4 bis 9 Centimeter gearbeitet.

Fig. 3.

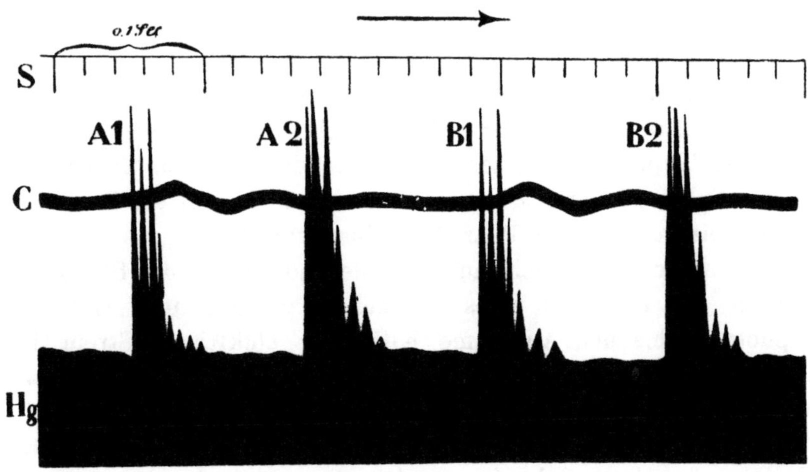

Herztöne des Kaninchens. *C* Cardiogramm. — *A1* und *B1* erste, *A2* und *B2* zweite Töne.

In Fig. 3 geben wir eine Abbildung [1]) der auf diese Weise registrirten Herztöne eines Kaninchens. Der Hartgummitrichter des Schlauchstethoscopes wird mit der Hand gegen die linke Brustwand des Thieres angedrückt, eine Kautschuktrommel gegen die rechte. Mit dieser letzteren ist ein Marey'scher Tambour verbunden, dessen Hebel eine Schattenlinie auf die lichtempfindliche Glasplatte schreibt. Bei *A1* und *B1* ist der erste, bei *A2* und *B2* der zweite Ton wiedergegeben; *C* ist das Cardiogramm und *S* die Linie der Secunden. Die Entfernung zweier Stimmgabelgipfel entspricht einer Zeit von 0,02 Secunden.

Schon bei einer oberflächlichen Betrachtung der die Herztöne wiedergebenden Figuren fällt es uns auf, dass sie nicht aus regelmässigen Schwingungen bestehen, was unmittelbar beweist, dass der Schall des Herztones kein einfacher Ton ist, sondern den Character eines Geräusches besitzt.

Genaue Messungen gewähren hierüber näheren Aufschluss So finden wir bei dem hier abgebildeten ersten Herztone *A1* die Zeit zwischen dem Anfange des Tones und dem ersten Rückstoss = 24, zwischen diesem und dem zweiten = 32, zwischen dem zweiten und dem dritten 22 und so weiter 39, 24, 40, 10, 44 Zehntausendstel einer Secunde. Wäre der Schall ein einfacher Ton gewesen, so hätten alle obengenannten Zeitintervalle einander gleich sein müssen.

Trotz dieser unregelmässigen Schwankungen wird die graphische Abbildung des Schalles durch etwas sehr typisches characterisirt. Man sieht in der Figur leicht den Unterschied zwischen dem Typus des ersten und dem des zweiten Tones, der noch deutlicher hervortritt, wenn man sich nicht auf die Beobachtung von einem einzigen Paar Töne beschränkt.

Man achte z. B. auch auf nachstehende Figur 4. Sie giebt gleichfalls die Herztöne eines Kaninchens wieder, aber während der photographischen Aufnahme hatte der elektrische Strom im Capillarelectrometer eine der Figur 3 entgegengesetzte Richtung. Sind also die Gipfel der Figur 3 nach der Schwefelsäure hin gerichtet, in Figur 4 weisen sie nach dem Quecksilber hin. Es darf nicht erwartet werden, dass die ersten Töne in allen Details,

1) Wir sind gern bereit den Fachgenossen auf Anfrage Copien unserer ursprünglichen Negative zu übersenden.

in allen feinen, den Klang characterisirenden Nuancen mit einander übereinstimmen, und doch gleichen die systolischen Töne der Fig. 4 einander so sehr und zugleich so sehr denjenigen der Fig. 3,

Fig. 4.

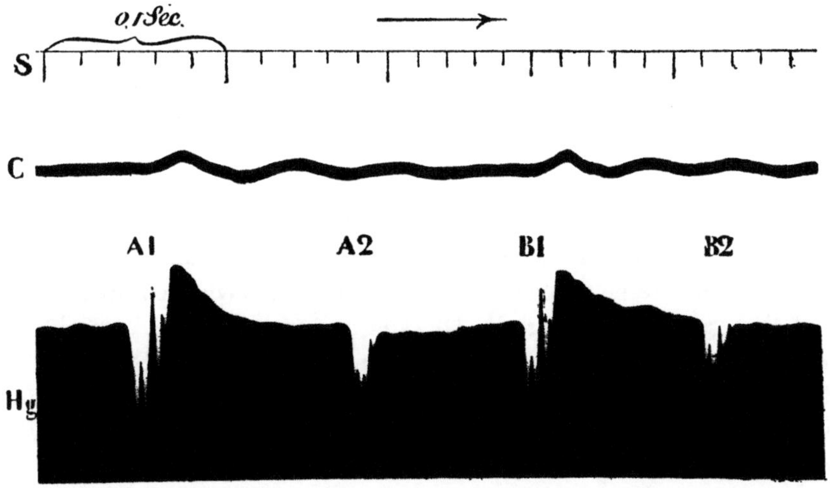

Herztöne des Kaninchens. Der Strom im Capillarelectrometer hat eine andere Richtung als diejenige der Fig. 3. Sonst kommen die Figuren 3 und 4 mit einander überein.

dass man sie ohne aufmerksame Betrachtung für Copien und Negative von einander halten könnte. Dasselbe gilt von den diastolischen Tönen.

Wir hoffen später den Typus jedes der beiden Herztöne des Kaninchens im Vergleich mit dem der Herztöne einiger anderen Thiere ausführlicher zu beschreiben, und sagen jetzt nur noch einige Worte über die Dauer der Töne.

Mit grosser Genauigkeit — bis auf einige Zehntausendstel einer Secunde — kann der Anfang jedes Tones bestimmt werden; das Ende kann jedoch wieder nicht scharf angegeben werden, weil die Intensität des Schalles gegen das Ende sehr langsam abnimmt, viel langsamer noch, als dies beim Metronomschlage der Fall war.

Wenn die die Töne registrirenden Apparate empfindlicher sein werden, wird man wahrscheinlich die Dauer der Töne etwas länger finden.

In Figur 3 dauert der kräftigste Theil des ersten Tones — die Zeit des Zustandekommens der ersten vier Gipfel — 0,023 Secunde; der folgende Theil — die Zeit des Zustandekommens der letzten vier Gipfel — 0,026 Secunde; der ganze erste Ton 0,049 Secunde. Auch der zweite Ton kann in zwei Theile getrennt werden, einen kräftigeren aus drei Gipfeln bestehenden ersten Theil, und einen schwächeren, zwei Gipfel besitzenden zweiten Theil. Die Dauer des ersten Theiles ist 0,028, des zweiten Theiles 0,011, des ganzen zweiten Tones 0,039 Secunde. Das Intervall zwischen dem Anfange des ersten und dem Anfange des zweiten Tones, d. h. die Dauer der Systole, beträgt 0,118 Secunde.

Menschliche Herztöne.

Das Registriren menschlicher Herztöne gelang uns bis jetzt nicht [1]) ohne eine mechanische Verbindung zwischen Brustwand und Microphon anzubringen. Die von uns angewendete Vorrichtung ist jedoch so, dass ebensowohl wie beim Registriren der Herztöne des Kaninchens das Microphon vollkommen gegen Stösse geschützt und nur durch Schall in der Form von Luftschwingungen in Wirkung gesetzt wird.

Fig. 5.

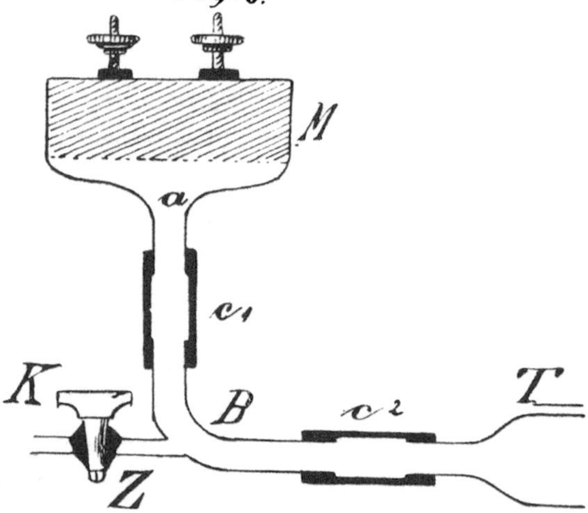

Apparat zur Registrirung der menschlichen Herztöne. *M* Microphon. — *T* Stethoscoptrichter.' — Siehe weiter den Text.

Figur 5 giebt eine schematische Darstellung des Apparates. *B* ist eine metallene Röhre mit einem Querstücke *Z*, worin sich

1) Wir haben einigen Grund, zu erwarten, dass weitere Bemühungen bessere Resultate ergeben werden.

der Hahn *K* befindet. Die Röhre *B* ist fest mit einem isolirten steinernen Pfeiler verbunden. Mit ihrem einen Ende ist sie durch ein Kautschukröhrchen C_1 an dem Microphon *M* befestigt, der ebenso wie bei der schon erwähnten Vorrichtung für Hunde und Kaninchen auf einen schweren, durch vier Stücke Kautschuk isolirten Quaderstein festgeklemmt ist. Mit ihrem anderen Ende ist sie durch das Kautschukröhrchen C_2 mit dem Trichter eines Stethoscopes verbunden. Namentlich das letztgenannte Kautschukröhrchen muss schlaff und dünnwandig sein, um zu verhüten, dass geringe, unvermeidliche Bewegungen des Stethoscoptrichters den Microphon in Wirkung setzen. Zum letzterwähnten Zwecke ist auch der Hahn *K* construirt. Bleibt dieser geschlossen und wird der Stethoscoptrichter gegen die Brustwand angedrückt, so wird der Raum in der Röhre *B* von der Luft abgeschlossen. Unter diesen Umständen wird ein Zusammenpressen oder Ausziehen der Kautschukröhren den Druck im Microphontrichter *a* beeinflussen und der Microphon reagirt auf nicht allzuträge Luftdruckänderungen nahezu ebenso stark wie auf Schälle. Hat man den Stethoscoptrichter an einer Stelle angelegt, wo der Ictus cordis fühlbar ist, so wird dieser rhythmische Luftdruckschwankungen im Microphontrichter hervorrufen. Der Microphon reagirt hierauf ebensowohl wie auf die Herztöne selbst und so wird es klar, dass der Capillarelectrometer, wenn der Hahn *K* geschlossen ist, nicht nur die Herztöne, sondern auch das Cardiogramm registrirt.

Wir besitzen einige Photogramme, welche bei geschlossener Kautschukverbindung zwischen Microphon und Stethoscop angefertigt sind und deren Bedeutung wir anfangs nicht verstanden. Sie geben sehr complicirte Bewegungen des Quecksilbers im Capillarelectrometer an, welche jedoch vollkommen regelmässig sind und denselben Rhythmus wie die Herzschläge zeigen. Erst als wir die Ursache dieser complicirten Bewegungen erkannten, brachten wir das Querstück *Z* und den Hahn *K* an. Sobald der Hahn *K* genügend geöffnet wird, bleiben die Effekte des Ictus Cordis zurück und werden nur die Töne fortgepflanzt[1]).

---

1) Als wir zur Controlle unserer Meinung bei unseren Versuchen mit Kaninchen eine geschlossene Verbindung zwischen Stethoscop und Microphon darstellten, erhielten wir, wie zu erwarten war, dieselbe Complication. Sogar die Athembewegungen des Thieres traten sehr deutlich auf dem Photogramm hervor.

In den Figuren 6 und 7 geben wir eine Abbildung menschlicher Herztöne, wie sie mit dem Stethoscope an der Herzspitze gehört werden. Die photographische Aufnahme wurde hier ebenso wie bei den folgenden Versuchen nur dann gemacht, wenn zuvor

Fig. 6.

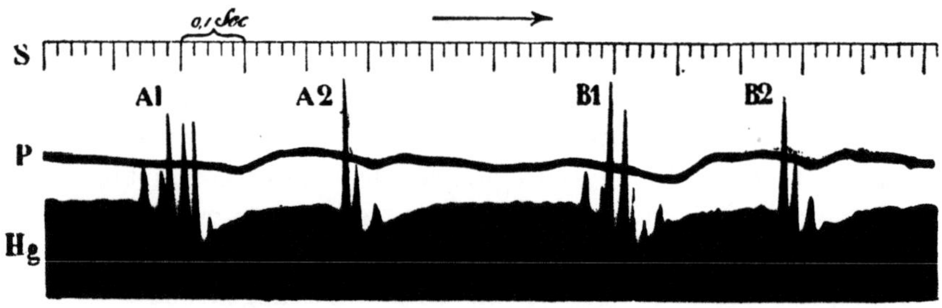

Menschliche Herztöne. Das Stethoscop ist an der Herzspitze angelegt. — *A1* und *B1* erste, *A2* und *B2* zweite Töne. — *P* Puls der A. carotis sin.

Fig. 7.

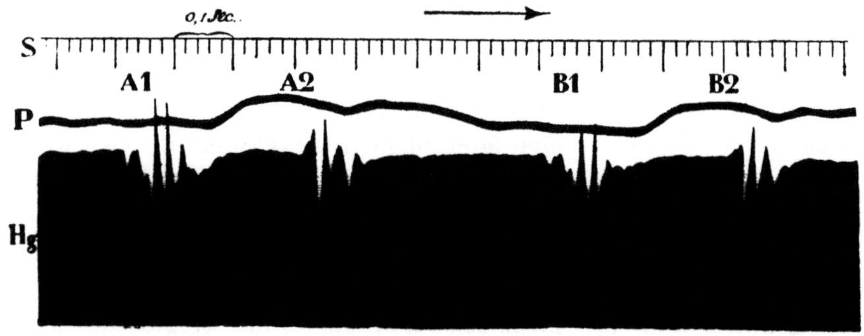

Menschliche Herztöne. Der Strom im Capillarelectrometer hat eine andere Richtung als diejenige der Fig. 6. Sonst kommen die Figuren 6 und 7 mit einander überein.

eine absichtlich gemachte Untersuchung gezeigt hatte, dass eine übertriebene Nachahmung des Spitzenstosses durch Zusammenpressen und Ausziehen der Kautschukröhre C_2 (siehe Fig. 5) den Quecksilbermeniscus unbewegt liess. In Fig. 6 hat der Strom die entgegengesetzte Richtung von derjenigen in Fig. 7. Beide Figuren zeigen bei *A1* und *B1* den ersten, bei *A2* und *B2* den zweiten Herzton. Ueber den Tönen ist der Puls der A. carotis sin. als eine schwarze Schattenlinie sichtbar.

Ebenso wie beim Kaninchen sehen wir beim Menschen, dass jeder der beiden Töne an der Herzspitze einen eigenthümlichen

Character hat. Legen wir den Stethoscop auf anderen Stellen der Brust an, so erleidet der Character der Töne gewöhnlich eine starke Veränderung; dies braucht uns aber nicht zu wundern, wenn wir nur an die Möglichkeit denken, dass dann auch andere Töne in den Vordergrund treten und die Spitzentöne überstimmen könnten.

Fig. 8.

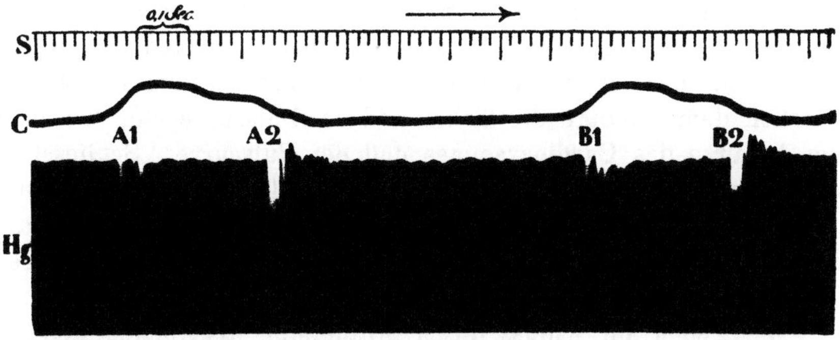

Menschliche Herztöne (Aortatöne). Das Stethoscop ist im zweiten rechten Intercostalraum angelegt. *A1* und *B1* erste, *A2* und *B2* zweite Töne. — *C* Cardiogramm.

Fig. 9.

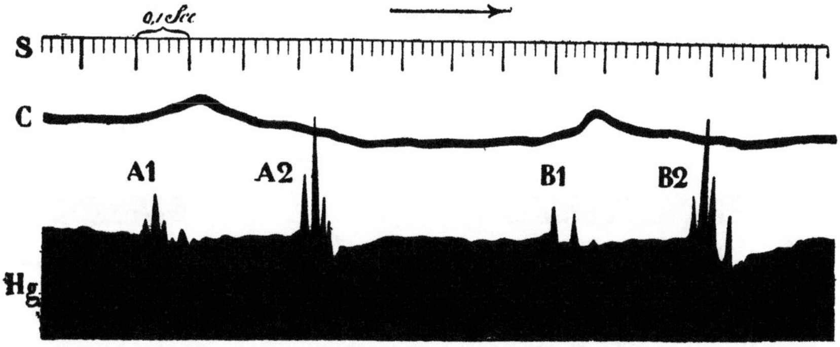

Menschliche Herztöne (Pulmonaltöne). Das Stethoscop ist im zweiten linken Intercostalraum angelegt. Der electrische Strom hat eine andere Richtung als diejenige der Fig. 8. Die Buchstaben haben dieselbe Bedeutung wie die in Fig. 8.

Fig. 8 giebt eine Abbildung der mit dem Stethoscope im rechten zweiten Intercostalraum gehörten Aortatöne; Fig. 9 giebt die Pulmonaltöne mit dem Stethoscop im linken zweiten Intercostalraum. Die schwarze Linie *C* giebt in beiden Figuren das

Cardiogramm, die übrigen Buchstaben haben dieselbe Bedeutung wie in den Figuren 6 und 7. Die Stromrichtung in Fig. 8 ist derjenigen in Fig. 9 entgegengesetzt.

Wenn wir die nähere Beziehung der Töne unter einander, ihr Verhältniss zum Cardiogramm und zur Pulscurve kennen zu lernen wünschen, so sind wir genöthigt, wieder genaue Zeitmessungen zu machen. Ausser der Dauer jedes der beiden Töne und ihrem gegenseitigen Abstande muss überdies noch der Zeitunterschied gemessen werden zwischen dem Auftreten des ersten Tones und der ersten Erhebung des Cardiogrammes. Ebenso zwischen dem Anfange des Tones und der Pulscurve und zwischen dem Anfange des Cardiogrammes und der Pulscurve. Schliesslich muss noch der Zeitunterschied zwischen der electrischen Fortpflanzung des Schalles durch den Microphon nach dem Capillarelectrometer einerseits und dem Lufttransport des Spitzenstosses nach der Registrirtrommel andererseits bestimmt werden.

Wir geben am Schluss dieser Mittheilung als Anhang die gefundenen Werthe in Zahlen wieder, während wir die Messungsergebnisse hier in einer Zeichnung verdeutlichen.

Fig. 10.

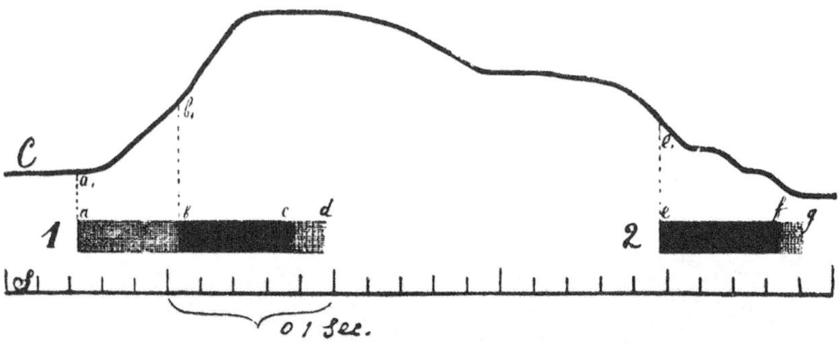

Menschliches Cardiogramm. *C* Cardiogramm. — *1* erster Ton. — *2* zweiter Ton. — Bei *a* fängt der erste Spitzenton an, bei *b* der erste Arterienton. Siehe weiter den Text.

Die Curve *C* der Fig. 10 stellt das menschliche Cardiogramm dar, *S* ist die Zeitlinie, deren jede Abtheilung 0,02 Secunden entspricht. Die breiten Streifen 1 und 2 bedeuten den ersten und zweiten Herzton. Der erste Ton tritt eher an der Herzspitze als im zweiten Intercostalraum hervor: bei *a* fängt der erste Spitzenton an, bei b der erste Aorta- und Pulmonalton[1]). Weder vom ersten noch vom zweiten Ton kann der genaue Zeitpunkt angegeben werden, worauf sie endigen; dieser Zeitpunkt muss irgendwo in den schraffirten Stücken *cd* und *fg* gefunden werden.

An der Herzspitze ist der erste Ton schon vorhanden — bei aa_1 — vor dem Anfange des Cardiogrammes. Dieses Ergebniss könnte auf verschiedene Weise gedeutet werden, wir gehen jedoch nicht näher darauf ein hauptsächlich, weil das Zeitintervall nur klein ist[2]). Eine grössere Bedeutung hat die Thatsache, dass im zweiten Intercostalraum der erste Ton in dem Augenblick anfängt, wo ungefähr die Hälfte des anakroten Theiles des Cardiogrammes vollendet ist (bb_1).

Wenn wir uns die Frage stellen, welchem Umstande es zugeschrieben werden muss, dass der erste Ton als Aorta- oder Pulmonalton so viel später als der erste Spitzenton anfängt, so erblicken wir zwei Möglichkeiten. Entweder man hört im 2. Intercostalraum als ersten Ton einen andern Schall als an der Herzspitze — und zwar hervorgerufen durch die plötzliche Spannung der Arterienmembranen — oder die Semilunarklappen verhindern — so lange sie noch geschlossen sind — die Fortpflanzung des Tones von den Ventrikeln nach den Arterien[3]). In beiden Fällen wird der erste Ton im zweiten Intercostalraum anfangen müssen in dem Augenblick, wo die Semilunarklappen sich öffnen, und daraus folgt, dass der Anfang dieses Tones ein ausgezeichnetes Mittel darbietet, diesen Zeitpunkt zu bestimmen (siehe das Cardiogramm b_1).

Der Anfang des zweiten Tones liegt im Cardiogramm bei e_1 und giebt hier den Zeitpunkt an, wo die Semilunarklappen geschlossen werden. Die ganze Herzsystole muss also in zwei Perioden getheilt werden, die erste $a_1 b_1$ — durchschnittlich 0,061 Sec. andauernd — worin der Druck in den Ventrikeln sich erhöht aber doch noch ungenügend bleibt, das Blut in die Arterien zu

1) Das Zeitintervall zwischen dem Auftreten des ersten Tones im zweiten rechten und im zweiten linken Intercostalraum ist so klein, dass wir es hier nicht in Rechnung bringen. Siehe den Anhang.

2) Siehe den Anhang.

3) Der Abstand zwischen der Herzspitze und dem 2. Intercostalraum ist nur klein, so dass wir die gewöhnliche Fortpflanzungsgeschwindigkeit des Schalles ausser Rechnung lassen können.

treiben — die zweite $b_1 e_1$, die Austreibungsperiode des Blutes, anfangend mit der Oeffnung, endigend mit der Schliessung der Semilunarklappen.

Wir erachten es für überflüssig, hier an das Bedürfniss einer entscheidenden Deutung des Cardiogrammes zu erinnern. Nicht lange her noch hat Léon Fredericq[1]) scharf ins Licht gestellt, wie sehr die Meinungen der verschiedenen Forscher sogar in den Hauptsachen auseinander gehen. Wir begnügen uns darum, darauf hinzuweisen, dass unsere Ergebnisse zweifelsohne die alten Vorstellungen von Chauveau und Marey über die ziemlich lange Dauer der Systole bestätigen.

Im Anhang geben wir die Resultate der Messung von 15 Herzperioden eines gesunden 18-jährigen jungen Mannes, der während des Registrirens seiner Herztöne eine sitzende Haltung angenommen hatte. Der Natur der Sache nach hat die Dauer der Systole und die der Diastole einen wechselnden Werth. Wir unterlassen es darum Mittelwerthe zu berechnen und begnügen uns mit der Erwähnung der gefundenen Aeussersten.

Die Dauer der Systole wechselte von 0,312 bis 0,346 Sec.
„ „ „ Diastole „ „ 0,385 „ 0,518 „
„ „ „ Systole, in Procenten der Herzperiode ausgedrückt, wechselte von . . . . . . 39,2 bis 45,3 %.

Unsere Ergebnisse stimmen sehr gut mit denjenigen, welche Donders nach seiner Methode des indirecten Registrirens erhalten hat, überein[2]).

Was die Vertheilung der Systole in zwei Perioden anbelangt, bemerken wir noch, dass Hürthle[3]) und Fredericq[4]) bei Hunden auf ganz anderm Wege als dem unsrigen zu übereinstimmenden Resultaten gekommen sind.

Wir endigen unsere kurze Mittheilung über die Registrirung der Herztöne mit der Abbildung eines Herzgeräusches.

---

1) Siehe verschiedene Abhandlungen von Léon Fredericq im Centralbl. f. Physiol. Bd. V, VI und VII.

2) A. a. O.

3) Dr. K. Hürthle, Beiträge zur Hämodynamik. Dieses Arch. 1891. Bd. 49. S. 86.

4) Léon Fredericq, Ueber die Zeit der Oeffnung und Schliessung der Semilunarklappen. Centralbl. für Physiol. 1892. Bd. VI. S. 257.

Bei einem Hunde wurden die Aortaklappen mit Hülfe einer in die A. carotis eingeführten Sonde durchstossen. Das hierdurch entstandene diastolische Geräusch ist in Fig. 11 abgebildet; zur

Fig. 11.

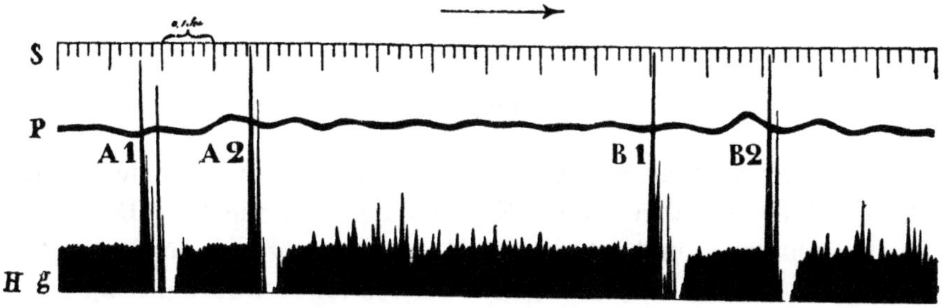

Herzgeräusch eines Hundes mit Aorteninsufficienz. *A1* und *B1* erste, *A2* und *B2* zweite Töne. — *P* Puls der A. cruralis.

Fig. 12.

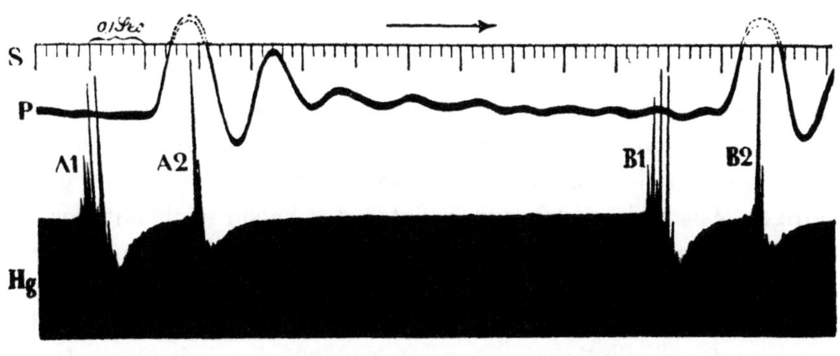

Herztöne eines Hundes mit normalem Herzen. Die Buchstaben haben dieselbe Bedeutung wie in Fig. 11.

Vergleichung sind in Fig. 12 die Herztöne eines Hundes mit normalem Herze registrirt.

Die Curve P. giebt den Puls der A. carotis dextra an. Die Ausschläge des Hebels waren in Fig. 12 übermässig gross, in Fig. 11 sehr klein, in beiden jedoch genügend, den Zeitpunkt zu markiren, wo die Pulswelle die A. carotis erreicht.

Wir sehen beim normalen Herzen — Fig. 12 — während der Diastole keine nennenswerthen Oscillationen hervortreten, beim Hunde mit Aorteninsufficienz hingegen — Fig. 11 — in grosser Zahl. Diese Oscillationen zeigen uns mehr als das alleinige Dasein des Geräusches. Es zeigt sich zum Beispiel recht deutlich, wie im Anfange der Diastole das Geräusch ganz durch den noch kräftigen Klappenton überstimmt wird und wie später Perioden grösserer und geringerer Intensität auftreten, welche — wahrscheinlich mit Schwankungen im arteriellen Blutdruck zusammenhängend — uns an die Form einer Pulscurve erinnern.

Anhang.

Zu der Ausführung der Messungen wurde eine von der Firma Dr. Carl Zeiss angefertigte Netztheilung verwendet[1]). Das Netz ist 300 mm lang und 50 mm breit und besteht aus quadratischen Feldern von 1 mm^2. Von dieser Netztheilung wurde ein Diapositiv angefertigt, das mit der Gelatineseite auf die Gelatineseite des auszumessenden Photogrammes festgeklemmt wurde.

Die beiden fest auf einander geklemmten Gläser wurden mit Hülfe eines Microscopes mit beweglichem Ocularmicrometer ausgemessen.

Während der photographischen Aufnahme der Herztöne wurde durch eine Stimmgabel von 50 ganzen Schwingungen in der Secunde eine Schattenlinie auf das lichtempfindliche Glas geschrieben. Die feinen und scharfen Gipfel dieser Curve hatten einen gegenseitigen Abstand, welcher der Natur der Sache nach mit der Bewegungsgeschwindigkeit des Glases wechselte. Wir wendeten meistentheils eine Geschwindigkeit von 60 bis 80 mm pro Secunde an, konnten jedoch für genaue Zeitmessungen mit gutem Erfolg grössere Geschwindigkeiten, z. B. von 200 mm pro Secunde benutzen.

Das Bild der Spaltöffnung — bei still stehender Glasplatte erhalten — war 0,075 mm breit. Nimmt man an, dass die Bewegung des lichtempfindlichen Glases zwischen zwei Stimmgabelgipfeln gleichmässig ist, so lässt sich die Genauigkeit der Zeitmessung aus obenstehenden Daten berechnen. Der Fehler braucht nicht grösser als $\frac{0,075}{200} = 0,00037$ Secunden zu sein und könnte

1) Siehe W. Einthoven, Lippmann's Capellarelectrometer zur Messung schnell wechselnder Potentialunterschiede. Pflüger's Archiv f. d. ges. Physiol. Bd. 56. S. 528.

II
Ueber das normale menschliche Elektrokardiogramm und über die capillair-elektrometrische Untersuchung einiger Herzkranken

G.J. Burch published in 1892 his analysis of curves obtained with the capillary electrometer, using it to reconstruct the records of action currents from the frog's gastrocnemius as published by Burdon Sanderson. Einthoven quoted Burch in a paper (19) in which he described his own (different) analysis and method of correction. He himself was the first to apply his correction to the electrocardiogram. In 1895 he published both the form of the directly recorded and of the corrected normal human electrocardiogram (26). The paper which follows here, contains a more exhaustive description of the normal electrocardiogram in its corrected form. The time relations, height and shape of the corrected electrocardiogram (called P,Q,R,S,T, in contrast to A,B,C,D, of the recorded tracing) are measured and discussed. It is thought likely that P and Q are caused by atrial contraction and RST by the ventricle. The length of the systolic period is established and compared with findings in the literature; the influence of the heart rate on duration of systole and on the shape of the individual waves is discussed. Particular attention is given to the positioning of the leads and its effect on potential differences (favourable and unfavourable combinations, according to Waller), and to the influence of the position of the body.

For the first time two pathological electrocardiograms are also shown and discussed (2 patients with aortic insufficiency and T wave changes). Some details about their phonocardiograms are also given, in particular about the division of the mechanical systole in an ejection period and a first systolic part (i.e. isometric period), as described in the preceding paper (1). The isometric period is found absent in the 2 cases of aortic insufficiency.

Equally for the first time, electrocardiograms were taken after exercise. This investigation was carried out in order to study the effect of increased heart rate. In retrospect it is interesting but misleading, that in the recorded tracing the main changes appeared in what now is called the ST segment (between the C and D waves); after correction of the electrocardiogram, mainly slight changes in the height of the peaks (from then on called PQRST) were found.

(Physiologisches Laboratorium in Leyden.)

Ueber das normale menschliche Elektrokardiogramm und über die capillar-elektrometrische Untersuchung einiger Herzkranken.

Von

W. Einthoven und **K. de Lint.**

(Hierzu Tafel II und III und 1 Textfigur.)

Um die Form des normalen menschlichen Elektrokardiogrammes kennen zu lernen, haben wir mittelst des Capillarelektrometers bei einer Anzahl von Personen in verschiedenen Umständen die elektromotorischen Bewegungen registrirt, welche in mehreren Körpertheilen im selben Rhythmus wie die Herzschläge constatirt werden können[1]). Manche Einzelheiten dieser Untersuchung findet man ausführlich an anderer Stelle beschrieben[2]). Hier beschränken wir uns auf die Mittheilung und die Erklärung der Resultate, denen wir das Ergebniss der capillar-elektrometrischen Untersuchung einiger Herzkranken hinzufügen.

Man muss einen scharfen Unterschied machen zwischen den direct registrirten Elektrokardiogrammen und denjenigen, welche durch Construction erhalten sind. Von den ersteren sind ein Dutzend Beispiele gegeben in Tafel II, die eine photographische Reproduction[3]) in ungefähr 65 % der natürlichen Grösse der ursprünglichen Curven darstellt. Die Spitzen *A*, *C* und *D* weisen auf eine zeitweilige Negativität der

1) Siehe Aug. D. Waller, Philosoph. transact. of the Royal Soc. of London vol. 180 (1889) B, p. 169. — Bayliss and Starling, Internat. Monatsschr. für Anat. und Physiol. Bd. 9 S. 256, 1892. — W. T. de Vogel, Inaug.-Dissert. 1893. Leyden. — W. Einthoven, Dieses Archiv Bd. 60 S. 101, 1895. — Die beiden Letzteren auch in Onderzoekingen Physiol. Laborat. Leyden R. 2 Dl. I und II.

2) K. de Lint, Inaug.-Dissert. Leyden 1896. — Auch in Onderzoekingen Physiol. Laborat. Leyden R. 2 Dl. III.

3) Die Copien der ursprünglichen Negative, welche ungleich deutlicher und schärfer als die Tafel sind, werden wir gern auf Anfrage den Fachgenossen übersenden.

Herzbasis gegen die Herzspitze hin, während B und C_1 einen zeitweiligen Potentialunterschied in entgegengesetztem Sinne andeuten.

Auf Tafel III findet man die construirten Elektrokardiogramme, bei denen eine Ordinatlänge von 10 Millivolt einer Abscissenlänge von 1 Secunde gleichgemacht ist. Die Dimensionen für die Construction sind aus den direct registrirten Elektrokardiogrammen von Tafel II berechnet worden. Die zwölf Nummern von Tafel II entsprechen den zwölf Figuren von Tafel III. Nur diese construirten Curven sind der genaue Ausdruck der Schwankungen des Potentialunterschiedes. In jedem construirten Elektrokardiogramm unterscheiden wir fünf Spitzen (siehe Tafel III Fig. 1), von denen P, R und T eine Negativität der Herzbasis gegen die Herzspitze und Q und S eine Negativität der Herzspitze gegen die Basis angeben.

Wir stellen uns die Frage, welche Unterschiede das normale Elektrokardiogramm in der Höhe, der Schärfe und der Dauer dieser Spitzen zeigen kann.

Es wurden 17 Personen in möglichst gleichen Umständen untersucht. Jede von ihnen sass während des Registrirens ruhig auf einem Stuhle und liess die beiden Arme schlaff am Körper herunterhängen. Jede Hand war bis über den Puls in eine grosse, mit einer 1 %igen Kochsalzlösung gefüllte Thonzelle getaucht, die selbst in einem gläsernen Cylinder stand. Letzterer war mit einer gesättigten Lösung von Sulfas zinzicus gefüllt, worin sich ein Blatt aus amalgamirtem Zink befand, das mit einem der Pole des Capillar-Elektrometers leitend verbunden war. Die Messungsergebnisse [1]) sind in den nachfolgenden Tabellen 1 und 2 zusammengestellt.

Das in der dritten Spalte nebenstehender Tabelle 1 erwähnte Alter ist für viele der untersuchten Personen, welche hierüber nicht speciell befragt worden sind, geschätzt. Diese Schätzung kann selbstverständlich nur ungenau sein, aber eine grosse Genauigkeit scheint hier ganz und gar überflüssig zu sein, weil wir bei unseren Messungen keine Beziehung zwischen dem Alter und der Form des Elektrokardiogrammes haben entdecken können.

Wir sehen, dass die grösste Spitze R, welche eine Negativität der Herzbasis gegen die Herzspitze andeutet, bei den 17 unter-

1) Unter die oben erwähnten Messungsergebnisse sind nicht die zwölf Elektrokardiogramme von Tafel II aufgenommen, weil diese nicht bei Stromableitung von den beiden Händen erhalten sind.

Tabelle 1.

Name	Geschlecht	Alter (Jahr)	Nummer der Platte	Die Werthe der verschiedenen Spitzen, ausgedrückt in Millivolt: P Die Herzspitze ist positiv	Q Die Herzspitze ist negativ	R Die Herzspitze ist positiv	S Die Herzspitze ist negativ	T Die Herzspitze ist positiv
v. d. W. .	m.	53	213	0,31	— 0,48	1,46	— 0,26	0,33
Bm. . . .	„	20	216	0,21	— 0,17	0,83	— 0,81	0,36
d. Gr. . .	„	23	298	0,13	— 0,30	0,86	— 0,45	0,44
d. Jg. . .	„	22	300	0,07	— 0,06	0,45	— 0,44	0,21
Wr. . . .	„	22	302	0,07	— 0,13	0,66	— 0,45	0,22
Fs.	„	22	303	0,13	— 0,14	1,28	— 0,78	0,42
v. d. L. . .	„	24	304	0,07	— 0,11	1,00	— 0,23	0,15
L. N. F. .	„	23	305	0,13	— 0,17	0,95	— 0,30	0,41
J. L. . . .	„	22	308	0,13	— 0,22	0,92	— 0,34	0,38
A. Ws. . .	„	50	309	0,09	— 0,12	0,76	— 0,13	0,25
Kg. . . .	„	25	310	0,11	— 0,14	1,11	— 0,26	0,34
P. L. . . .	„	22	312	0,12	— 0,22	1,09	— 0,41	0,38
W. E. . .	„	35	316	0,075	— 0,12	0,75	— 0,19	0,20
M. A. J. G.	„	32	317	0,11	— 0,17	0,86	— 0,09	0,53
J. E. . . .	„	33	325	0,13	— 0,145	1,08	— 0,54	0,33
R. Ws. . .	„	9	332	0,13	— 0,60	1,13	— 0,18	0,39
W. Ws. . .	„	4	333	0.12	— 0,33	1,10	— 0,39	0,34
Durchschnittlich:				0,125	— 0,21	0,96	— 0,37	0,33

Tabelle 2.

Name	Nummer der Platte	Dauer der verschiedenen Theile, ausgedrückt in Secunden: P	Q	R	S	T	Erster Theil (bis zum Anfang von R)	Zweiter Theil (bis zum Ende von T)
v. d. W. .	213	0,04	0,035	0,02	0,10	0,125	0,11	0,305
Bm. . . .	216	0,04	0,025	0,03	0,08	0,125	0,11	0,30
d. Gr. . .	298	0,04	0,03	0,03	0,075	0,12	0,11	0,31
d. Jg. . .	300	0,04	0,02	0,03	0,08	0,12	0,13	0,31
Wr. . . .	302	0,04	0,02	0,02	0,06	0,12	0,12	0,31
Fs.	303	0,05	0,04	0,03	0,06	0,16	0,16	0,32
v. d. L. . .	304	0,03	0,03	0,03	0,08	0.12	0,12	0,30
L. N. F. .	305	0,04	0,03	0,02	0,075	0,16	0,11	0,31
J. L. . . .	308	0,04	0,02	0,02	0,08	0,16	0,12	0,34
A. Ws. . .	309	0,04	0,03	0,02	0,055	0,12	0,16	0,32
Kg. . . .	310	0,04	0,03	0,02	0,08	0,14	0,12	0,32
P. L. . . .	312	0,045	0,04	0,02	0,09	0,16	0,13	0,35
W. E. . .	316	0,04	0,04	0,03	0,075	0,12	0,13	0,33
M. A. J. G.	317	0,04	0,02	0,03	0,08	0,16	0,12	0,36
J. E. . . .	325	0,04	0,04	0,02	0,085	0,14	0,13	0,30
R Ws. . .	332	0,04	0,02	0,02	0,075	0,16	0,16	0,31
W. Ws. . .	333	0,04	0,02	0,02	0,08	0,14	0,14	0,30
Durchschnittlich:		0,04	0,03	0,02	0,08	0,13	0,12	0,32

suchten Individuen zwischen einem Betrag von 0,45 bis 1,46 Millivolt schwankt und durchschnittlich 0,96 Millivolt beträgt. Die andern Spitzen sind kleiner und zeigen, in absolutem Maasse ausgedrückt, weniger Unterschied.

P schwankt zwischen 0,07 und 0,31 und beträgt durchschnittlich 0,125 Millivolt;

Q schwankt zwischen — 0,06 und — 0,60 und beträgt durchschnittlich — 0,21 Millivolt;

S schwankt zwischen — 0,09 und — 0,81 und beträgt durchschnittlich — 0,37 Millivolt;

T schwankt zwischen 0,15 und 0,53 und beträgt durchschnittlich 0,33 Millivolt.

Achten wir, statt auf die absoluten, auf die relativen Unterschiede, so ist *R* die constanteste Spitze; darauf folgt *T* und dann kommen *P*, *Q* und *S*, wie aus der folgenden Tabelle, in welcher der grösste und der kleinste Betrag jeder Spitze in Procenten des Durchschnittswerthes angegeben werden, ersichtlich ist.

Tabelle 3.

	Grösster Betrag in Procenten des Durchschnittswerthes	Kleinster Betrag in Procenten des Durchschnittswerthes
P	248,00	56,00
Q	228,57	28,57
R	152,08	46,87
S	218,91	24,32
T	160,60	45,45

Da also *R* nicht allein die höchste, sondern auch die constanteste Spitze ist, darf sie als die wichtigste angesehen werden.

Die Form der Spitze wird, ausser durch ihre Höhe, auch noch durch ihre Dauer bestimmt. Die Dauer von

P schwankt zwischen 0,045 und 0,03 Sec. und beträgt durchschnittlich 0,04 Sec.;

Q schwankt zwischen 0,02 und 0,04 Sec. und beträgt durchschnittlich 0,03 Sec.;

R schwankt zwischen 0,02 und 0,03 Sec. und beträgt durchschnittlich 0,02 Sec.;

S schwankt zwischen 0,055 und 0,10 Sec. und beträgt durchschnittlich 0,08 Sec.;

T schwankt zwischen 0,12 und 0,16 Sec. und beträgt durchschnittlich 0,13 Sec.

Hieraus sehen wir, dass *Q* und *R* von kürzerer Dauer, also schärfer, *P*, *S* und *T* von längerer Dauer, also stumpfer sind.

Der Einfluss der Frequenz des Herzschlages auf die Form des Elektrokardiogrammes.

Es wurde ein Elektrokardiogramm registrirt von einer Person, welche längere Zeit geruht hatte. Sie musste darauf schwere Gewichte heben, schnell laufen, schnell und wiederholt Treppen steigen, — welche letztere Bewegung die grösste Wirkung hatte — und unmittelbar darauf wieder dieselbe Haltung annehmen, in der sie sich befand beim Schreiben des Elektrokardiogrammes vor der Ausführung der Körperbewegung. Nun wurde wieder ein Elektrokardiogramm registrirt.

Um die Unterschiede zwischen den Curven so deutlich wie möglich in's Auge springen zu lassen, legten wir die Elektroden an diejenigen Stellen des Körpers an, welche die grössten Schwankungen des Potentialunterschiedes zeigen. Wie noch eingehender dargelegt werden wird, müssen als solche betrachtet werden auf der einen Seite die Brustwand nahe bei dem Apex cordis, auf der anderen Seite die rechte Schulter oder der rechte Arm. Die zu untersuchende Person tauchte den rechten Arm in die mit Kochsalzlösung gefüllte Thonzelle der oben erwähnten unpolarisirbaren Elektrode. Als zweite Elektrode wurde zuerst eine mit Zinksulfatlösung gefüllte Thonzelle gebraucht, deren Boden mit Sämischleder bedeckt war. Letzteres war in einer Kochsalzlösung getränkt worden, während ein Stab aus amalgamirtem Zink in die Zinksulfatlösung getaucht und mit einem von den Polen des Capillar-Elektrometers leitend verbunden war. Diese Vorrichtung hatte den grossen Uebelstand, dass kleine Verschiebungen an der Brustwand Schwankungen im Potentialunterschiede zur Folge hatten, womit die rhythmischen Wellen des Elektrokardiogrammes complicirt wurden. Namentlich wenn die Person, welche untersucht wurde, starke Körperbewegung verrichtet hatte und demzufolge tief und frequent athmete, zeigten sich rhythmische Schwankungen des Elektrokardiogrammes. Diese hatten dieselben Frequenzen wie die Athembewegungen und mussten durch letztere verursacht sein.

Wir halfen obenerwähntem Uebelstande dadurch gründlich ab, dass wir von der folgenden Vorrichtung Gebrauch machten. Ein gläserner Trichter, dessen Rand mit einem Kautschukring umgeben war, wurde mit einer 1 %igen Kochsalzlösung gefüllt und gegen die Regio cordis gehalten. Der Trichterrand hatte einen Durchmesser von 9,5 cm. Mittelst des Kautschukrings war es möglich, den Trichter, ohne Schmerz zu verursachen, fest gegen die Brustwand zu drücken und eine wasserdichte Verbindung zu erhalten. Eine gleichfalls mit einer Kochsalzlösung gefüllte, 85 cm lange, 13 mm weite Kautschukröhre verband den Hals des Trichters mit der Thonzelle einer unpolarisirbaren Elektrode, welche, um unnöthige Druckunterschiede zu vermeiden, auf ungefähr dieselbe Höhe wie der gläserne Trichter gestellt wurde. Um die Füllung des Trichters zu erleichtern, war in demselben eine Seitenöffnung angebracht worden, welche mit einem Korke geschlossen werden konnte. Man konnte den Trichter bewegen, die Kochsalzlösung schütteln und verschieben, ohne dass dadurch merkliche elektromotorische Kräfte erweckt wurden; auch hatten unter diesen Umständen die tiefsten Athmungen keinen Einfluss mehr auf die Form des Elektrokardiogrammes.

Während des Photographirens war der gläserne Trichter mit einem Bande um die Brust befestigt.

Die registrirten Curven.

Wir verfügen über 51 photographische Platten mit Elektrokardiogrammen, welche genommen worden sind, um den Einfluss erhöhter Pulsfrequenz zu untersuchen. Von diesen sind 12 zum Theil auf Tafel II abgebildet. Die Figuren 1, 3, 5, 7, 9 und 11 sind Elektrokardiogramme von 6 verschiedenen Personen, welche untersucht wurden, bevor sie Körperbewegung verrichtet hatten; die Figuren 2, 4, 6, 8, 10 und 12 sind Elektrokardiogramme derselben 6 Personen nach der Körperbewegung.

Es ist leicht, einen regelmässig vorkommenden Unterschied zwischen der ersten und der zweiten Gruppe zu constatiren, und zwar in dem Theil der Curve, welcher zwischen den Spitzen C und D liegt. Ohne Ausnahme wird hier, bei C_1, die Herzbasis, wo sie negativ gegen die Spitze war, weniger negativ oder sogar positiv (siehe die Figuren 1 und 2, 5 und 6, 7 und 8, 11 und 12), und wo sie schon positiv war, stärker positiv (siehe die Figuren 3 und 4, 9 und 10).

Bei grosser Pulsfrequenz scheinen die Elektrokardiogramme in einander zu laufen (siehe Fig. 10). Dies gilt aber nur von den direct registrirten Curven; die methodische Construction kann lehren, dass die Schwankungen im Potentialunterschiede nahezu vollständig von einander getrennt bleiben.

Ferner sehen wir, dass bei einigen Personen die Spitze *D* bei Körperbewegung an Grösse zunimmt (siehe z. B. Tafel II, Fig. 5 und 6), dagegen bei andern abnimmt (siehe z. B. Fig. 7 und 8, 9 und 10, 11 und 12). Die übrigen 39 nicht abgebildeten Tafeln stimmen mit den abgebildeten im Wesentlichen überein.

Die construirten Elektrokardiogramme.

In untenstehender Tabelle stellen wir die Ergebnisse der Messung von 20 Elektrokardiogrammen zusammen. Sie stimmt in der Form mit der ersten Tabelle überein, nur sind Geschlecht und Alter nicht angegeben. Statt dessen wird angedeutet, wie gross die Frequenz des Herzschlages war und ob das Elektrokardiogramm vor oder nach der Körperbewegung genommen worden ist. Zudem ist noch in den letzten drei Spalten die Dauer des ersten Theiles, des zweiten Theiles und des ganzen Elektrokardiogrammes angegeben.

Tabelle 4.

Name	Zahl der Herzschläge per Minute	Vor der Körperbew. = *v*; danach = *n*	Nummer der Platte	Die Werthe der verschiedenen Spitzen, ausgedrückt in Millivolt					Dauer in Secunden des		
				P	*Q*	*R*	*S*	*T*	ersten Theiles (bis zum Anfang von *R*)	zweiten Theiles (bis zum Ende von *T*)	Ganzen
d. Lt. .	62	*v*	238	0,30	— 0,23	1,60	— 1,40	0,65	0,13	0,34	0,47
d. Lt. .	83	*n*	240	0,25	— 0,23	2,00	— 1,70	0,74	0,13	0,33	0,46
d. Lt. .	67	*v*	282	0,19	— 0,08	1,77	— 0,53	0,48	0,13	0,32	0,45
d. Lt. .	114	*n*	284	0,11	— 0,24	1,71	— 1,04	0,88	0,13	0,30	0,43
Bl. . .	98	*v*	250	0,23	— 0,58	2,04	— 0,71	0,68	0,14	0,32	0,46
Bl. . .	104	*n*	252	0,24	— 0,61	2,73	— 1,17	1,04	0,14	0,32	0,46
Bl. . .	104	*n*	253	0,19	— 0,66	2,66	— 0,96	0,82	0,14	0,28	0,42
Bm. . .	90,5	*v*	255	0,29	— 0,405	2,03	— 1,69	1,03	0,15	0,31	0,46
Bm. . .	95	*n*	256	0,28	— 0,50	1,60	— 2,47	1,27	0,15	0,31	0,46
Gn. . .	85	*v*	261	0,12	— 0,16	1,16	— 0,57	0,73	0,12	0,29	0,41
Gn. . .	104	*n*	264	0	— 0,33	1,07	— 0,86	1,04	0,12	0,28	0,40
Vs. . .	67	*v*	270	0,12	— 0,42	3,55	— 0,35	0,94	0,12	0,34	0,46
Vs. . .	67	*v*	271	0,11	— 0,36	2,51	— 0,52	0,97	0,11	0,36	0,47
Vs. . .	102	*n*	272	0,08	— 0,43	3,11	— 0,81	0,80	0,13	0,29	0,42
Vs. . .	102	*n*	273	0,11	— 0,47	3,24	— 0,67	0,71	0,13	0,31	0,44
Bs. . .	90,5	*v*	288	0,14	— 0,14	2,00	— 1,38	1,22	0,14	0,32	0,46
Bs. . .	106	*n*	289	0,13	— 0,30	2,10	— 1,70	0,80	0,14	0,29	0,43
v. d. W.	67	*v*	292	0,21	— 0,33	1,90	— 0,45	0,58	0,15	0,30	0,45
v. d. W.	67	*v*	293	0,22	— 0,34	1,85	— 0,46	0,67	0,14	0,32	0,46
v. d. W.	88	*n*	294	0,14	— 0,50	1,80	— 0,91	0,36	0,14	0,32	0,46

Vorstehende Tabelle gibt Anlass zu verschiedenen Bemerkungen, welche man aber leichter verstehen kann, wenn wir die erhaltenen Ziffern auf andere Weise gruppiren.

In der folgenden Tabelle 5 haben wir nur die Unterschiede in den Werthen der Spitzen und in der Dauer des Elektrokardiogrammes angegeben. In der zweiten Spalte findet man die Nummern der Platten: die Paare, welche durch Klammern verbunden sind, haben dazu gedient, Durchschnittswerthe zu berechnen, welche letzteren in die Tabelle aufgenommen worden sind. In den Spalten 4 bis 8 sind die in Millivolt ausgedrückten Höhenunterschiede der Spitzen angegeben. Wenn nach der Körperbewegung die Höhe zugenommen hat, wird der Unterschied positiv, wenn die Höhe abgenommen hat, negativ genannt, während unter Höhe der Abstand bis zur Abscissenachse verstanden wird, gleichgültig, ob die Spitze über oder unter der Achse liegt. Dagegen nennen wir den Unterschied in Dauer positiv, wenn durch die Körperbewegung die Dauer abgenommen, negativ, wenn sie zugenommen hat (siehe die Spalten 9, 10 und 11). Die Bedeutung der übrigen Spalten ist in der Tabelle selbst schon angegeben und bedarf hier keiner weiteren Erklärung.

Wir lernen aus der Tabelle, dass die Spitzen *R* und *T* bei beschleunigter Herzthätigkeit bald vergrössert, bald verkleinert werden. Berechnet man den Durchschnittsbetrag der Veränderung, so zeigt sich, dass *R* vergrössert wird mit einem Betrag von durchschnittlich 0,10 Millivolt und dass *T* vergrössert wird mit einem Betrag von durchschnittlich 0,16 Millivolt.

Die Spitzen *P*, *Q* und *S* werden auf constante Weise verändert: ohne Ausnahme wird *P* stets verkleinert und werden *Q* und *S* stets vergrössert.

Die Verkleinerung von	*P*	beträgt maximal	0,12,	durchschn.	0,05 Milliv.
„ Vergrösserung „	*Q*	„ „	0,17,	„	0,11 „
„ „ „	*S*	„ „	0,78,	„	0,41 „

Die Vergrösserung von *S* erreicht den höchsten Betrag und muss als die wichtigste Veränderung bezeichnet werden, welche durch eine beschleunigte Herzthätigkeit in der Form des Elektrokardiogrammes hervorgerufen wird. Dies konnte schon bei der Betrachtung der direct registrirten Curven vor der Messung vermuthet werden.

Aus Tabelle 5 ist nicht zur Genüge ersichtlich, ob überhaupt Beziehung besteht zwischen dem Betrag der Frequenzveränderung

Tabelle 5.

Name	Nummern der Platten	Unterschied in Frequenz des Herzschlages	Unterschied in Höhe der verschiedenen Spitzen, ausgedrückt in Millivolt					Unterschied in Dauer, ausgedrückt in Secunden		
			P	*Q*	*R*	*S*	*T*	Erster Theil	Zweiter Theil	Das Ganze
d. Lt. . . .	238 und 240	83 — 62 = 21	— 0,05	0	0,40	0,30	0,09	0	0,01	0,01
d. Lt. . . .	282 „ 284	114 — 67 = 47	— 0,08	0,14	— 0,06	0,51	0,40	0	0,02	0,02
Bl.	250 „ {252, 253}	104 — 98 = 6	— 0,015	0,055	0,655	0,355	0,25	0	0,02	0,02
Bm.	255 „ 256	95 — 90 = 5	— 0,01	0,095	— 0,43	0,78	0,24	0	0	0
Gn.	261 „ 264	104 — 85 = 19	— 0,12	0,17	— 0,09	0,29	0,31	0	0,01	0,01
Vs.	{270, 271} „ {272, 273}	102 — 67 = 35	— 0,02	0,06	0,145	0,305	— 0,2	— 0,015	0,05	0,035
Bs.	288 „ 289	106 — 90,5 = 15,5	— 0,01	0,16	0,1	0,32	0,42	0	0,03	0,03
v. d. W. . .	{292, 293} „ 294	88 — 67 = 21	— 0,075	0,165	0,075	0,455	— 0,265	0,005	— 0,01	— 0,005

Tabelle 6.

Name	Rechtsseitige Lage = *r*, linksseitige Lage = *l*	Nummer der Platte	Die Werthe der verschiedenen Spitzen, ausgedrückt in Millivolt				
			P	*Q*	*R*	*S*	*T*
d. Lt.	*r*	224	0,17	— 0,32	1,21	— 0,50	0,41
	l	225	0	0	0,655	— 0,655	0,37
v. d. W.	*r*	226	0,18	— 0,44	1,25	— 0,17	0,41
	l	227	0,15	— 0,26	1,06	— 0,34	0,33
Bm.	*r*	230	0,15	— 0,21	0,79	— 0,46	0,32
	l	231	0	0	0,74	— 0,76	0,29

und dem Betrag der Veränderung der verschiedenen Spitzen. Man würde diesen Punkt nur dann mit einiger Genauigkeit beurtheilen können, wenn man über eine grössere Anzahl von Wahrnehmungen zu verfügen und die Elektrokardiogramme einiger Personen ausgemessen hätte, welche jede für sich bei einer Anzahl verschiedener Pulsfrequenzen untersucht worden wären. In unserer Tabelle verkehrt nur d. Lt. in diesem Falle, und bei ihm sehen wir die Vermuthung bestätigt, dass bei stärkerer Zunahme der Frequenz die Zunahme der regelmässig sich verändernden Spitzen P, Q und S auch vergrössert wird.

Unsere Bemerkungen über die Veränderung in der Dauer der beiden Theile des Elektrokardiogrammes können kurz sein. Die Tabelle zeigt deutlich, dass der erste Theil fast immer unverändert bleibt, der zweite Theil dagegen bei gesteigerter Herzfrequenz fast immer verkürzt wird. All' diese Ergebnisse sind in Uebereinstimmung mit dem, was uns auf Tafel III durch die Constructionen veranschaulicht wird.

Der Einfluss der Körperhaltung.

Um den Einfluss der Körperhaltung auf die Form des Elektrokardiogrammes zu untersuchen, leiteten wir den Strom von den beiden Armen einer Person ab, die sich erst auf die linke, danach auf die rechte Seite gelegt hatte.

Drei Personen unterwarfen sich einer Untersuchung und lieferten jede zwei Reihen von Elektrokardiogrammen.

Die direct registrirten Curven zeigten schon gleich einen deutlichen Einfluss der Körperhaltung. Bei der Lage auf der linken Seite sind die Spitzen A und B viel kleiner als bei der Lage auf der rechten Seite, ja, sie verschwinden beinahe ganz, während der Theil der Curve zwischen C und D, der oberhalb der Abscissenachse gelegen ist, sich senkt.

Die Resultate der Messungen und der methodischen Constructionen findet man in den beiden untenstehenden Tabellen, die, was ihre Einrichtung betrifft, völlig mit den beiden vorigen übereinstimmen, zusammengestellt. Sie bedürfen kaum einer weiteren Erklärung.

Nur sei bei Tabelle 7 erwähnt, dass wir die Untersuchung stets mit der rechtsseitigen Lage der Person anfingen. Wenn eine Spitze bei der Wälzung der Person auf die linke Seite an Höhe zunimmt, nennen wir den Unterschied positiv, wenn sie abnimmt, negativ.

Tabelle 7.

Name	Nummern der Platten	Unterschied in Höhe der Spitzen, ausgedrückt in Millivolt				
		P	*Q*	*R*	*S*	*T*
d. Lt. . .	224 und 225	—0,17	—0,32	—0,555	0,155	—0,04
v. d. W. .	226 „ 227	—0,03	—0,18	—0,19	0,17	—0,08
Bm. . . .	230 „ 231	—0,15	—0,21	—0,05	0,30	—0,03

Wir sehen, dass die Messungsergebnisse die Vermuthung, welche durch die directe Betrachtung der registrirten Curven erweckt wurde, vollkommen bestätigen.

Die Spitzen *P* und *Q* des construirten Elektrokardiogrammes verschwinden beinahe ganz, wenn die in Untersuchung befindliche Person auf der linken Seite liegt, während die Spitze *S* an Grösse zunimmt. Die zwei Spitzen *R* und *T* werden verkleinert, aber verhältnissmässig viel weniger als *P* und *Q*.

Die Dauer des Elektrokardiogrammes wird durch einen Lagewechsel von der rechten auf die linke Seite nicht verändert.

Der Einfluss der Stellen, von denen der elektrische Strom abgeleitet wird.

Waller[1]) unterscheidet günstige Combinationen von Körpertheilen, zwischen denen die rhythmischen Schwankungen im Potentialunterschiede gross und ungünstige Combinationen, bei denen die Schwankungen klein sind. Wir haben versucht, die Grösse dieser Schwankungen in Maass und Zahl auszudrücken. Dazu leiteten wir den Strom bei einigen Personen von sehr verschiedenen Stellen des Körpers ab. Die Elektroden waren stets nach dem Princip von E. du Bois-Reymond eingerichtet und hatten die verschiedenen Formen, wie diese auf den vorigen Seiten beschrieben worden sind[2]).

Die 23 Platten mit Reihen von Elektrokardiogrammen, welche uns zur Verfügung stehen, bestätigen im Wesentlichen Waller's Wahrnehmungen.

1) Aug. D. Waller, a. a. O.

2) Bei Ableitung von dem Munde wurde das mit einer Kochsalzlösung getränkte Ende der Elektrode direct in den Mund genommen.

Wie er müssen wir im Allgemeinen zu den günstigen Combinationen rechnen: rechte Hand, rechte Scapula, Stirn und Mund auf einer Seite gegenüber dem Apex cordis, der linken Hand, dem linken Fuss, dem rechten Fuss auf der anderen Seite, während durch jedes Paar Stellen, welche wir zur selben Seite gerechnet haben, eine weniger günstige Combination gebildet wird.

Die direct registrirten Curven geben schon deutlich an, dass von den verschiedenen Combinationen, welche wir in Anwendung brachten, die der Herzspitze mit dem rechten Arme oder dem rechten Schulterblatte die günstigste und die der beiden Füsse die ungünstigste ist.

Ferner stellt es sich heraus, dass alle Spitzen ungefähr gleichmässig grösser oder kleiner werden, sodass die Form des registrirten Elektrokardiogrammes im grossen Ganzen ungefähr dieselbe bleibt. Die Unterschiede, welche sich hierbei noch zeigen, betreffen im Wesentlichen die weniger constanten Spitzen A und B und die inconstante Spitze C_1, welche letztere sich in den Elektrokardiogrammen von zwei der drei untersuchten Personen, jedesmal wenn der Strom von einem Paar der günstigsten Stellen abgeleitet wird, deutlich zeigt.

Tabelle 8.

Name	Nummer der Platte	Combination	Die Werthe der verschiedenen Spitzen, ausgedrückt in Millivolt				
			P	Q	R	S	T
d. Lt. . .	238	rechte Hand — Herzspitze	0,30	— 0,23	1,75	— 1,09	0,65
d. Lt. . .	232	rechte Scapula — Herzspitze	0,11	— 0,10	0,90	— 0,42	0,42
d. Lt. . .	322	rechte Hand — linker Fuss	0,15	— 0,09	0,92	— 0,39	0,26
d. Lt. . .	324	rechte Hand — rechter Fuss	0,13	— 0,12	0,87	— 0,34	0,23
d. Lt. . .	336	linke Hand — Stirn	0,11	— 0,07	0,87	— 0,21	0,34
d. Lt. . .	337	linker Fuss — Stirn	0,11	— 0,06	0,88	— 0,21	0,27
d. Lt. . .	338	linker Fuss — Mund	0,13	— 0,05	0,83	— 0,17	0,26
d. Lt. . .	320	linke Hand — rechter Fuss	0,14	— 0,23	0,82	— 0,39	0,14
d. Lt. . .	323	linke Hand — linker Fuss	0,09	— 0,15	0,79	— 0,29	0,14
d. Lt. . .	321	rechte Hand — linker Fuss	0	0	0,17	— 0,11	0,09
d. Lt. . .	335	Stirn — rechte Hand	0	0	0,19	— 0,22	0,07
v. d. W. .	292	rechte Hand — Herzspitze	0,21	— 0,33	1,90	— 0,45	0,58
v. d. W. .	219	rechte Scapula — Herzspitze	0,30	— 0,50	1,90	— 1,20	0,55
v. d. W. .	217	rechte Hand — linker Fuss	0,27	— 0,59	1,20	— 0,29	0,36
v. d. W. .	295	rechte Hand — linke Hand	0,15	— 0,71	1,51	— 0,42	0,29
v. d. W. .	297	linke Hand — Herzspitze	0,10	— 0,30	1,10	— 0,14	0,29
Bm. . . .	255	rechte Hand — Herzspitze	0,29	— 0,405	2,03	— 1,69	1,03
Bm. . . .	220	rechte Scapula — Herzspitze	0,28	— 0,35	1,50	— 2,38	0,58
Bm. . . .	236	rechte Hand — linke Hand	0,25	— 0,15	1,02	— 0,64	0,44
Bm. . . .	218	rechte Hand — linker Fuss	0,35	— 0,40	1,50	— 1,04	0,43

In nebenstehender Tabelle sind die Ergebnisse der Messungen von 20 Elektrokardiogrammen zusammengestellt. Die Zahlen bestätigen die Bemerkungen, welche wir oben schon bei der Beschreibung der registrirten Curven machten.

Die günstigste Combination ist also die der Herzspitze mit dem rechten Arme, Nr. 238, 292, 255, oder die der Herzspitze mit der rechten Scapula, Nr. 232, 219, 220.

Die ungünstigste ist die der beiden Füsse, Nr. 321.

Ferner zeigt die Tabelle deutlich, dass die Spitzen *R* und *T* ihr Verhältniss zu einander besser bewahren als die weniger constanten Spitzen *P*, *Q* und *S*.

Allgemeine Betrachtungen.
Die Erklärung und die Bedeutung des Elektrokardiogramms.

Die Kenntniss des Zeitpunktes, in dem die rhythmische Schwankung des Potentialunterschiedes anfängt, und des Zeitpunktes, in dem dieselbe endet, ist von grosser Bedeutung für die Erklärung des Elektrokardiogramms. Wir haben desshalb einige Zeitmessungen vorgenommen und das Elektrokardiogramm mit dem gewöhnlichen Kardiogramm verglichen.

Von einer Person, Bm., wird auf die gewöhnliche Weise ein Elektrokardiogramm geschrieben durch Stromableitung von der Regio cordis nahe beim Apex und von dem rechten Arme. Zu gleicher Zeit wird sein Ictus cordis registrirt.

Dazu wird ein Luftkissen gegen den Thorax gehalten, an der Stelle, wo der Ictus cordis am besten zu fühlen ist, während eine Kautschukröhre die Bewegungen des Luftkissens nach einer Registrirtrommel fortpflanzt. Der Hebel dieser letzteren befindet sich dicht vor der Spalte, auf welche das Bild der Haarröhre des Capillarelektrometers projicirt ist, und schreibt eine schwarze Schattenlinie auf die empfindliche Platte.

Wenn wir den Zeitpunkt, in dem das gewöhnliche Kardiogramm anfängt, vergleichen mit dem Anfang der Spitze *R* im Elektrokardiogramm, so sehen wir, dass dieser stets früher erscheint als jener. Der Unterschied betrug bei zehn verschiedenen Messungen durchschnittlich 0,0502 Secunden (*A*). Dieser Betrag kann den gesuchten Unterschied nicht genau angeben, weil der Lufttransport des Herzstosses nach der Registrirtrommel eine grössere Verzögerung erleidet als der elektrische Transport von den Elektroden nach dem Capillar-Elektrometer. Der Unterschied in der Verzögerung muss gesondert gemessen werden. Wir befestigten dazu auf die Kautschukmembran des Luftkissens einen kupfernen Knopf und schlossen, indem wir mit einem Metallstift gegen den Knopf drückten, plötzlich eine Kette, in der sich ein Daniell-Element befand. Auf diese Weise wurde ein Strom — dessen Stärke mittelst eines Nebenschlusses in einem Widerstandskasten zweckmässig gewählt worden war — durch den Capillar-Elektrometer geleitet.

Der Druck gegen das Luftkissen wurde durch dieselbe Kautschukröhre, welche beim Registriren des Ictus cordis gebraucht worden war, nach der Registrirtrommel fortgepflanzt. Es zeigte sich, dass der Hebel dieser letzteren erst einige Zeit nach dem Quecksilberfaden des Capillar-Elektrometers sich zu bewegen anfing.

Der Zeitunterschied betrug in sechs verschiedenen Fällen durchschnittlich 0,0203 Secunden (B).

Der wirkliche Zeitunterschied zwischen dem Anfang der Spitze R und dem Anfang des Ictus cordis beträgt also

$$A - B = 0{,}0299 \text{ Secunden.}$$

Wie muss dieser Zeitunterschied erklärt werden, und zu welchen Schlüssen kann er uns führen?

An erster Stelle wird durch unsere Zeitmessungen der Ausspruch Waller's bestätigt, dass die rhythmischen Schwankungen im Potentialunterschied, welche das Elektrokardiogramm bilden, nicht durch den arteriellen Puls verursacht werden. Letzterer kommt erst viel später in den verschiedenen Körpertheilen an. So kommt z. B. der Carotispuls bei derselben Person Bm. 0,124 Secunden nach dem gewöhnlichen Kardiogramm [1]), also 0,154 Secunden nach dem Elektrokardiogramm. Ferner können wir wahrscheinlich die Vorkammersystole als die Ursache des ersten Theiles des Elektrokardiogrammes — die Spitzen P und Q — betrachten, während die Kammersystole dem zweiten, aus den Spitzen R, S und T bestehenden Theile entspricht. Zwar fängt das Elektrokardiogramm noch ungefähr 0,03 Secunden vor dem Anfang des Ictus cordis an, aber es ist leicht zu begreifen, dass die Contraction des Kammermuskels erst bis zu einem gewissen Grade vorgeschritten sein muss, bevor der Herzstoss sich als solcher geltend macht, während doch die ersten Spuren von

1) Siehe „Die Registrirung der Herztöne". Dieses Arch. 1894 Bd. 57 S. 617.

Contraction schon unmittelbar elektromotorische Kräfte hervorrufen, welche im Elektrokardiogramm zum Ausdruck kommen.

Wir stellen uns bei dieser Erklärung auf den Standpunkt jener Physiologen, welche keinen Unterschied im latenten Stadium zwischen den elektrischen Erscheinungen und dem Contractionsvorgang eines Muskels annehmen, wollen aber nicht unterlassen, zu erwähnen, dass man, auch wenn man einen anderen Standpunkt einnimmt, dennoch dieselbe Erklärung beibehalten kann. Man hat dann den Zeitunterschied von 0,03 Secunden entweder ganz oder zum Theil als den Unterschied im obenerwähnten latenten Stadium aufzufassen.

Die Dauer der zwei Theile des Elektrokardiogrammes ist in guter Uebereinstimmung mit der von uns gegebenen Erklärung, 0,13 Secunden für die Vorkammer- und 0,32 Secunden für die Kammersystole. Marey[1]) gibt für die Vorkammersystole des Pferdes 0,17, für die Kammersystole 0,45 Secunden an. Diese Zeiten sind von uns aus den von ihm publicirten Curven berechnet worden; sie sind ein wenig länger als dieselben Stadien des menschlichen Herzschlages.

Für die Kammersystole fand

Volkmann[2]) bei einer Pulsfrequenz von 84 Schlägen per Min. 0,375 Sec.;

Donders[3]) bei einer Pulsfrequenz von 74—94 Schlägen per Min. 0,327—0,301 Sec.;

Landois bei einer Pulsfrequenz von 55—65 Schlägen per Min. 0,327—0,300 Sec.;

Edgren bei einer Pulsfrequenz von 70 Schlägen per Min. 0,379 Sec.;

Thurston bei einer Pulsfrequenz von 47—128 Schlägen per Min. 0,347—0,256 Sec.;

Einthoven und Geluk[4]) bei einer Pulsfrequenz von 70 bis 85 Schlägen per Min. 0,346—0,312 Sec.

---

1) Marey, La circulation du sang à l'état physiologique et dans les maladies 1881 p. 96.

2) Die Angaben von Volkmann, Landois, Edgren und Thurston sind nach Tigerstedt angeführt. Lehrbuch der Physiologie des Kreislaufes S. 127 ff. 1893.

3) F. C. Donders, De rhythmus der hartstonen. Nederl. Arch. v. Genees. en Natuurk. 1866 Dl. 2 p. 139.

4) Die Registrirung der Herztöne, a. a. O.

Bei erhöhter Pulsfrequenz fanden wir die Dauer des ersten Theiles des Elektrokardiogrammes, welcher der Vorkammersystole entspricht, nahezu unverändert, die Dauer des zweiten Theiles, welcher der Kammersystole entspricht, ein wenig verkürzt.

Gehen wir jetzt über zur Erklärung der verschiedenen Spitzen, jede für sich. Im Allgemeinen können wir unsere Betrachtungen auf die Anwesenheit einer Contractionswelle basiren, welche von der Herzbasis nach der Herzspitze fortschreitet. Eine derartige Welle muss erst in den Vorkammern vorhanden sein, um sich dann in den Kammern zu zeigen. Schon die Vorkammerwelle an und für sich verursacht eine fortschreitende Negativität, welche von der Herzbasis (*P*) ausgeht und nach der Spitze (*Q*) gerichtet ist. Darauf kommt die Welle in die Kammern und fängt nach Bayliss und Starling[1]) auch hier bei der Basis an, schreitet nach der Spitze fort, hat aber in der Basis selbst eine so lange Dauer, dass sie da noch vorhanden ist, wenn sie in der Spitze schon zu bestehen aufgehört hat. So werden die Spitzen *R* und *T* gebildet. Die Spitze *S* verdient noch eine eingehendere Besprechung. Sie lässt sich vielleicht aus dem Unterschied erklären, der zwischen der rechten und der viel kräftigeren, den eigentlichen Apex bildenden linken Kammer besteht. Werden die beiden Herzhälften gleichmässig in ihrer Function verändert, so wird das Elektrokardiogramm auch in all' seinen Theilen gleichmässig verändert werden; wenn aber die Thätigkeit des linken Herzmuskels durch irgend eine Ursache mehr als die des rechten erhöht wird, so müssen einige Spitzen des Elektrokardiogrammes mehr als andere vergrössert werden. Wir haben alle Ursache, zu erwarten, dass bei grösserer Pulsfrequenz in Folge von Körperbewegung die Contractionen der linken Kammer am meisten an Kraft zugenommen haben, und hiermit in Uebereinstimmung sehen wir bei grösserer Pulsfrequenz die Spitze *S* regelmässig grösser werden, und zwar mehr zunehmen als die anderen Spitzen des Elektrokardiogrammes.

Auch die Veränderung der Körperhaltung lehrt von dieser Spitze etwas Besonderes. Legt man sich wagerecht hin und wälzt man sich von der rechten Seite auf die linke, so werden bei Stromableitung von den beiden Händen alle Spitzen des Elektrokardiogrammes — zumal die Spitzen *P* und *Q* — kleiner, mit Ausnahme der Spitze *S*.

---

1) A. a. O.

Dies lässt sich erklären, indem man annimmt, dass das Herz im Thorax eine kleine Drehung erleidet, sodass der Einfluss des Potentials des linken Herzens auf die linke Körperhälfte vergrössert wird.

Einfluss der Stellen, von denen der Strom abgeleitet wird, und das Erkennen der Lageabweichungen des Herzens.

Schon Waller bemerkte, dass man mittelst des Elektrokardiogrammes in einem bestimmten Falle im Stande sei, eine Lageabweichung des Herzens kennen zu lernen. Denn beim Situs inversus viscerum sind im Gegensatz zur normalen Erscheinung die Schwankungen im Potentialunterschiede gross, wenn der Strom von dem Munde und dem rechten Arme, klein, wenn derselbe von dem Munde und dem linken Arme abgeleitet wird.

Dies ist in Uebereinstimmung mit der Theorie, dass der ganze Körper bei jedem Herzschlage durch eine Fläche, welche senkrecht durch die Mitte der Herzachse geht, in zwei Theile getheilt wird. Der eine Theil, in dem die Spitze des Herzens gelegen ist, nimmt den Potential dieser Spitze, der andere den Potential der Basis des Herzens an. Aus derselben Theorie leiten wir ab, dass auch kleine Lageabweichungen, ja sogar die normalen Unterschiede in der Lage des Herzens mittelst des Elektrokardiogrammes entdeckt werden können.

Vergleichen wir einige in Tabelle 8 näher beschriebene Elektrokardiogramme, welche bei Stromableitung von verschiedenen Körpertheilen registrirt worden sind, z. B. das bei Ableitung vom Apex cordis und der rechten Scapula erhaltene Elektrokardiogramm von v. d. W. mit dem vorigen, wobei die Stromableitung vom Apex cordis und der rechten Hand stattgefunden hat.

Die wichtigste Spitze *R* ist bei beiden Combinationen gleich gross, 1,9 Millivolt. Dagegen verhält sich die Sache bei d. Lt. anders. Bei der Combination: Herzspitze und rechte Hand ist die Spitze *R* des Elektrokardiogrammes beinahe zwei Mal so gross, 1,75 Millivolt, als bei der Combination: Herzspitze und rechtes Schulterblatt. Wir können hieraus wohl schliessen, dass bei v. d. W. die Herzachse mehr von hinten nach vorn gerichtet ist als bei d. Lt.

Vergleichen wir v. d. W. mit Bm., so sehen wir, dass bei jenem eine stärkere Schwankung im Potentialunterschied erfolgt, wenn der

Strom von den beiden Händen abgeleitet wird, als wenn die Elektroden an die rechte Hand und an einen der Füsse angelegt werden.

Bei Bm ist es gerade umgekehrt, und die Unterschiede zwischen diesen beiden Personen sind in dieser Hinsicht auffallend gross. Sie können, unseres Erachtens, wohl nicht anders erklärt werden, als indem wir annehmen, dass bei Bm die Herzachse mehr von oben nach unten und weniger von rechts nach links gerichtet ist als bei v. d. W.

Es hat sich herausgestellt, dass die allgemeine Form des Elektrokardiogramms sehr constant ist, und es leidet keinen Zweifel, dass wir in ihr ein sehr schätzenswerthes Mittel zur Beurtheilung der Herzthätigkeit besitzen. Weder verschiedene Pulsfrequenzen, noch Unterschied in Haltung, noch Unterschied im Anlegen der Elektroden führt irgend eine principielle Veränderung in derselben herbei.

Wohl kann man von günstigen und ungünstigen Combinationen sprechen, allein auch bei den ungünstigsten Combinationen zeigt es sich, dass das Elektrokardiogramm, obgleich die Schwankungen im Potentialunterschied bedeutend verkleinert sind, ungefähr dieselbe typische Form besitzt wie bei den günstigsten Combinationen, während auch die Elektrokardiogramme aller von uns untersuchten Personen, 17 an der Zahl, im Wesentlichen mit einander übereinstimmen. Pathologische Fälle dagegen weisen deutliche Abweichungen auf.

Zwei kranke Herzen.

Durch die Freundlichkeit des Herrn Professors Rosenstein wurde uns die Gelegenheit gegeben, ein Paar Herzkranker mit dem Capillar-elektrometer zu untersuchen. Die Krankheitsdiagnose beider Patienten, R. und v. H., war „Aorteninsufficienz". Der erstere Patient, R., hatte eine bedeutende Hypertrophie des linken Herzens. Sowohl bei der Herzspitze wie im zweiten Intercostalraum rechts und links wurden Geräusche statt der normalen systolischen und diastolischen Töne gehört. Der zweite Patient, v. H., hatte eine geringe linke Herzhypertrophie. An die Stelle der systolischen Töne waren Geräusche getreten, während die diastolischen Töne schwach waren und im zweiten rechten Intercostalraum ein deutliches diastolisches Geräusch hörbar war.

Wir haben von beiden Kranken sowohl die Elektrokardiogramme wie die Herztöne und -geräusche registrirt. Die ersteren wurden erhalten durch Stromableitung von den beiden Händen und können also unmittelbar mit den normalen Elektrokardiogrammen der Tabellen 1 und 2 verglichen werden.

In der untenstehenden Tabelle 9 sind die Werthe der verschiedenen Spitzen in Millivolts wiedergegeben.

Tabelle 9.

Bezeichnung der Spitzen	Patient R.	Patient v. H.
P	0,1 Millivolt	0,2 Millivolt
Q	— 0,2 "	— 0,1 "
R	1,4 "	1,5 "
S	— 0,35 "	— 0,35 "
T	0,05 "	— 0,3 "
R (Dauer):	0,04 Secunden	0,045 Secunden

Es zeigt sich, dass die Höhe der Spitzen *P*, *Q*, *R* und *S* bei den beiden Patienten innerhalb der Grenzwerthe fällt, welche die Untersuchung von 17 normalen Herzen ergeben hat. Dahingegen ist die Dauer der Spitze *R* verlängert und zeigt die Höhe der Spitze *T* eine bedeutende Abweichung. Während diese letztere bei den 17 normalen Elektrokardiogrammen zwischen + 0,15 und + 0,53 Millivolt abwechselt, ist sie beim Patienten R. so klein, dass sie innerhalb der durch die Wahrnehmungsfehler bedingten Grenze fällt; bei v. H. hat sie sogar eine entgegengesetzte Richtung. Wie die Verringerung und Umkehrung der Spitze *T* zu erklären seien und ob diese Abweichungen die Natur der Herzkrankheit „Aorteninsufficienz" kennzeichnen, kann erst nach ausführlicheren Untersuchungen entschieden werden.

Wir haben wohl Grund, zu erwarten, dass die Grenzen, zwischen welchen die Dimensionen des normalen Elektrokardiogrammes variiren, nicht zu sehr von den in den Tabellen I und II verzeichneten abweichen.

Von den vielen von uns registrirten, scheinbar normalen Elektrokardiogrammen zeigte nur ein einziges eine bedeutende Abweichung, was unmittelbar zur Vermuthung, dass wir es hier mit einer abnormalen Herzwirkung zu thun hatten, Anlass gab. Die Vermuthung wurde durch die später angestellte Auscultation bestätigt; der Capillar-Elektrometer hatte also zur Entdeckung der Abnormität geführt. Zu unserem Bedauern fehlte uns die Gelegenheit zu einer ausführlichen Untersuchung.

Die Photogramme der Herztöne beider Patienten zeigten das Vorhandensein von Geräuschen deutlich. Ausserdem blieb aber ein kräftiger erster Ton sichtbar, welcher sowohl an der Herzspitze wie im zweiten Intercostalraum vorhanden war, während er doch bei der Auscultation nicht bemerkt wurde. Den zweiten Ton konnte man nicht oder kaum im Geräusche erkennen.

Werthvoller als die Untersuchung der Form der registrirten Töne erscheint uns die Messung des Zeitunterschiedes zu sein zwischen dem Anfange des ersten Tones und dem Anfange des Carotispulses.

Beim Patienten R. betrug dieser Zeitunterschied:

zwischen dem Anfange des 1. Spitzentones und dem Anfange des Carotispulses im Mittel 0,0671 Sec.;

zwischen dem Anfange des 1. Pulmonaltones und dem Anfange des Carotispulses im Mittel 0,0670 Sec.;

zwischen dem Anfange des 1. Aortentones und dem Anfange des Carotispulses im Mittel 0,0765 Sec.

Beim Patienten v. H. betrugen die bezüglichen Werthe:

0,0592 Sec.
0,0673 „
0,0597 „

Bei obenstehenden Messungen ist der Verzögerung Rechnung getragen, welche der Transport des Pulses nach dem Marey'schen Tambour hin erleidet.

Der Zeitunterschied zwischen dem Auftreten der ersten Töne an der Herzspitze und im zweiten Intercostalraum ist gering und kann ausser Betracht gelassen werden. Er beträgt kaum mehr als die bei einigen Messungsreihen erhaltene mittlere Abweichung des Mittelwerthes. Das durch diese mittlere Abweichung erreichte Maximum war 0,008 Secunden.

In untenstehender Figur 1 ist das Zeitintervall zwischen dem Anfange der verschiedenen Herztöne bei einem gesunden Individuum und bei den zwei Patienten graphisch verzeichnet.

S ist die Zeitlinie, *B* bezieht sich auf die Herztöne eines gesunden Individuums, *R* und *v. H* auf diejenigen des untersuchten Kranken. *s* bedeutet den Anfang des Spitzentones, *a* denjenigen der Arterientöne und *c* den Anfang des Carotispulses.

Die drei Linien *B*, *R* und *v. H* sind so unter einander gesetzt, dass der Anfang des Carotispulses für alle in denselben Zeitpunkt fällt.

Wir sehen, dass der Spitzenton beim gesunden Individuum *B* einen Zeitunterschied von 0,061 Secunden mit den Arterientönen zeigt, während sie beim Patienten *R* sowohl wie bei *v. H* zusammenfallen.

In einer früheren Abhandlung über die Registrirung der Herztöne[1]) wurde die Kammersystole in zwei Perioden eingetheilt. Die erstere Periode fängt mit dem ersten Spitzenton an und endigt mit dem Beginn des ersten Arterientones. Während dieser Periode bleibt das Ostium Aortae geschlossen. Die zweite Periode fängt mit der

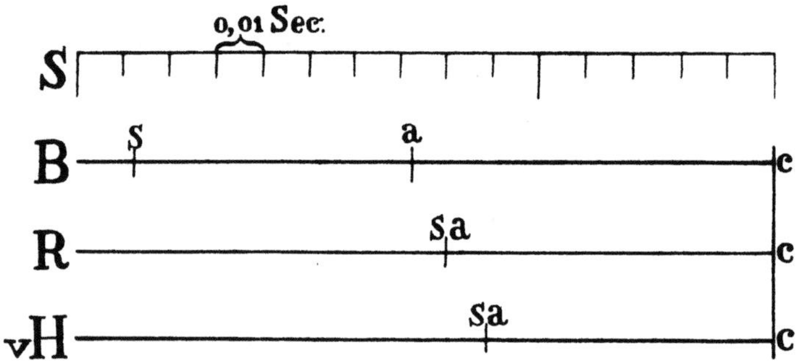

Fig. 1.

Oeffnung des Ostium Aortae und der Austreibung des Blutes aus den Kammern an. Wenn die Aortenklappen insufficient sind, kann diese Eintheilung in zwei Perioden nicht mehr durchgeführt werden. Das Ostium Aortae bleibt fortwährend geöffnet, so dass das Blut schon beim Anfange der Kammersystole nach den Arterien getrieben und der erste Aortenton zur selben Zeit wie der erste Spitzenton gehört wird. Diese Erklärung liegt so auf der Hand, dass man beim Zusammenfallen vom ersten Spitzenton mit dem ersten Aortenton mit grosser Wahrscheinlichkeit das Vorhandensein von Aorteninsufficienz anzunehmen berechtigt ist.

Der Kürze wegen nannten wir oben immer den ersten Ton im zweiten linken Intercostalraum ersten Pulmonalton, aber das starke systolische Geräusch macht es unmöglich, an der erwähnten Stelle

1) A. a. O.

einen reinen ersten Pulmonalton zu hören. Man darf also aus dem Zusammenfall des ersten Spitzentones und des ersten Tones im zweiten linken Intercostalraum nicht auf das Vorhandensein einer Pulmonalinsufficienz schliessen.

Bei den beiden kranken Herzen ist der Abstand zwischen dem ersten Aortenton und dem Carotispuls ungefähr ebenso gross wie beim normalen Herzen; der Spitzenton hat sich also in dem kranken Herzen dem Carotispuls angenähert. Auch dieses letztere lässt sich aus dem Wegfall der ersten Periode der Kammersystole ohne Weiteres erklären.

Erklärung der Tafeln.

Tafel II. Phothographische Reproduction in ungefähr 65 % der natürlichen Grösse einer Anzahl von Elektrokardiogrammen, die alle mit Hülfe der Capillare *G. 116* registrirt worden sind. Die Copien der ursprünglichen Negative, welche ungleich deutlicher und schärfer als die Tafel sind, werden wir gern auf Anfrage den Fachgenossen übersenden. Das Bild der Capillarröhre wurde bei 800facher Vergrösserung projectirt, während die empfindliche Platte sich mit einer Geschwindigkeit von 25 mm in der Secunde fortbewegte.

Unter den Elektrokardiogrammen sind die Stimmgabelspitzen sichtbar; die Stimmgabel machte 50 ganze Schwingungen in der Secunde.

Der Schwefelsäurepol des Capillar-Elektrometers war mit der Brustwand in der Gegend des Apex cordis verbunden und der Quecksilberpol mit dem rechten Arme. Die zwölf Elektrokardiogramme gehören sechs verschiedenen Personen an, welche alle erst im Ruhezustand — siehe die ungeraden Nummern — und dann unmittelbar nach der Verrichtung kräftiger Körperbewegung — siehe die geraden Nummern — untersucht wurden. Die zu jeder der untersuchten Personen gehörenden Photogramme sind mit auf einander folgenden Ziffern numerirt. Für nähere Auskunft sehe man den Text.

Tafel III. Construirte Elektrokardiogramme, bei denen eine Ordinatlänge von 10 Millivolt einer Abscissenlänge von 1 Secunde gleichgemacht ist. Die Dimensionen für die Construction sind nach den direct registrirten Elektrokardiogrammen von Tafel II berechnet. Die zwölf Nummern von Tafel II entsprechen den zwölf Figuren von Tafel III.

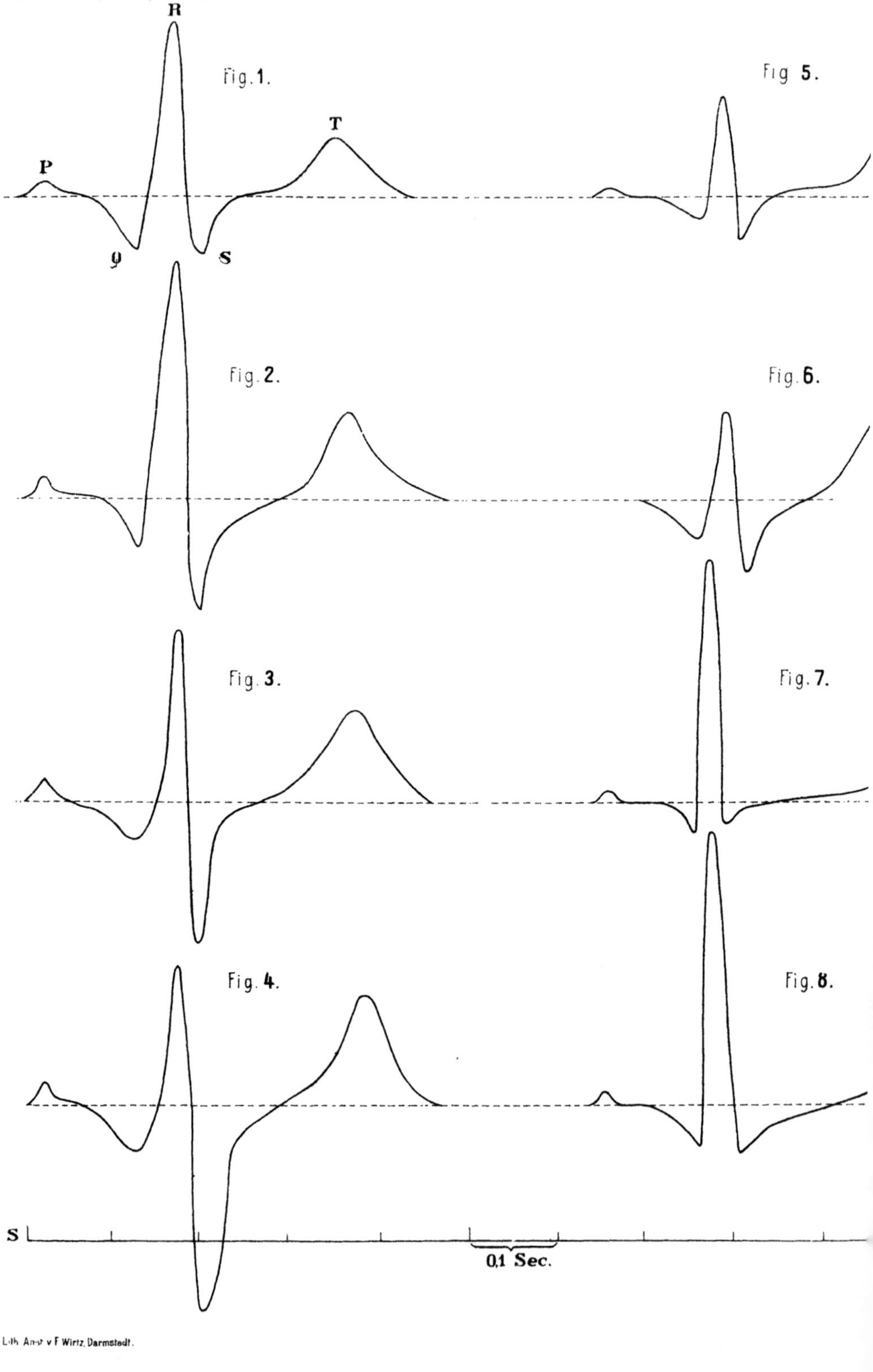

Lith. Anst. v. F. Wirtz, Darmstadt.

Fig. 9.

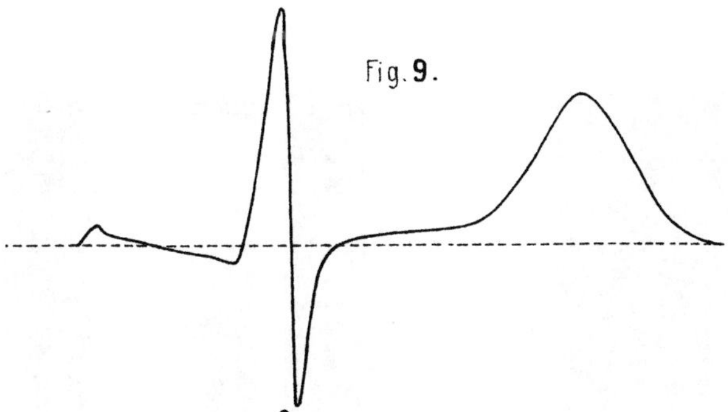

Fig. 10.

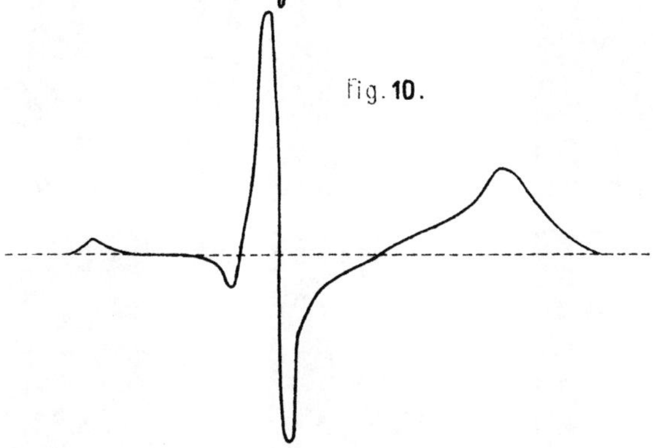

Fig. 11.

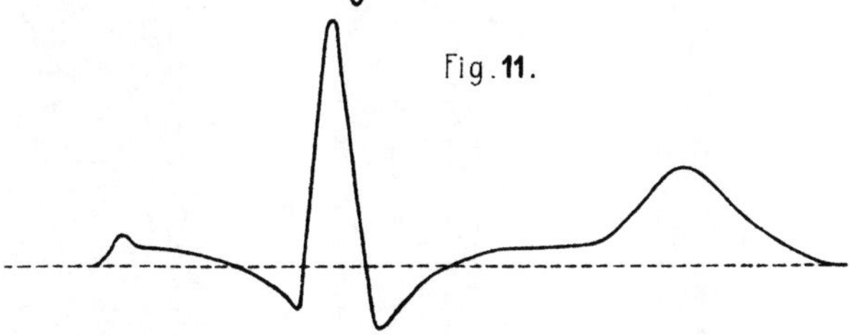

Fig. 12.

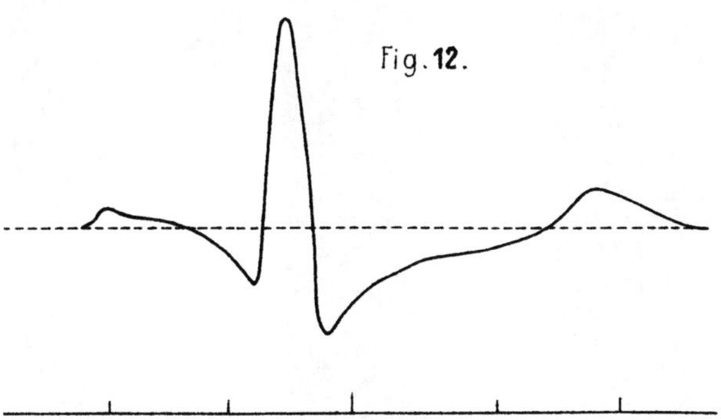

Verlag v. Emil Strauss Bonn.

Tafel III.

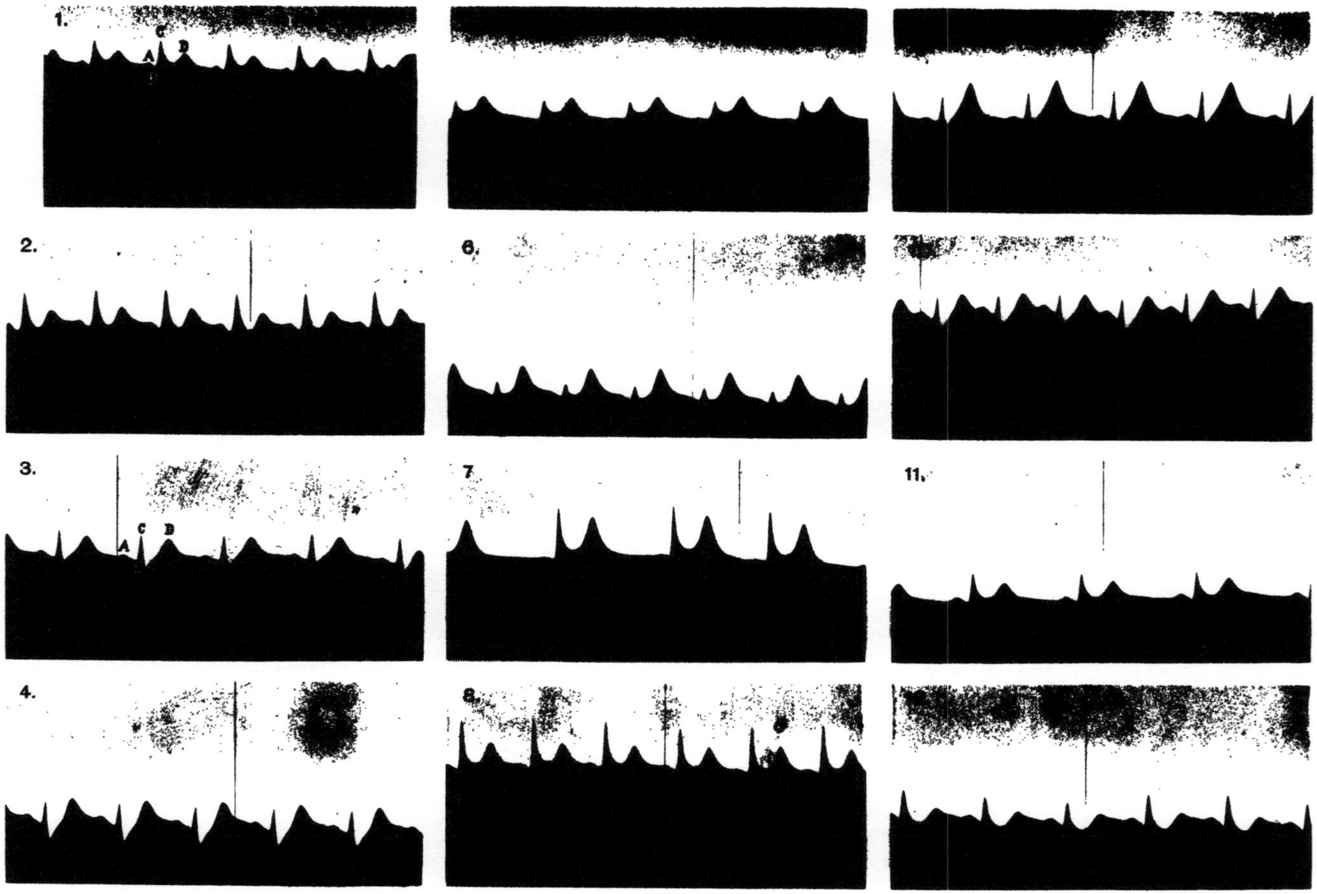

III
Un nouveau galvanomètre

This paper from 1901 contains the first description of the string galvanometer. It is usually assumed, that this galvanometer was first published in 1903. In fact there were then two publications (58, 59*) dealing chiefly with the applications to electrocardiography, while the other was concerned with physical and technical details (60). An following reprint gives a brief historical review and thereafter exposes the basic problems in constructing a galvanometer with improved sensitivity and speed, and appropriate damping. As mentioned in chapter 1, the calculated profit of maximal reduction of windings (of the coil of a Deprez-d'Arsonval galvanometer) led to the use of a string, which had to have such a small diameter however, that Einthoven had to make it in his own laboratory. This was done in the first model by coating a thread of quartz with silver.

Reference is made to Ader's string receiver for use in telegraphy (see also ch. 1).

* reprint IV

UN NOUVEAU GALVANOMÈTRE

PAR

W. EINTHOVEN.

Depuis la publication de la thèse [1]) de M. BOSSCHA „De galvanometro differentiali", la technique de la mesure des courants a fait bien des progrès. On distingue actuellement un grand nombre de types de galvanomètres, qui sont non seulement utiles aux recherches faites au laboratoire de physique mais dont l'électrotechnique, l'électrophysiologie et la pratique de la médecine tirent aussi du profit. Et presque chacun de ces nombreux modèles a des avantages spéciaux pour le but qu'on a en vue en construisant l'instrument.

L'instrument, dont nous allons parler dans ces pages et qu' on pourrait nommer „galvanomètre à corde", servira principalement dans les recherches électrophysiologiques. En examinant les phénomènes électriques des muscles, des glandes, des nerfs, des organes des sens, bref de presque tous les tissus et organes vivants, on doit tenir compte de leur grande résistance. Les forces électromotrices produites n'étant en outre qu' assez faibles, il faudra le plus souvent se servir de galvanomètres très sensibles et d'une grande résistance intérieure, permettant des mesures de courants de 10^{-9} et 10^{-10} ampères.

Au moyen de plus d'un galvanomètre usuel on peut facilement faire ces mesures. Cependant la propriété commune à tous c'est que le mouvement du système d'aiguilles et du miroir qui y est attaché se fait lentement. Si le mouvement est oscillatoire, la durée d'une oscillation est de quelques secondes au moins, et quand on rend le mouvement à peu près apériodique en appliquant un grand amortissement, la durée de la déviation est encore considérablement prolongée.

---

[1]) Leyde, 1854.

Le galvanomètre cuirassé astatique au système d'aiguilles petites de du Bois et Rubens, représentant un des plus sensibles si pas le plus sensible des instruments usuels, peut servir d'exemple. Les auteurs donnent comme *sensibilité normale* [1]) de leur instrument le nombre 1000. On entend par *sensibilité normale* la déviation en millimètres sur une échelle placée à un mètre du miroir. On pose pour l'intensité du courant 10^{-6} amp., pour la résistance intérieure du galvanomètre 1 ohm et pour la durée d'une oscillation 5 secondes. On admet que la déviation est proportionnelle à l'intensité du courant. Puis on suppose que pour une intensité de courant donnée la déviation est en raison directe de la racine carrée — ou, ce qui est souvent plus exact, de la $\frac{2}{5}$ puissance — de la résistance. Enfin la deviation est proportionelle au carré de la durée de l'oscillation.

On en déduit qu' avec la plus grande résistance intérieure de 8000 ohms que MM. du Bois et Rubens ont donné à leur galvanomètre, un courant de 10^{-10} amp. produit une déviation de 1 mm. sur une échelle placée à un mètre de distance, si la durée d'une oscillation est de 2,6 sec. Le petit poids et la grande mobilité du système d'aiguilles, joints à l'exiguité du miroir, ne permettent guère dans ces conditions d'observer avec précision des déviations beaucoup plus petites q'un mm. Aussi peut on admettre la dite mesure comme limite d'une déviation facile à observer.

En amortissant le mouvement du systéme d'aiguilles jusqu' à produire l'apériodicité on prolonge la durée de la déviation. Cette durée devient infiniment longue en théorie mais dans la pratique on peut régler l'amortissement en sorte qu'au bout de 5 secondes au plus après le commencement du mouvement toute la déviation soit à peu près terminée. Il est vrai qu' une durée de 5 secondes pour une déviation galvanométrique n'offre pas d'inconvénients pour beaucoup de mesures, mais il n'en est pas de même pour toutes. Pour maintes observations électrophysiologiques la dite durée est beaucoup trop longue. Les forces électromotrices produites dans les tissus vivants par leur réaction sur plusieurs excitations, sont généralement d'une durée très courte et pour la plus grande partie épuisées au bout d'une petite partie d'une seconde.

Il est vrai qu' il y a des galvanomètres avec une durée d'oscillation

---

[1]) H. du Bois et H. Rubens. Panzergalvanometer. Zeitschr. f. Instrumentenkunde 1900, S. 77.

plus courte que la susdite mais ceux-ci ne sont pas assez sensibles pour les expériences physiologiques. J'ai particulièrement en vue l'instrument construit par MM. DEPREZ et D'ARSONVAL où un cadre mobile est suspendu entre les pôles d'un aimant fixe. [1])

Les dits oscillographes, dont celui de M. DUDDELL est certainement le plus connu, ont une très courte durée d'oscillation: celle-ci peut être réduite à 0,0001 sec. L'instrument, qui est utile à l'électrotechnique ne peut pas servir aux mesures physiologiques, n'étant sensible qu' à des courants assez intenses. L'échelle étant à une distance de 50 cm., la déviation pour un ampère entier est de 290 mm.

Ce que nous nous sommes proposé en construisant le galvanomètre à corde, c'est de joindre une sensibilité permettant des mesures électrophysiologues à une grande rapidité de déviation. L'instrument se compose principalement d'un conducteur mobile, c'est à dire d'une corde, tendue d'une manière convenable entre les pôles d'un électroaimant. Nous exposerons le plus facilement les raisons qui nous ont amené à construire cet instrument, en partant d'une forme actuelle du galvanomètre de DEPREZ-D'ARSONVAL et en nous demandant quelles modifications nous pourrions y apporter à son profit.

Nous devons considérer en premier lieu la *sensibilité normale*. Nous avons déjà expliqué ce terme plus haut. On ne pourra jamais modifier la sensibilité normale en changeant la force directrice du fil de suspension, pas plus qu' en augmentant ou diminuant le nombre des tours, *si le poids et les dimensions du cadre sont conservés*. Par contre elle augmentera proportionnellement à l'intensité du champ magnétique, et les modifications apportées dans les dimensions du cadre ne manqueront pas non plus d'exercer une influence déterminée. Seulement cette dernière influence doit être examinée de plus près.

Maintenons provisoirement la forme du cadre et posons nous comme première question: „Quelle sera la conséquence de la suppression de quelques tours, *si l'on n'agrandit pas le diamètre du fil pour suppléer à la diminution de poids et de dimensions du cadre?*"

En supprimant tant de tours que le nombre en est n fois plus petit,

---

[1]) La maison SIEMENS et HALSKE fournit un modèle de ce galvanomètre, au moyen duquel on peut mesurer des courants très faibles. Cependant il n'a plus l'avantage de la courte durée de l'oscillation.

le cadre devient n fois plus léger et le moment d'inertie est également n fois plus petit, de sorte que la durée d'une oscillation devient $\sqrt{n}$ fois plus courte. La résistance est n fois plus faible et la déviation pour la même intensité de courant n fois plus petite.

Il résulte de ces changements de durée d'oscillation, de résistance et de déviation que la sensibilité normale augmente $\sqrt{n}$ fois. Pour l'augmenter autant que possible il faut donc laisser sur le cadre **aussi peu de tours que possible.** S'il n'y avait pas d'inconvénients pratiques le cadre à un seul tour offrirait le plus d'avantages.

Nous devons nous demander en second lieu: „Quel changement subira la sensibilité normale à la suite de la modification du diamètre du fil?" Si le diamètre du fil devient m fois plus petit, le moment d'inertie diminue m^2 fois. Il en résulte que la durée de l'oscillation devient m fois plus courte. La déviation pour une intensité donnée reste la même, mais la résistance du fil devient m^2 fois plus grande. On déduira des changements de la durée de l'oscillation et de la résistance, que la sensibilité normale augmente m fois. C'est pourquoi il sera nécessaire de se servir d'un fil *au plus petit diamètre possible.*

Quant aux deux susdites modifications, il s'agit de diminuer autant que possible le poids et en conséquence le moment d'inertie du cadre. Il va de soi qu' on ne pourra en tirer profit que si le poids du miroir peut être négligé.

On peut aussi supprimer le miroir et observer directement les oscillations du fil au moyen d'un microscope. Enfin il ne faut qu' un pas pour passer du cadre ne portant qu' un seul tour de fil très fin, à la corde tendue. [1])

Outre la grosseur la longueur de la corde influe aussi sur la sensibilité normale du galvanomètre. Si la corde est p fois plus courte, la sensibilité normale est $\sqrt{p}$ fois plus grande.

La matière dont on construit la corde doit avoir à côté d'une grande conductibilité L un petit poids spécifique S. Si $\frac{S^2}{L}$ est un minimum, les conditions les plus favorables au sujet de la matière sont réalisées.

---

[1]) M. ADER construisit déjà un instrument avec une corde tendue entre les pôles d'un aimant. C'était un récepteur pour la télégraphie. Au moyen d'une gaine en moelle de plume on grossissait la corde au milieu, c'est à dire à l'endroit où ses mouvements étaient photographiés. Comptes Rendus de l'Ac. d. Sc. 1897, T. 124, p. 1440.

Mais comment mesurer la sensibilité normale d'un galvanomètre sans miroir et dont la partie mobile est observée au moyen d'un microscope? Le terme „sensibilité normale" n'a été employé jusqu' ici que pour des instruments où la lecture se faisait par la méthode du miroir, et ce qu' il y a de singulier, c'est qu' on n'a jamais tenu compte de la grandeur du miroir. Un miroir de 3 mm. de diamètre, employé dans le système d'aiguilles léger d'un galvanomètre cuirassé de DU BOIS et RUBENS produit de chaque point de l'échelle se trouvant à 5 mètres de distance un cercle de diffraction d'environ 1 mm. de diamètre. Sans compter l'éclairage faible, il sera donc très difficile d'observer une déviation d'une petite fraction d'un millimètre. En employant un plus grand miroir le cercle de diffraction variera en raison inverse du diamètre du miroir. Aussi il me semble, qu' il vaudra mieux tenir compte du diamètre du miroir en donnant la sensibilité normale d'un instrument.

Si nous prenons comme base du calcul de la sensibilité normale un rayon de miroir de 1 mm., la valeur que MM. DU BOIS et RUBENS donnent pour leur galvanomètre cuirassé à système d'aiguilles léger, s'élève de 1000 à 1500.

La portée de la „sensibilité normale", exprimée de cette manière, se maintient, quand on remplace l'observation faite au moyen d'un miroir par l'observation microscopique. Car le grossissement convenable obtenu à l'aide d'un microscope est limité par la même diffraction de la lumière que la réduction du rayon du miroir ou l'augmentation de la distance de l'échelle. Ainsi pour comparer la sensibilité il faut appliquer un grossissement microscopique tel, que les cercles de diffraction deviennent aussi grands que si l'on s'était servi du miroir. La valeur du grossissement est alors exprimée par

$$v = N \times \frac{d}{2r},$$

où v représente le grossissement de l'image microscopique, N l'ouverture numérique de l'objectif, r le rayon du miroir et d la distance de l'échelle jusqu' au miroir.

L'ouverture numérique des meilleurs objectifs à sec est de 0,95. Si l'on prend comme base du calcul de la sensibilité normale $d = 1000$ et $r = 1$, le grossissement admissible est de $v = 475$.

Qu' il nous soit permis maintenant d'ajouter aux observations théoriques précédentes quelques remarques pratiques. Quelque grande que puisse être la sensibilité normale d'un galvanomètre, celui-ci ne servira pas à notre but s'il ne permet pas de mesurer un courant très faible, la déviation n'étant que médiocrement rapide. Puis l'amortissement doit répondre à certaines conditions, car une oscillation non amortie anéantirait tout l'avantage d'une déviation rapide.

Les déviations sont elles bien proportionnelles aux intensités du courant? L'observateur ne sera-t il pas gêné pendant ses mesures par les vibrations du sol et par des courants d'air, au point qu'il ne pourra pas se servir de l'instrument? Et quelle est en somme la sensibilité normale qu' on pourra atteindre?

Comme nous l'avons exposé plus haut le diamètre de la corde est un des éléments les plus importants. Des fils ou des rubans métalliques, dont on pourrait se servir et qui seraient assez fins pour le but que nous nous sommes proposé, ne se vendent pas. On doit donc les préparer soi même et on pourra non sans succès se servir d'aluminium en feuilles de livret. Une feuille d'aluminium, qui, comme on le pourra constater facilement au moyen de la balance, n'est épaisse que de 0,75 μ, est coupée en bandes de la façon dont un relieur coupe les feuilles d'or pour la dorure des livres. On colle une bande de quelques millimètres de largeur au moyen de vernis sur une plaque de verre, et on la divise ensuite avec un couteau bien tranchant en bandes étroites. Nous n'avons pas réussi à tendre dans le galvanomotre de bandes plus étroites que de 0,3 ou 0,4 mm., mais avec celles-ci nous avons déjà obtenu des résultats assez satisfaisants.

En se servant des fils de quartz rendus conductibles par l'argenture, on arrive à une amélioration assez considérable. Voici en quelques mots les resultats de quelques unes de nos expériences.

Un fil de quartz argenté, de 2,1 μ de diamètre et long de 13 cm., est tendu dans un champ magnétique très intense, évalué à plus de 30000 C. G. S. La résistance s'élève à 20300 ohms. Les mouvements grossis 400 fois, sont projetés sur une fente, derrière laquelle on fait passer une plaque photographique. A coté de la fente se trouve une échelle divisée en millimètres et permettant de mesurer les déviations pendant qu' on photographie les mouvements de la corde.

On commence par tendre la corde faiblement. Un courant de 10^{-8} amp. produit une déviation de 5,6 mm. Les déviations sont proportionnelles aux intensités des courants et égales à droite et à gauche en tant qu' elles se bornent aux dimensions de l'échelle. L'instrument est placé sur un pilier et bien que nous n'ayons pas pris d'autres mesures pour mettre l'appareil à l'abri des vibrations du sol, et que nous n'ayons par conséquent pas appliqué la méthode de suspension de M. Julius ou la méthode de faire flotter l'instrument sur du mercure, la corde ne montre pas la moindre vibration. Nous avons aussi garanti l'appareil des courants d'air et le zéro semble être absolument constant. Une déviation de 0,1 mm. pouvant encore être observée, un courant de $1{,}79 \times 10^{-10}$ amp. se mesure également. Ainsi l'instrument doit être rangé parmi les plus sensibles galvanomètres.

On doit considérer que nous ne communiquons ici que quelques observations préliminaires et qu' il n'est pas douteux que les expériences poursuivies nous apprendront que les mesures pourront se faire avec un fil de quartz encore plus fin et moins tendu, de sorte qu' on pourra démontrer des courants bien plus faibles.

Les mouvements du fil peu tendu subissent à un haut degré l'influence de l'amortissement produit par l'air; plus le fil est fin plus l'amortissement est intense. Car le poids du fil varie en raison directe du carré du diamètre, tandis que la résistance de l'air est proportionnelle à cette dimension. Avec la susdite tension de corde, un courant de 10^{-8} amp. produisant une déviation de 5,6 mm., le mouvement est absolument apériodique. La courbe tracée sur la plaque photographique est la

G

T

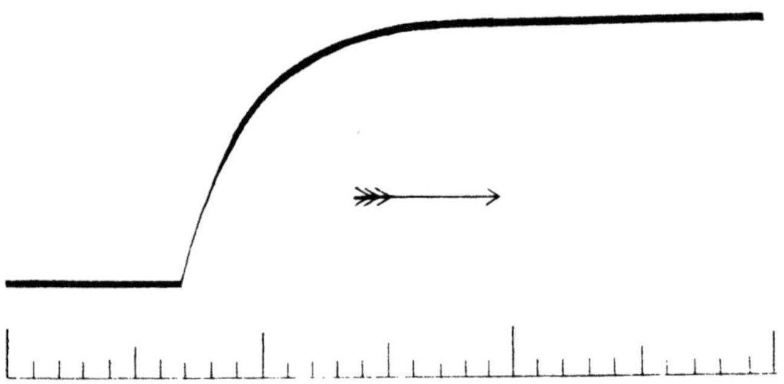

Fig 3.

A peu près 2,5 fois plus grande que le photogramme primitif. Le fil de quartz n'est tendu que très faiblement. Une résistance de 1 mégohm est montée en série dans le circuit du galvanomètre.

G = Courbe, tracée par le fil de quartz pendant qu' on y fait passer subitement un courant de 2×10^{-8} amp.

T = Temps en centièmes de seconde.

représentation graphique d'une fonction exponentielle, v. fig. 1, et est conforme à la *courbe normale*, tracée par l'électromètre capillaire de M. LIPPMANN. [1]) La vitesse de l'image du fil de quartz est de 35 cm. par seconde au moment où elle se trouve à 1 cm. de sa position d'équilibre.

Pour le susdit exemple l'amortissement électromagnétique ne comptait pas, parceque une résistance de 1 mégohm etait montée en série dans le circuit du galvanomètre. L'amortissement électromagnétique se fait cependant valoir perceptiblement, quand on intercale une petite résistance entre les deux extrémités de la corde. L'amortissement total est alors augmenté, l'amortissement électromagnétique étant ajouté à l'amortissement produit par l'air. La courbe, tracée sur la plaque photographique, est encore la représentation graphique d'une fonction exponentielle. Cependant il se trouve que la vitesse de l'image du fil de quartz au moment où celle-ci est à 1 cm. de sa position d'équilibre, se réduit à 25 cm. par seconde.

Si la corde est tendue plus fortement, il faut une plus grande intensité du courant, pour obtenir la même déviation, mais la rapidité de la déviation augmente. L'amortissement a moins d'influence et même, avec une tension suffisante, le mouvement de la corde devient oscillatoire. L'expérience suivante pourra servir d'exemple.

Entre les extrémités du fil de quartz assez fortement tendu, on a intercalé une petite résistance. On fait passer subitement un courant de

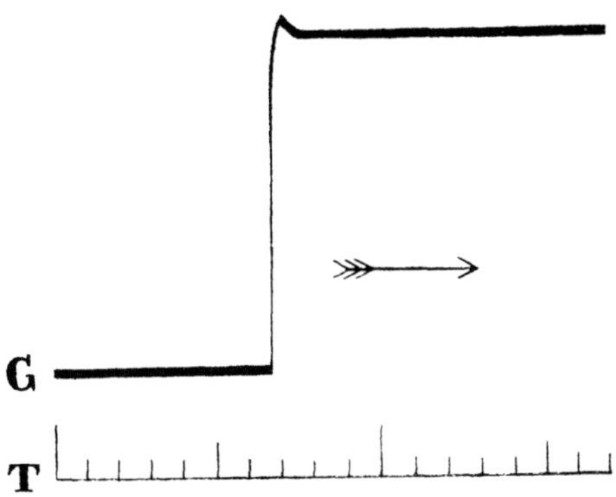

Fig. 2.

A peu près 2,3 fois plus grande que le photogramme primitif. Le fil de quartz est assez fortement tendu. Une petite résistance a été intercalée entre les extrémités du fil.

G = Courbe tracée par le fil de quartz pendant le passage subit d'un courant de un micrampére.

T = Temps en centièmes de seconde.

[1]) Voir plusieurs articles dans PFLÜGER's Arch. f. d. gesammte Physiol. Bd. 56, 60 et 79, ainsi que dans „Onderzoekingen'' Physiol. laborat, Leiden, II, T. 1—4.

1 micrampère par le galvanomètre. L'image du fil de quartz marque une déviation permanente de 14,4 mm., de sorte que la déviation pour un courant égal est devenu $\frac{560}{14,4} = 39$ fois plus petit.

Le mouvement, quoique fort amorti, est encore oscillatoire, v. fig. 2. Une oscillation s'accomplit en 0,003 sec. et le décrément logarithmique est de 3,09.

Si l'on monte en série dans le circuit du galvanomètre une résistance de 1 mégohm, l'influence de l'amortissement électromagnétique est à peu près nul. Seul l'amortissement produit par l'air reste. Avec la même tension de fil la déviation permanente se maintient pour un micrampère, mais la durée d'une oscillation est un peu raccourcie et le décrément logarithmique est réduit de 3,09 à 2,2.

La sensibilité normale de l'instrument est évaluée à 6×10^5.

IV

The string galvanometer and the human electrocardiogram

Two years after the initial and provisional report (III), this paper goes into more details about the string galvanometer and gives much information concerning the technique of registration, including the adjustment of sensitivity and damping. The experience obtained in applying the string galvanometer to the action currents of the heart, is described. Recalling the discovery by A.D. Waller* of the electrocardiogram, the correction of the tracings taken with the capillary electrometer and the subsequent development of the string galvanometer are discussed. The confrontation of an earlier, corrected, electrocardiogram with a recent one of the same person, obtained by means of the new instrument, offers proof both of the validity of the correction and of the accuracy of the string galvanometer.

The constancy of the electrocardiogram of each individual in the course of time is commented upon. Small irregular vibrations are demonstrated, which must be caused within the body because all external causes can be excluded (tremor as a cause is not yet mentioned).

* The date of Waller's paper in the Philosoph. Transactions is given in Einthoven's paper as 1899. This should be 1890 (read June 21, 1888, inserted in Transactions Series B for the year 1889).

Physiology. — *The string galvanometer and the human electrocardiogram.* By Professor W. EINTHOVEN. (Physiological laboratory at Leyden.)

In the Bosscha-celebration volume of the "Archives Néerlandaises" [1]) the principle of a new galvanometer was mentioned and the theory of the instrument dealt with. The practical usefulness of the instrument especially for electrophysiological measurements may be judged from what follows.

It may be remembered that the instrument consists principally of a silvered quartz thread which is stretched like a string in a strong magnetic field. When an electric current is passed through the thread, this latter deflects perpendicularly to the direction of the magnetic lines of force and the amount of the deflection can directly be measured by means of a microscope with an eye-piece micrometer.

What is the sensitiveness that can be obtained in this manner?

Since the above-mentioned publication a number of material improvements have been made in the instrument by which it is possible, for instance, to give a very feeble tension to the string, now a quartz thread 2.4 μ thick, with a resistance of 10 000 Ohms. If the tension is so regulated that a deflection takes place in from 10 to 15 seconds depending on its amount, every millimetre of the displacement of the image of the string corresponds to a current of 10^{-11} Amp. when a 660-fold magnification is used. As under these circumstances a

1) W. EINTHOVEN. Un nouveau galvanomètre. Archives Néerlandaises des sciences exactes et naturelles. Sér. II. Tome VI. p. 625. 1901.

displacement of 0,1 mm. is still noticeable, as will appear from the discussion of the plates, currents of 10^{-12} Amp. can consequently be detected.

As far as is known to the writer, no other galvanometer is capable of demonstrating with certainty such feeble currents. In practical work the string galvanometer must consequently be placed on a line with the most sensitive galvanometers of other construction and must be distinguished from so-called oscillographs which only react on much stronger currents.

The force which deflects the string in a field of 20 000 C. G. S. with a current of 10^{-12} Amp. is very small and works out for a length of 12.5 cm. at 2.5×10^{-11} grammes i. e. four times less than one ten millionth part of a milligramme.

By giving the string a greater tension its movements become quicker but its deflections for equal currents less. It is easy to give the string exactly such a tension that a current of given intensity causes a predetermined deflection, as may appear from the photograms of the two accompanying plates. These photograms were obtained in the same way as the formerly described capillary-electrometric curves [1]).

The 660-fold enlarged image of the middle part of the string is projected on a slit, perpendicular to the image. Before the slit a cylindrical lens is placed, the axis of which is parallel to it; behind it a sensitive plate is moved in the direction of the image of the string. While the movements of the string are thus registered, at the same time a system of coordinates is projected on the sensitive plate by the excellent method of GARTEN [2]). Of these coordinates the horizontal lines are obtained by mounting a glass millimetre-scale close before the sensitive plate so that the sharp shadows of the scale-divisions fall on the plate, while the vertical lines owe their origin to a uniformly rotating spoked disc which intermittently intercepts the light falling on the slit. The distance of the vertical as well as of the horizontal lines has in our photograms been taken about one millimetre, every fifth line being somewhat thicker. This latter peculiarity can easily be introduced into the coordinate system by drawing every fifth line in the glass millimetre-scale before the sensitive plate slightly thicker and by also making every fifth spoke of the rotating disc somewhat broader.

---

[1]) See various essays in "PFLÜGER's Arch. f. d. gesammte Physiol." and in "Onderzoekingen physiol. laborat. Leyden." 2nd series.

[2]) DR. SIEGFRIED GARTEN. Ueber rhythmische elektrische Vorgänge im quergestreiften Skeletmuskel. Abhandl. der Königl. Sächs. Gesellsch. der Wissensch. zu Leipzig. Mathem. phys. Classe, Bd. 26, No. 5. S. 331. 1901.

The first photogram, fig. 1 plate I represents the deflections of the string when currents of 1,2 and 3×10^{-9} Amp. are successively passed through the galvanometer. In the coordinate system a length of 1 mm. of the abscissae has a value of 0.1 second, an ordinate of 1 mm. representing 10^{-10} Amp. Although the image of the string has considerable breadth and has no perfectly sharp outlines — as must be expected with a magnification of 660 times — yet its displacement in the coordinate system can easily be determined with an accuracy of 0.1 mm. For if one of the margins of the image before and after the deflection is observed, observation with the unaided eye or with a magnifying-glass will show that the deflection differs from the tabulated amount by less than 0.1 mm. Hence the currents are measured in the photogram with an accuracy of 10^{-11} Amp.

One notices that the deflections are accurately proportional to the intensity of the current, that they are dead-beat and that they are accomplished in 1 to 2 seconds according to their magnitude. The strong damping must be ascribed to the resistance of the air, for during the registering of the curves a resistance of one Megohm was put into the galvanometer circuit by which the ordinary electromagnetic damping was almost entirely suppressed.

If the tension of the string is made ten times less, the galvanometer becomes ten times more sensitive and, as stated above, currents of 10^{-12} Amp. may still be observed. But with this greater sensitiveness the deflections are no longer proportional to the current and the movements of the string are difficult to record, as the quartz thread no longer moves exactly in a plane. Yet the instrument can still be used then for direct observation with the microscope.

Figure 2 plate I shows that the deflections to the right and to the left — in the figure corresponding to upward and downward deflections, are equal. The velocity of the sensitive plate has remained the same so that again an abscissa of one millimetre corresponds to a time of 0.1 second. But the tension of the string is 200 times stronger so that one millimetre of the ordinates represents 2×10^{-8} Amp. A current of 4×10^{-7} Amp. is alternately sent in opposite directions through the galvanometer and hence causes deviations of 20 mm. to the right and also to the left. It is easy to ascertain that these deviations are equal to each other up to 0.1 millimetre.

The movement of the string is very quick so that during the deflection the string can only cast a feeble shadow on the sensitive plate. The ascending and descending nearly vertical lines which in the original negative are still visible as very thin streaks have become invisible in the reproduced photogram.

In fig. 3 plate 1 a movement of the string is represented when a current of 3×10^{-8} Amp. is suddenly made and broken. The sensitive plate has been moved along with a tenfold velocity and the string has ten times more tension than in fig. 1, consequently one mm. absc. = 0.01 second and one mm. ord. = 10^{-9} Amp. The galvanometer circuit contains again one Megohm so that the same causes of damping exist as in fig. 1. The movement is still dead-beat, but on account of the 10 times greater force on the string it is 10 times quicker, as can easily be ascertained by comparing the great descending curve of fig. 1 with one of the curves of fig. 3 or better still by superposing diapositives of the curves of both figures. They will then be seen to cover each other exactly and since in one figure the velocity of the moving plate is ten times greater than in the other, the deflection of the string must in one case take place ten times more quickly than in the other. At the same time the resistance of the air is proved in our case to increase proportionally to the velocity of the string itself.

In recording the curves of fig. 4 and 5 of plate I the velocity of the moving plate has been increased to 250 mm. per sec. so that 1 mm. of the abscissae is 0.004 sec. The plate at first moves slowly and reaches the mentioned velocity only when it has travelled through a distance of 4 or 5 centimetres, whereas the spokes of the rotating disc always cast their shadows on the plate accurately every 0.004 second. Hence the coordinate system is in the first sixth part of the photogram compressed in the direction of the abscissae.

In fig. 4 one mm. ord. = 2×10^{-8} Amp., while in fig. 5 one mm. ord. = 3×10^{-8} Amp. These two figures together show us the limit-value of the sensitiveness for which the movement of the string is still dead-beat. In fig. 4 a current of 4×10^{-7} Amp., in fig. 5 a current of 6×10^{-7} Amp. has been transmitted through the galvanometer and interrupted. One sees that the deflection in fig. 4 is still dead-beat and is completed in about 0.009 sec., whereas in fig. 5 the motion begins to become oscillatory and for a single oscillation takes 0.006 sec. The sensitiveness with which the motion of the string is on the border between aperiodic and oscillatory motion is consequently such that a deflection of one millimetre corresponds to a current between 2 and 3×10^{-8} Amp.

In the tracing of fig. 4 and 5 only an insignificant resistance is put into the galvanometer circuit so that here besides the viscosity of the air also the ordinary electromagnetic damping checks the motion.

Now some particulars may be mentioned referring to the 5 photograms of plate 1 in common.

In order to obtain the image of the string equally sharp in all parts of the visual field, the string must move in a plane perpendicular to the optical axis of the projecting microscope. A displacement of the string of 0.5 μ in the direction of the optical axis suffices to cause a noticeable indistinctness of the image with the magnification used. The photograms show that such a displacement does not take place.

The great constancy of the zero point and the equality of the deflections deserve notice and also — which is especially important for practical work with the instrument in electro-physiological measurements — the possibility of accurately fixing beforehand the sensitiveness of the instrument. The unaided eye can already observe in nearly all the figures of plate I that this can be done successfully with an error of less than 0.1 mm. for deflections of 30 or 40 mm., i.e. with an error of less than 2.5 or 3 per thousand. Only fig. 5 shows a real deficiency of about 0.1 mm. which some greater care might have avoided.

It is hardly necessary to point out that the galvanometer is not affected by variations in the surrounding magnetic field. Moreover it is not to any extent affected by tremors of the floor. It stands on the same stone pillar on which a large tin disc with spokes is rapidly rotated by an electromotor. This electromotor is only at a few centimetres' distance from the galvanometer, while another motor, coupled with a heavy fly-wheel, for moving the sensitive plate, is clamped to the same pillar at a somewhat greater distance. Yet no trace of mechanical vibrations appears in the photograms.

The first electro-physiological investigation made with the string galvanometer was one concerning the shape of the human electrocardiogram discovered by Aug. D. Waller [1]). Until now this could only be obtained by means of the capillary electrometer. But the curve traced by that instrument gives, when superficially observed, a quite erroneous idea of the changes of potential differences actually occurring during the registering. In order to know these they have to be calculated from the shape of the recorded curve and the properties of the capillary used. This leads to the construction of a new curve, the form of which is the correct expression of the actual variations of potential.

---

1) Augustus D. Waller. On the electromotive changes, connected with the beat of the mammalian heart and of the human heart in particular. Philosoph. Transactions of the Royal Society of London, vol. 180 (1899), B, pp. 169—194.

An example may explain this [1]).

The following fig. 1 represents the curve traced for the electro-cardiogram of Mr. v. d. W. when the current was derived from

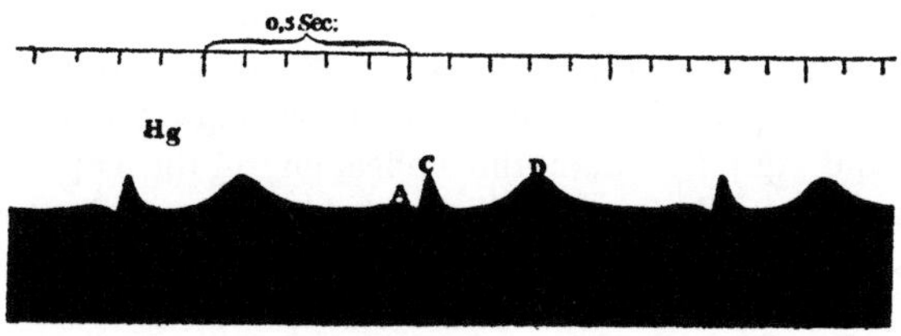

Fig. 1.

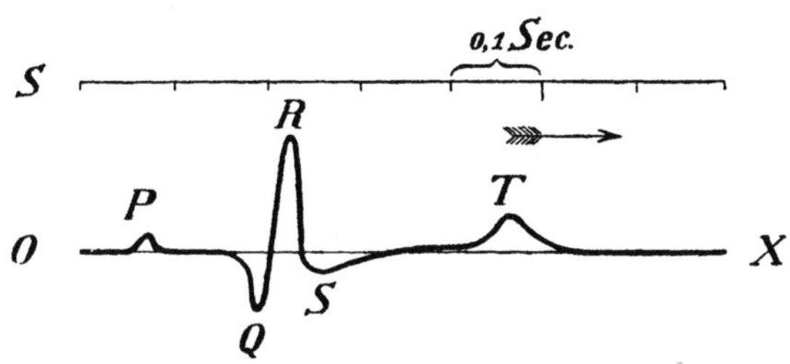

Fig. 2.

the right and left hands, whereas fig. 2 is the constructed curve. The differences are obvious. Especially the tops *C* and *D* in the registered curve should be compared with the corresponding tops *R* and *T* in the secondary curve which latter alone truly represents the ratio of the heights of the tops.

We shall now try to compare the string galvanometer as a research instrument with the capillary electrometer and must first of all bear in mind that the deflections of the string galvanometer measure a current, that of the capillary electrometer an electromotive force. But it must be remarked that whenever variations in current or tension are measured, the mercury meniscus as well as the string moves. And during this movement the capillary must be charged or discharged by an *electric current,* whereas the string in the magnetic field develops an opposed *electromotive force.* Moreover, when there is a constant considerable resistance with negligeable self-induction, such as commonly occurs in electro-physiological investigations, the

---

[1]) See Pflüger's Arch. Bd. 60. 1895 and "Onderzoekingen". Physiol. Laborat. Leyden. 2nd series, vol. 2.

intensity of the current will at any moment be proportional to the active electromotive force, so that the fundamental difference between the electrometer and the galvanometer is no obstacle to a comparison of both instruments.

The string galvanometer has several advantages over the capillary electrometer. First the deflection of the string galvanometer will in many cases and especially in the case of tracing a human cardiogram be greater and quicker than the deflection of the capillary electrometer. Then the capillary electrometer is less accurate in the constancy of its indications, their proportionality to the potential differences and their equality in opposed directions.

A highly magnified image of the mercury meniscus cannot be so sharply projected as that of a fine thread and one cannot regulate the sensitiveness of the capillary electrometer to a predetermined amount. The electrical insulation of the string galvanometer is much easier than of the capillary electrometer and a phenomenon like "creeping" does not occur with the galvanometer.

In the capillary electrometer the movement of the meniscus is damped by the friction of the mercury and sulphuric acid when streaming through a narrow tube. Invisibly small traces of impurities may hinder or even entirely stop the movement of the mercury meniscus. Many a capillary had after a relatively short time to be replaced by a new one because there was a "hitch" in the movement of the meniscus. In the string galvanometer, on the other hand, we have air-damping as well as electromagnetic damping, both of which work with perfect regularity. The electromagnetic damping can moreover be varied at will by changing the intensity of the field and the resistance in the galvanometer circuit.

Plate II contains the electrocardiograms of some six persons, traced by means of the string galvanometer. In the coordinate system an absciss of one millimetre has a value of 0.04 sec., while an ordinate of one mm. represents a P.D. of 10^{-4} Volts. By choosing these round numbers the curves satisfy generally the requirements of the international committee for the unification of physiological methods.

The movement of the quartz thread, as may be seen from the normal curves at the end of each photogram, was dead-beat and very quick, so that the traced electrocardiogram is a fair representation ot the oscillations in the potential difference existing between the right and left hands of the experimental person. As a rule this may be admitted for the lower tops P, Q, S and T without any noticeable error. But for the high and sharp top R a correction should be applied especially in photograms 8 and 9, a correction by which the extremity of the top would be shifted a little to the left and upwards. The necessary correction is small however and its amount may be approximately estimated at less than 0.2 mm. for the shifting to the left and less than one mm. for the shifting upwards.

Photogram 8 represents the electrocardiogram of the same person whose capillary-electrometric curve is shown in the text. When the registered curve of fig. 8 plate II is compared with the formerly plotted curve of fig. 2 in the text, it is evident that both curves have great similarity. The tops *P*, *Q*, *R*, *S*, and *T* are not only present in both curves, but have also the same relative height in both.

In the plotted curve 1 millivolt of ordinate has been made equal to 0.1 sec. of absciss, while in the galvanometer curve 1 millivolt of ordinate corresponds to 0.4 sec. of absciss. Hence the galvanometer curve is compressed in the direction of the abscissae, as a superficial inspection will reveal. Besides the galvanometer curve, on account of the gradual transitions of one top to another, gives the impression of being in its minor details a more faithful representation of nature than the plotted curve. It is obvious that of this latter curve only a limited number of points could be accurately calculated, while for the rest the calculated points had to be joined by the curve that fitted them best. But these small differences are immaterial.

It may give some satisfaction that the results formerly obtained by means of the capillary electrometer and more or less laborious calculation and plotting have been fully confirmed in a different and simple manner by means of the new instrument. For this affords us a twofold proof, first of the validity of the theory and of the practical usefulness of the formerly followed methods and secondly of the accuracy of the new instrument itself.

The six electrocardiograms of plate II were selected among a greater number and arranged after the dimensions of the downward top *S* (see the figure in the text). In 6 and 7 the curve remains, at the spot where *S* ought to be, above the zero-line of the diastole, in 8 and 9 *S* is only small, in 10 and 11 great. The numbers 6 and 11 mark in this respect the extremes which occur in our collection of electrocardiograms, whereas N°. 8, that of Mr. v. D. W. represents a sort of norm with which the other numbers may all be easily compared.

The constancy of shape of the curve for a certain person is remarkable. This shape seems even to change so little in course of time, that with some practice one may recognize many an individual by his electrocardiogram. We conclude this essay with a remark on the

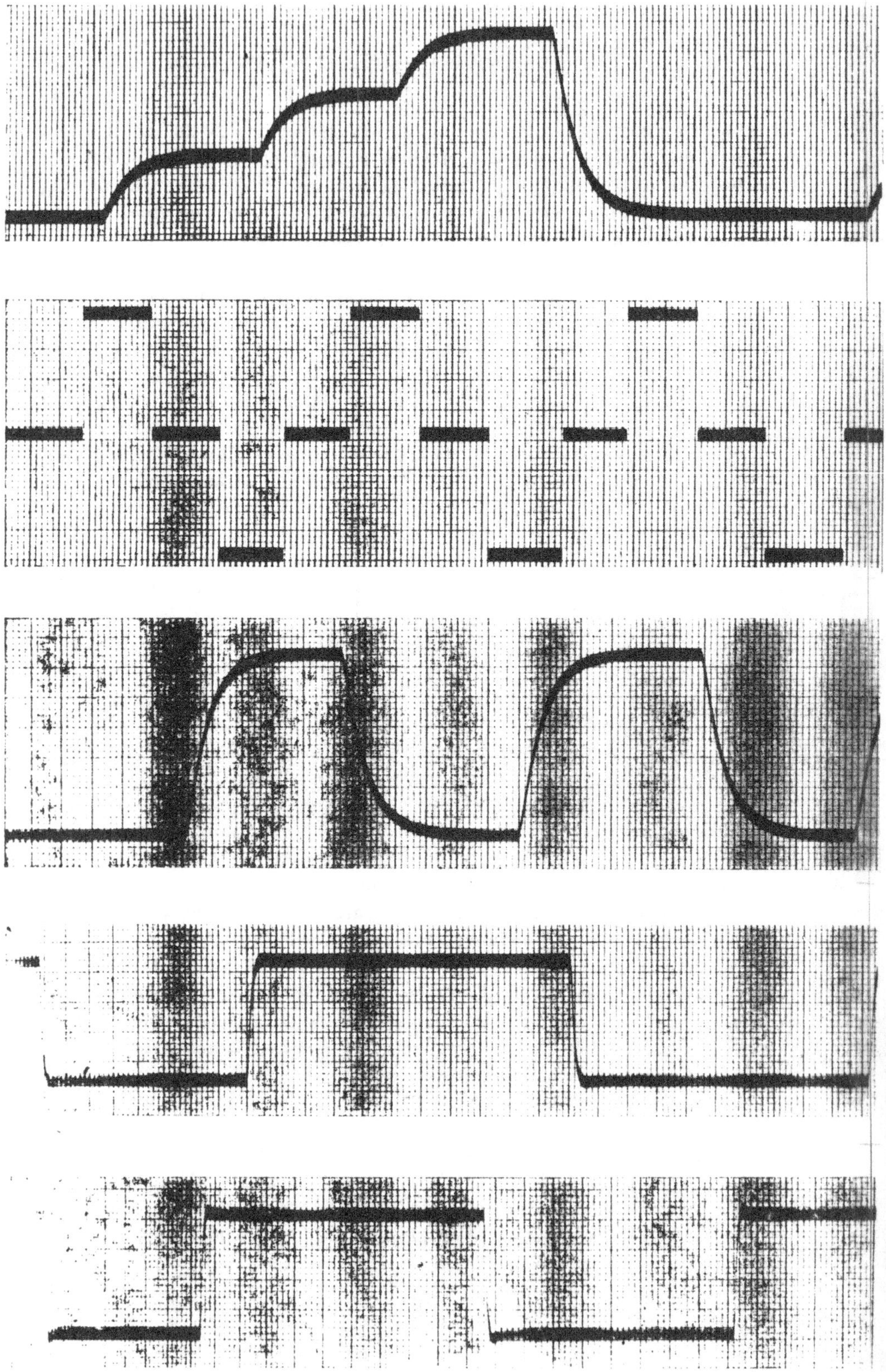

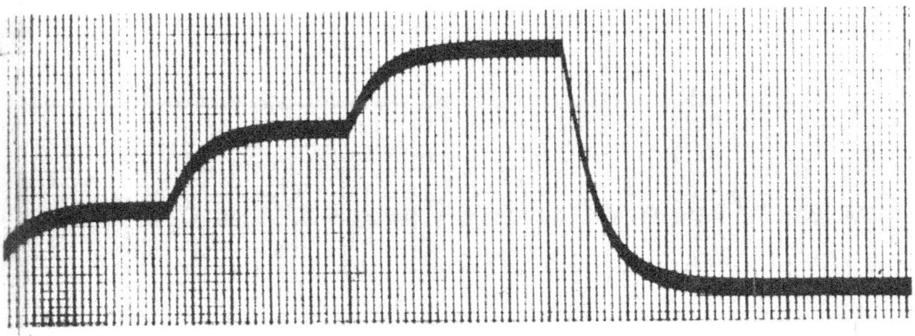

1.

Absc. 1 mm. = 0.1 Sec.

Ord. 1 „ = 10 ^{10} Amp

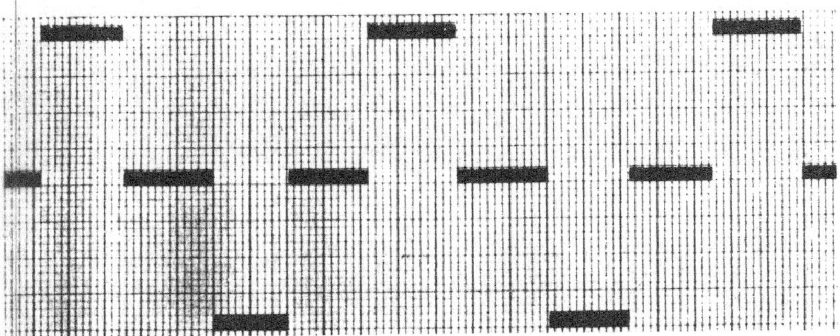

2.

Absc. 1 mm. = 0,1 Sec.

Ord. 1 „ = 2×10 ^{8} Amp

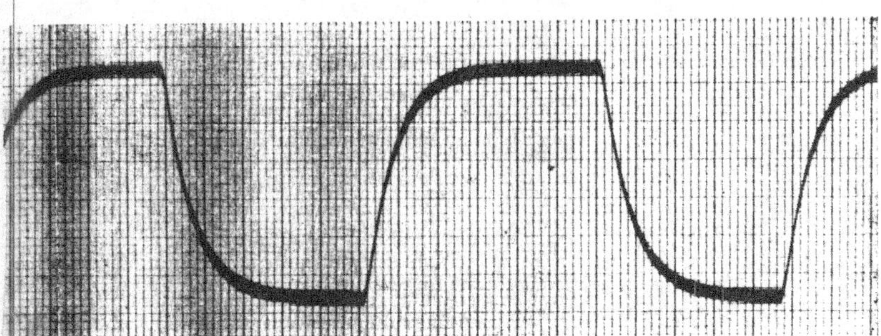

3.

Absc. 1 mm. = 0,01 Sec.

Ord. 1 „ = 10 ^{9} Amp.

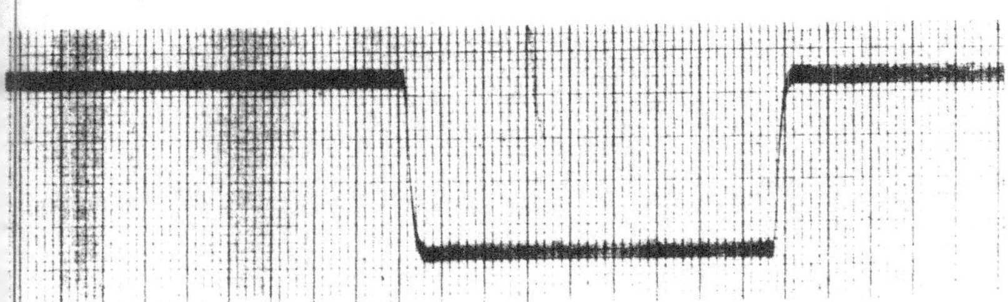

4.

Absc. 1 mm. = 0,004 Sec.

Ord. 1 „ = 2×10 ^{8} Amp.

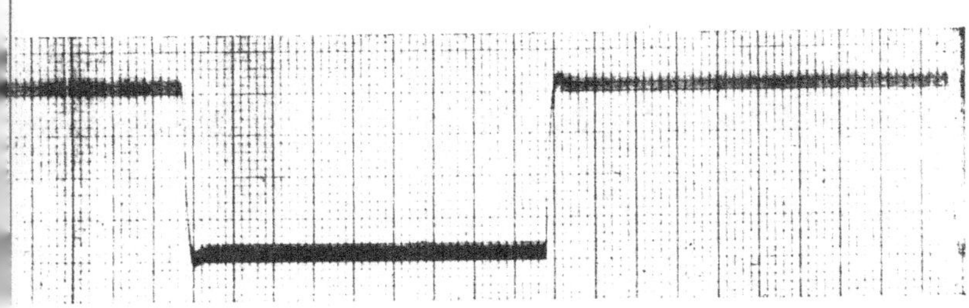

5.

Absc. 1 mm. = 0,004 Sec.

Ord. 1 „ = 3×10 Amp.

Absc. 1 mm. = 0,04 Sec. Ordin. 1 mm = 10^{-4} Volt.

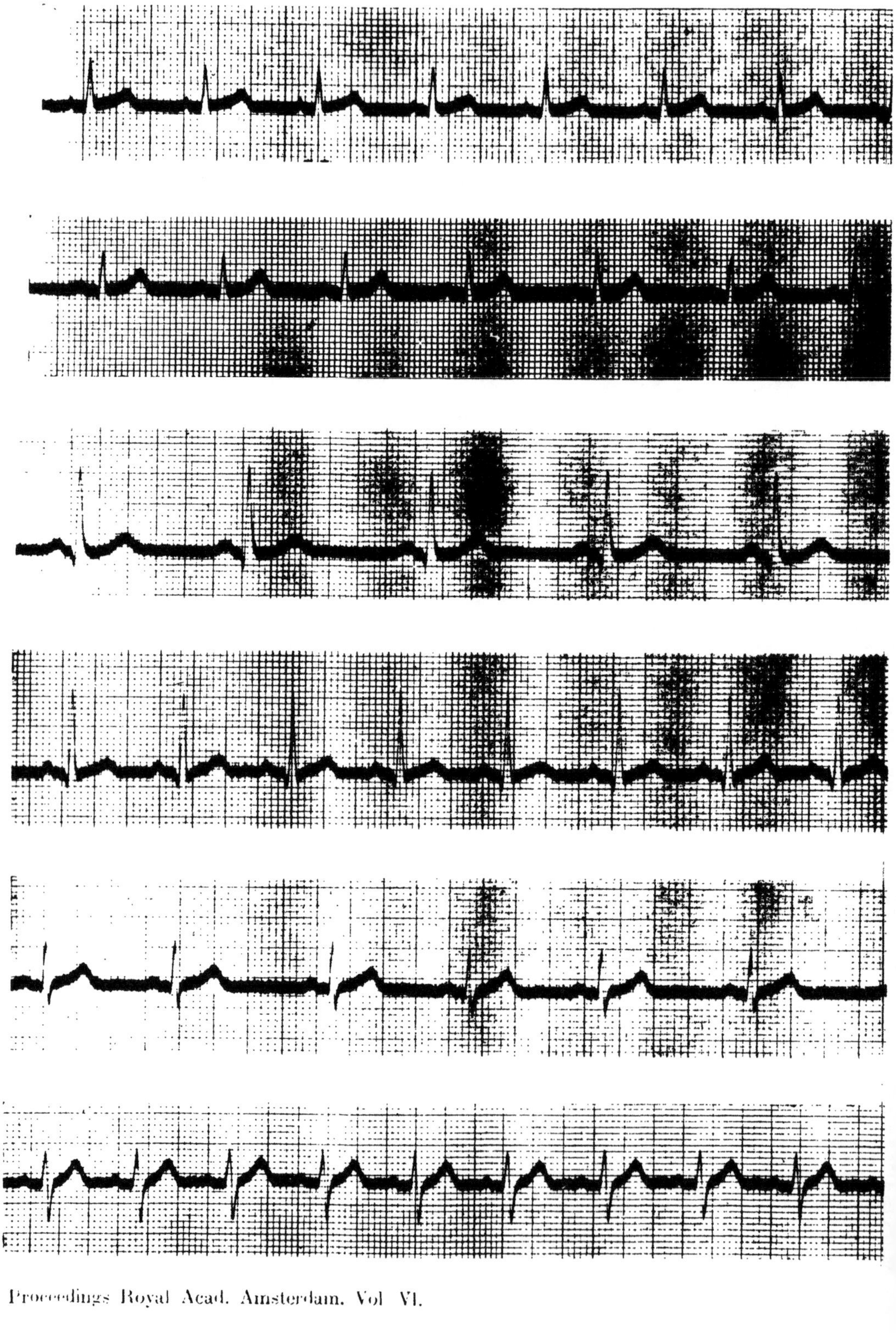

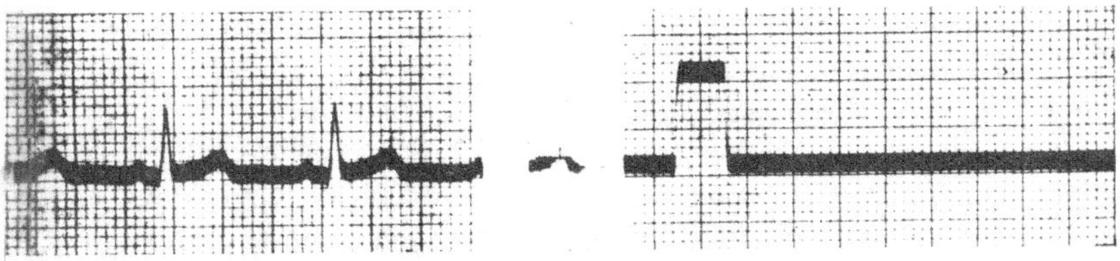

6.
Ad.

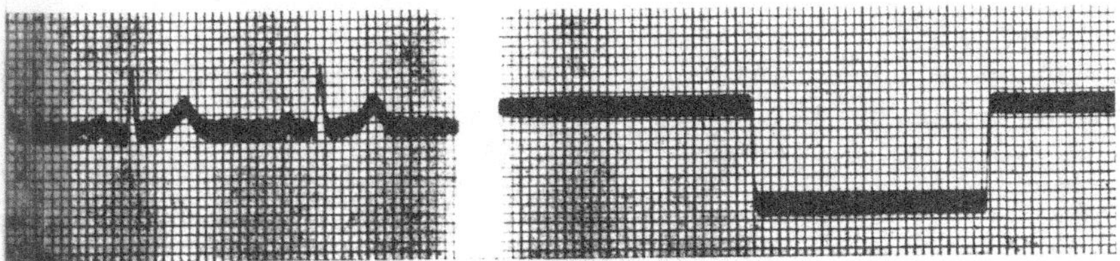

7.
Vr.

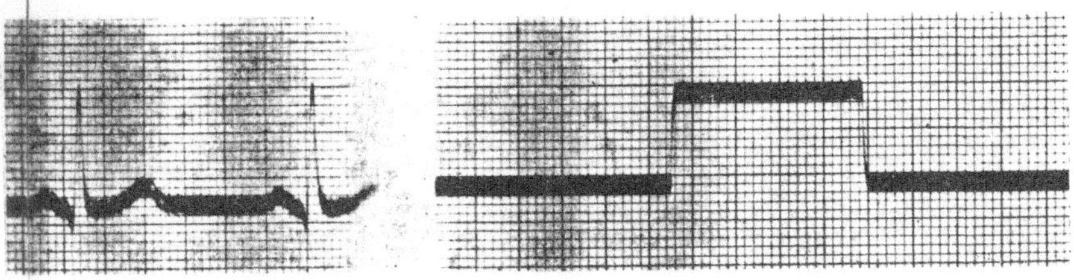

8.
v. d. W.

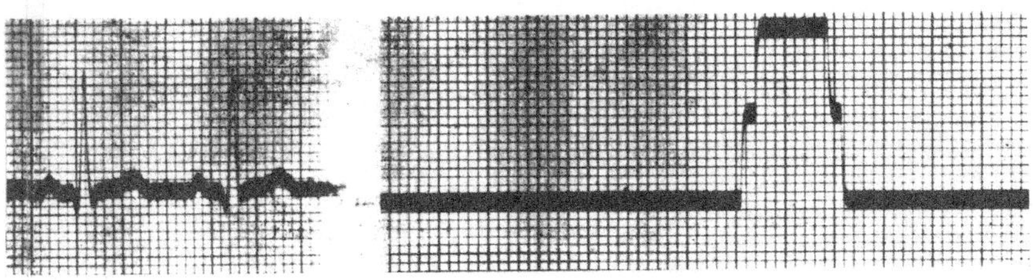

9.
Kr.

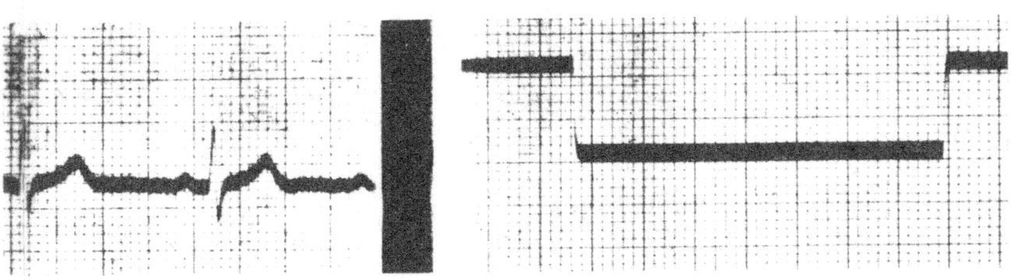

10.
Be.

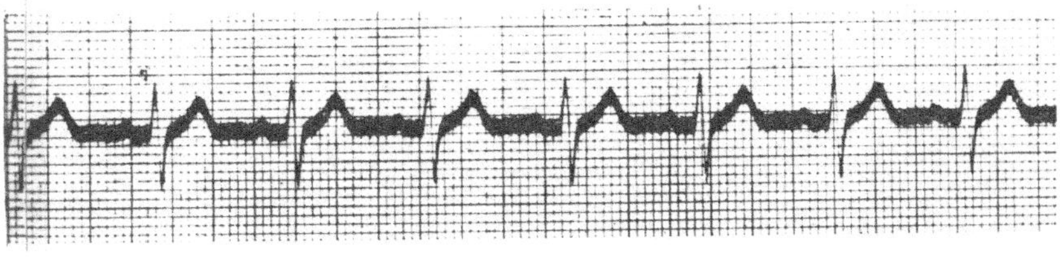

11.
Bi.

small irregular vibrations occurring in most electrocardiograms, where they sometimes reach a height of 0,1 to 0.5 mm. and more, but are sometimes entirely absent, as e.g. in N°. 6 of Mr. AD.

These vibrations are not caused by tremors of the floor or other irregularities which should be ascribed to an insufficient technique as is easily shown by the vibrationless normal curves at the end of almost every series of electrocardiograms. Hence they must be caused by electromotive agents in the human body itself and the question arises whether they find their origin in the action of the heart or of other organs. We may expect that an investigation undertaken with this object will give a definite answer to this question.

V

Le télécardiogramme

After a brief description of the string galvanometer, the electrocardiogram thereby obtained, is presented and found identical with the corrected tracing from the capillary electrometer. The leads used are from both hands and the left foot, immersed in saline. They conform to leads I, II and III, used ever since, but had not yet received that designation. It is noteworthy that the standard calibration of voltage and time has remained unchanged, as well as the background with its 1 mm quadrangles and the thickening of every fifth line. It is announced that in a forthcoming thesis (by Einthoven's assistant Vaandrager) the relation of the leads will be discussed, that is, the calculation of the third lead when the two others have been registered. It is added, that the waves of the same name in different leads are not quite identical.

Subsequently a long distance connection of the string galvanometer with the hospital is described together with the technical difficulties encountered in its construction. It is calculated that the distance (1,5 km) could have been enlarged 20 or even 40 times. It is mentioned however, that the resistance of the circuit cannot made too high, because it must remain low compared with that of extraneous leaks. It is easily seen from the calibration curve, shown in this paper, that the damping is slightly more than Einthoven recommended at other times.

However, the connection with the hospital yielded a rich harvest of abnormal electrocardiograms, most of which are shown in this paper for the first time. These concern in particular various types of arrhythmias but also normal rhythm in valvular disease, in which the electrocardiogram shows signs of ventricular hypertrophy (as in aortic insufficiency) or of atrial hypertrophy (as in mitral disease). Among the arrhythmias, premature beats occupy an important place. It is shown that the height of the following pulse depends on the timing of the extrasystole in the cardiac cycle. The peculiar circumstance, that Einthoven could warn the clinician in the hospital by telephone that an intermission of the pulse was forthcoming, is described; it has been referred to in chapter 1. Atrial flutter and fibrillation are shown as types of atrial tachycardia (much later (137), the same tracing of flutter was again reproduced with the correct interpretation). Special attention is given to heart block, both experimental in the dog from vagus stimulation and in a patient with a ventricular rate of 29, in whose electrocardiogram the P waves are clearly dissociated from the ventricular complexes.

The existence of an U wave is shown here for the first time (in a patient with "myocardial degeneration"). In a later paper (101) Einthoven described normal cases with U waves, although of lower voltage.

[612.172.4] [Q 4512.2]

LE TÉLÉCARDIOGRAMME,

par W. EINTHOVEN (1)

(34 fig., 1 pl.)

(Institut de physiologie. Leyde)

Messieurs,

L'EXAMEN des phénomènes, dont nous allons nous occuper aujourd'hui, repose sur l'emploi d'un instrument de mesure électrique, le galvanomètre à corde (2).

Cet instrument consiste essentiellement en un mince fil de quartz argenté ($\mathcal{A}\ \mathcal{A}_1$, fig. 1), tendu comme une corde de violon dans un champ magnétique très intense, formé entre les pièces polaires $\mathcal{P}\mathcal{P}_1$ d'un électro-aimant. Dès qu'un courant électrique est lancé à travers la corde, cette dernière subit un écart dans un sens perpendiculaire aux lignes de force, et la grandeur de cet écart est proportionnelle à l'intensité du courant.

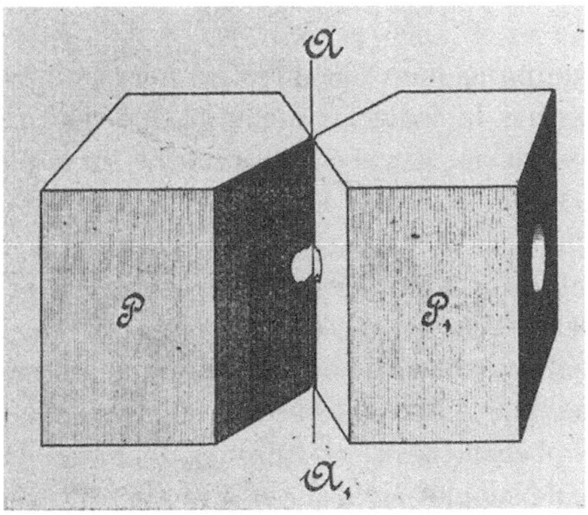

FIG. 1.

Pour permettre l'observation de cet écart, les pièces polaires sont percées

(1) Rédigé d'après deux conférences faites, l'une le 20 mai 1905 à l'Assemblée générale de la Société hollandaise des Sciences (voir le programme pour l'année 1905), l'autre le 7 novembre de la même année, à Amsterdam, à une réunion de la Société de physique, de médecine et de chirurgie (Genootschap voor natuur-, genees- en heelkunde).

(2) Pour les détails, voir *Arch. néerl. des sc. exact. et nat.* 1901 (2), VI, 625; 1904, IX, 186; 1905, X, 137; 1905, X, 414. Voir aussi *Annalen der Physik*, 1903-1905 et *Onderzoekingen physiol. laborat. Leiden*, 2e Reeks.

chacune d'une ouverture, par où passe un microscope; l'un des deux microscopes (𝔐, fig. 2) sert à concentrer la lumière sur le fil de quartz, tandis que l'autre ($\mathfrak{M}_1$) fournit une image fortement grossie du fil. Cette image, verticale comme le fil lui-même, est tournée de 90° autour de la ligne de foi du microscope de projection, au moyen d'un prisme de verre, taillé spécialement dans ce but; l'image prend ainsi une position horizontale. Elle est projetée sur un écran présentant une fente verticale, derrière laquelle une plaque photographique se meut avec une vitesse uniforme dans une direction horizontale. Le mince faisceau lumineux qui traverse la fente est rendu plus net encore par une lentille cylindrique, convenablement placée, qui projette sur la plaque une raie lumineuse, large de 0.05 mm. et haute de 50 mm. Cette raie est interrompue par un espace obscur, dont la hauteur, correspondant à la largeur de l'image de la corde, atteint 1.5 à 2 mm. Cet espace obscur, en se déplaçant vers le haut ou vers le bas, décrit les tracés que l'on veut obtenir et dont la netteté laisse fort peu à désirer, comme on peut en juger par les reproductions ci-jointes (1).

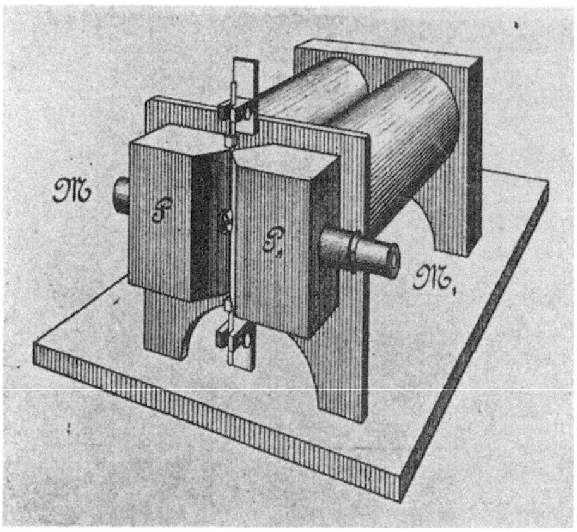

Fig. 2.

Mieux que tout autre instrument, le galvanomètre à corde nous permet d'étudier les phénomènes électriques du cœur humain. Le cœur, battant dans notre corps, développe à chaque contraction un courant électrique, qui est conduit vers toutes les parties de notre organisme, par ex. vers nos mains et vers nos pieds. Il suffit de raccorder le galvanomètre avec les deux mains, ou avec une main et un pied d'une personne, pour observer un écart de la corde à chaque battement du cœur.

(1) Les figures ont été reproduites par la photographie. Comme il est évident qu'au point vue de la finesse elles ne sauraient concourir avec les photographies originales, je donnerai volontiers des épreuves positives de ces dernières à quiconque m'en exprimera le désir.

On voit dans la fig. 3 une reproduction d'une courbe qui a été tracée par la corde, pendant que le galvanomètre était mis en communication avec les deux mains d'une personne. Cette courbe, qui est l'expression exacte du mouvement électrique dans le cœur et qui peut nous donner des renseignements sur la façon dont cet organe travaille, a reçu le nom d'*électrocardiogramme* (1).

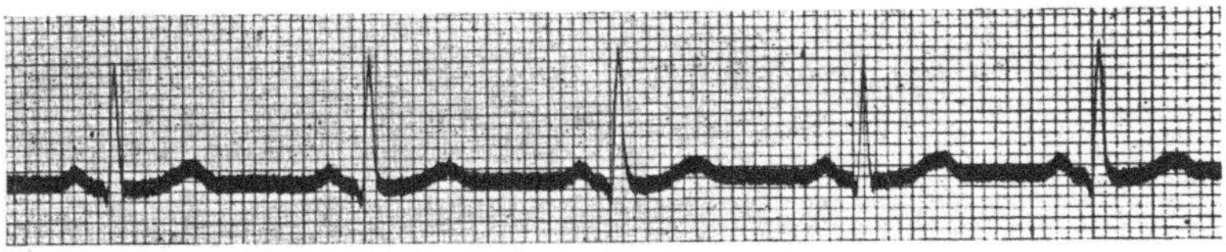

FIG. 3.

V. D. W. — Dérivation de la main droite à la main gauche.

Dans cette figure, l'électrocardiogramme est représenté dans un système de coordonnées (2), consistant en un réseau de millimètres carrés. Les traits horizontaux, ou abscisses, s'obtiennent en plaçant en avant de la plaque photographique, et tout près de celle-ci, une échelle en verre verticale, divisée en millimètres, de sorte que les ombres nettes des traits de division tombent sur la plaque; tandis que les traits verticaux, ou ordonnées, s'obtiennent par une espèce de roue, tournant d'un mouvement uniforme, dont les rayons interceptent par intermittences la lumière qui tombe sur la plaque. Dans nos photographies il est toujours fait en sorte que la distance des ordonnées soit à peu près la même que la distance des abcisses. De cinq en cinq les traits sont rendus un peu plus gros. Cette dernière particularité du système de coordonnées s'obtient aisément en renforçant quelque peu, de cinq en cinq, les traits sur l'échelle de verre disposée devant la plaque; de même les rayons du disque tournant sont rendus un peu plus épais de cinq en cinq.

(1) Les courants électriques accompagnant les battements d'un cœur de grenouille ont été démontrés pour la première fois par A. KÖLLIKER et H. MÜLLER; pour le cœur humain ils ont été montrés pour la première fois par AUG. D. WALLER. Pour de plus amples détails relatifs à la bibliographie ancienne, je renvoie à la dissertation de W. T. DE VOGEL, Leyden, 1893. On trouve des publications plus récentes dans *Archiv f. d. ges. Physiol.* 1895, 1900 et 1903, et dans *Onderzoekingen physiol. laborat. Leiden*, 2e Reeks.

(2) Voir S. GARTEN, *Abhandl. d. k. Sächs. Gesellsch. d. Wissensch. zu Leipzig, Math. phys. Kl.* 1901, XXVI, n° 5.

Dans la fig. 3 un mm. en abscisse correspond à 0.04 sec., et un mm. en ordonnée représente une différence de potentiel de 10^{-4} volts entre les pôles du galvanomètre (1).

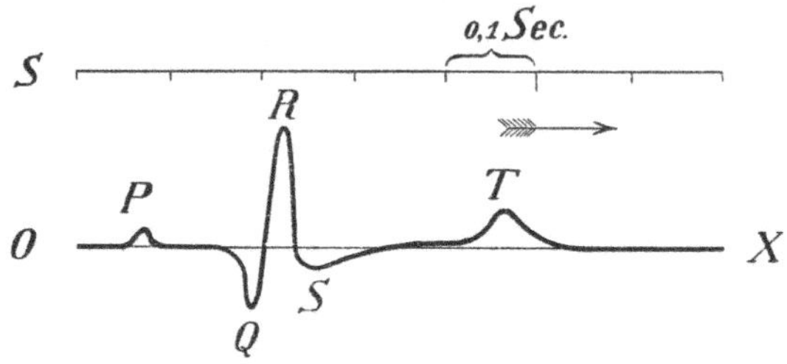

FIG. 4.

Afin de pouvoir discuter aisément la forme de l'électrocardiogramme, je représenterai par des lettres les divers sommets de la courbe. Dans la figure schématique fig. 4, nous distinguons les cinq sommets *P*, *Q*, *R*, *S* et *T*. Le premier sommet *P* correspond seul à la contraction des oreillettes, tandis que les quatre sommets suivants représentent le mouvement électrique produit par la systole des ventricules. Ces sommets peuvent différer assez notablement quant à la forme et à la hauteur, tant suivant le sujet examiné que suivant les endroits d'où dérive le courant.

Nous reproduirons maintenant quatre électrocardiogrammes, pris successivement chez une même personne, mais dans quatre circonstances différentes de dérivation du courant. Pour rendre comparables entr'elles les courbes ainsi obtenues, il a été fait en sorte que la partie du corps qui prend le potentiel de la base du cœur ou du cœur droit fût toujours reliée au même pôle du galvanomètre, et à l'autre pôle la partie du corps qui prend le potentiel de la pointe du cœur, ou du cœur gauche. Quand la première partie prend passagèrement une charge négative par rapport à l'autre il se forme dans l'électrocardiogramme un sommet dirigé vers le haut.

La vitesse du mouvement de la plaque photographique et la sensibilité du galvanomètre sont réglées de telle manière que, dans toutes les épreuves 1 mm. en abscisse correspond à 0.04 sec. et 1 mm. en ordonnée à une différence de potentiel de 0.1 millivolt.

(1) Sauf indication contraire, il en est de même pour toutes les autres figures.

Dans la fig. 5 j'ai reproduit le premier des quatre électrocardiogrammes; le courant venait des deux mains. Au premier coup d'œil, la fig. 5 ressemble à l'électrocardiogramme de la fig. 3; mais ils proviennent de personnes différentes, et, en y regardant de près, on reconnaît facilement des différences

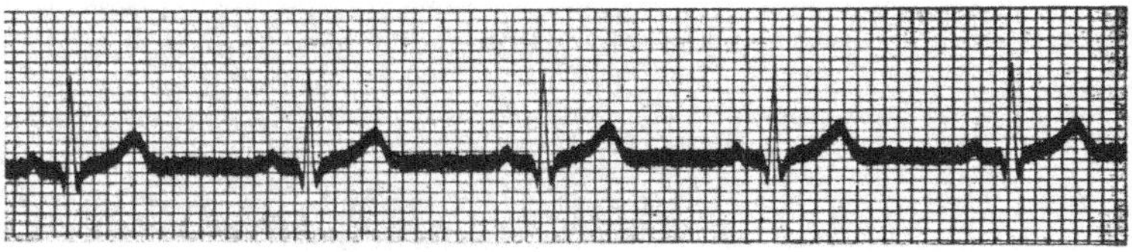

FIG. 5.

M. — Dérivation de la main droite à la main gauche.

entre les deux cardiogrammes. Ainsi p. ex. le sommet *T*, comparé au sommet *R*, est nettemement plus haut dans la fig. 5 que dans la fig. 3; dans la fig. 5 surtout, le sommet *S*, dirigé vers le bas, s'abaisse plus loin au-dessous de la position d'équilibre et il est beaucoup plus net que dans la fig. 3. En somme, avec un peu d'exercice, l'analyse quelque peu détaillée des courbes permet de distinguer les personnes par la forme de leur électrocardiogramme.

Je ne puis manquer d'attirer ici l'attention sur une particularité qui paraît se présenter dans tous les électrocardiogrammes, savoir, que dans le dernier sommet *T* la branche ascendante est moins abrupte que la branche descendante. Un sommet d'une telle forme ne s'observe ni dans un sphygmogramme, ni dans un myogramme, ni même, pour autant que je sache, dans aucune autre courbe physiologique.

Quand on obtient le courant en reliant les deux mains, la hauteur des divers sommets est assez grande. Par contre, quand on relie le galvanomètre aux deux pieds, les sommets sont beaucoup moins prononcés, comme on pouvait s'y attendre d'ailleurs. La fig. 6 prouve qu'on n'observe plus alors que deux sommets, dont l'un atteint une hauteur de 0.9 mm., et l'autre, à peine sensible, 0.1 mm.

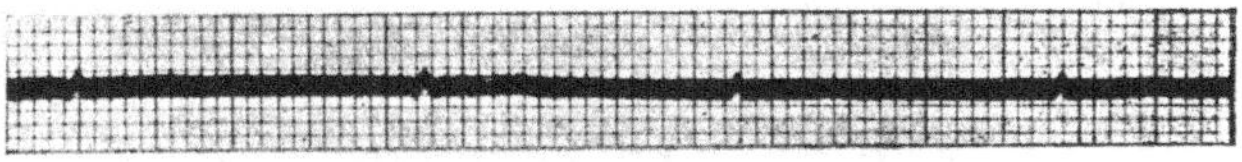

FIG. 6.

M. — Dérivation du pied droit au pied gauche.

Dans la troisième manière de dériver le courant, nous faisons usage de la main droite et du pied gauche. La fig. 7 représente l'électrocardiogramme obtenu dans ces conditions. En général les sommets sont plus élevés que dans la dérivation par les deux mains, et c'est de cette façon que l'on obtient d'ordinaire les plus belles courbes.

Une quatrième dérivation s'obtient en reliant le galvanomètre à la main gauche et au pied gauche. Dans ces conditions, les écarts sont généralement

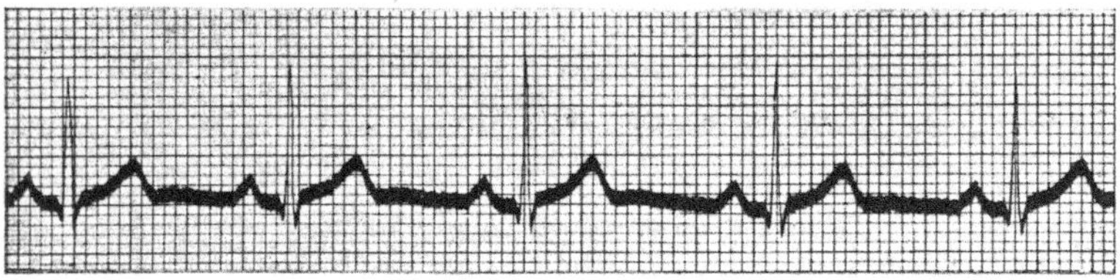

FIG. 7.

M. — Dérivation de la main droite au pied gauche.

plus petits, comme on peut le voir sur la fig. 8 ; mais ce qu'il y a de plus frappant c'est que la hauteur relative des divers sommets est modifiée. Le sommet S s'abaisse plus loin, tandis que le dernier sommet T a diminué dans une plus forte mesure que les autres. On peut même constater dans les électrocardiogrammes de plus d'une personne que le sommet T a totalement disparu ou est devenu négatif.

Une fois que l'on connaît les courbes obtenues 1° en reliant la main droite à la main gauche, 2° en reliant la main droite au pied gauche, il doit être possible de déduire de ces deux-là la courbe résultant d'une dérivation par la main gauche et le pied gauche. Ce calcul, qui est utile non seulement pour le contrôle de la précision des tracés, mais encore pour l'identification des

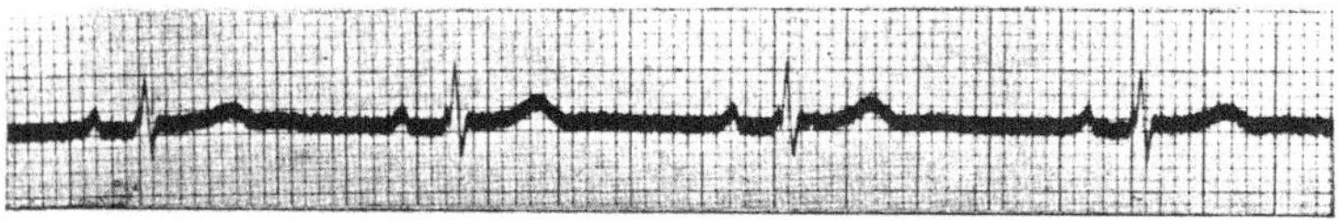

FIG. 8.

M. — Dérivation de la main gauche au pied gauche.

sommets qui ont été représentés par la même lettre dans les diverses courbes, sera traité bientôt, j'espère, dans la dissertation d'un de mes élèves. On y verra que les sommets de même nom ne sont pas absolument identiques, et que les écarts nous permettent de nous faire une idée de la façon dont les sommets prennent naissance.

Pour effectuer le calcul, nous nous servons de courbes enregistrées avec

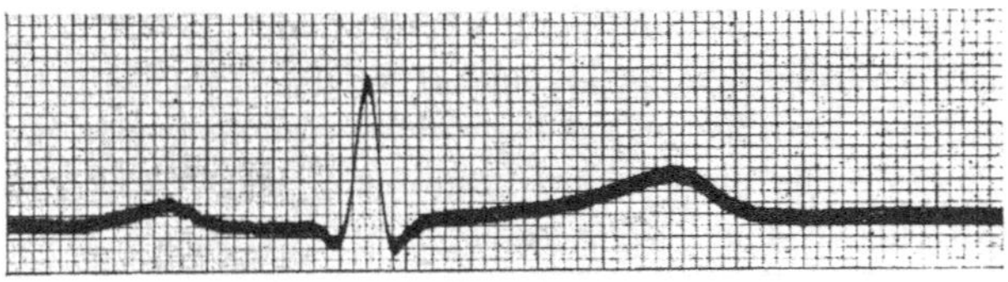

FIG. 9.

M. — Dérivation de la main droite au pied gauche.

Absc. 1 mm. = 0,01 sec. ; ordon. 1 mm. = 10^{-4} volts.

une vitesse du tableau d'enregistrement quatre fois plus grande. La fig. 9 représente une pareille courbe. Elle a été fournie par la même personne qui a donné les quatre-électrocardiogrammes précédents, en reliant la main droite au pied gauche. Ici encore 1 mm. en ordonnée correspond à 10^{-4} volts, mais 1 mm. en abscisse correspond maintenant à 0.01 sec. La distance des sommets *Q*, *R* et *S* est assez grande pour qu'il soit possible de déterminer avec une précision suffisante le moment exact de leur apparition.

La vitesse plus grande, dont la surface d'enregistrement est animée, nous permet aussi de mieux étudier la forme de chaque sommet en particulier. J'attire spécialement l'attention sur le relèvement accompagnant la contraction

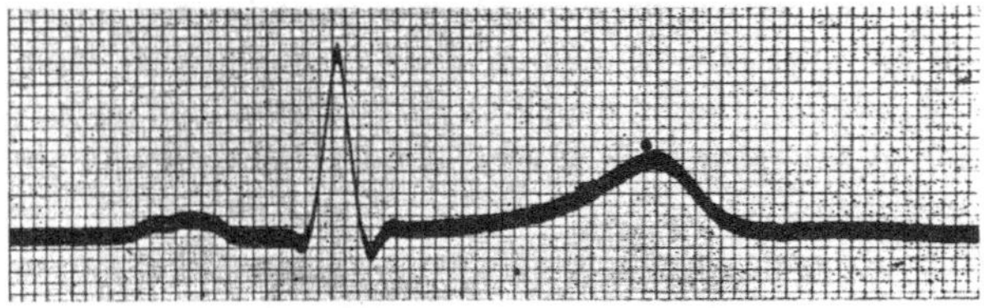

FIG. 10.

Th. — Dérivation de la main droite au pied gauche.

Absc. 1 mm. = 0.01 sec.; ordon. 1 mm. = 10^{-4} volts.

des oreillettes ; ce sommet est ici bien accusé, ainsi que cela s'observe très souvent. Par contre, dans la fig. 10, qui représente l'électrocardiogramme d'une autre personne, mais pris dans des conditions absolument les mêmes d'ailleurs, le sommet des oreillettes présente un plateau où l'on remarque encore une petite dépression.

On peut naturellement s'attendre à ce qu'un cœur malade trace un électrocardiogramme d'une autre forme qu'un cœur sain. Cette prévision a été directement confirmée par quelques observations préliminaires, faites dans mon laboratoire. Mais le nombre des cas ainsi examinés devait évidemment rester fort restreint, puisque le transport des malades au laboratoire de physiologie, surtout dans des cas graves, n'était pas sans difficulté. Pourtant il fallait multiplier le nombre des observations ; pour une étude quelque peu approfondie des maladies du cœur il est, en effet, nécessaire que les recherches s'étendent sur un grand nombre d'exemples.

C'est alors que M. BOSSCHA suggéra l'idée de relier, par des fils conducteurs, à l'hôpital de l'Université de Leyde, le laboratoire de physiologie, où est établi le galvanomètre difficilement transportable. De cette manière on rendrait possible l'examen des malades de l'hôpital au moyen du galvanomètre du laboratoire.

Afin d'établir jusqu'à quel point cette idée était susceptible d'une réalisation pratique, une expérience était nécessaire et M. le Prof. PLACE proposa d'employer pour cette expérience le subside que la Société Hollandaise des Sciences destine à une recherche de physiologie. La proposition de M. PLACE fut approuvée et l'expérience eut lieu.

A première vue la question du raccordement électrique paraît très simple. En effet, les courants électriques nous apportent journellement par le télégraphe des informations de tous les coins de la terre. Pourquoi les courants provenant du cœur ne pourraient-ils pas être conduits de l'hôpital au laboratoire ? En réalité, il n'y a aucune difficulté quant au principe; mais dans l'exécution des détails on se heurte pourtant à un certain nombre de difficultés d'ordre pratique.

Nous nous sommes servis d'une paire de fils du réseau téléphonique de Leyde, installé d'une façon parfaite par MM. RIBBINK et VAN BORK. Les fils de ce réseau s'étendent en partie sous le sol, en partie dans l'air. Tandis que les fils souterrains, fournis par la maison FELTEN ET GUILLEAUME à Mülheim s. l. Rhin, ne laissaient rien à désirer, nous avons reconnu que les raccords terminaux, tendus au-dessus du sol ne pouvaient être utilisés pour nos recherches.

Des fils tendus dans l'air ne sont jamais absolument immobiles. Ils sont toujours animés d'un léger mouvement d'oscillation, par lequel ils se rapprochent ou s'écartent irrégulièrement l'un de l'autre. Par là ils renferment dans leur circuit un nombre variable de lignes de force du champs magnétique terrestre, ce qui donne naissance à des courants rendant le galvanomètre instable.

Il est assez difficile de placer sous le sol les extrémités des fils conducteurs; nous les avons donc fait aboutir à des fils isolés, tordus ensemble de manière à occuper l'un par rapport à l'autre une position invariable, et entourés d'un manchon en plomb. Ce câble de plomb, lourd et flexible, ne saurait être tendu; voilà pourquoi nous l'avons suspendu dans l'air à un câble en acier (1). Même quand ce câble est agité par le vent, il n'en résulte aucune modification de l'indication du galvanomètre; nous avons donc vaincu ainsi une des difficultés que nous avons rencontrées au commencement.

Nous avons rencontré d'autres difficultés dans une isolation imparfaite et dans une induction réciproque des fils du réseau téléphonique. Chaque fois

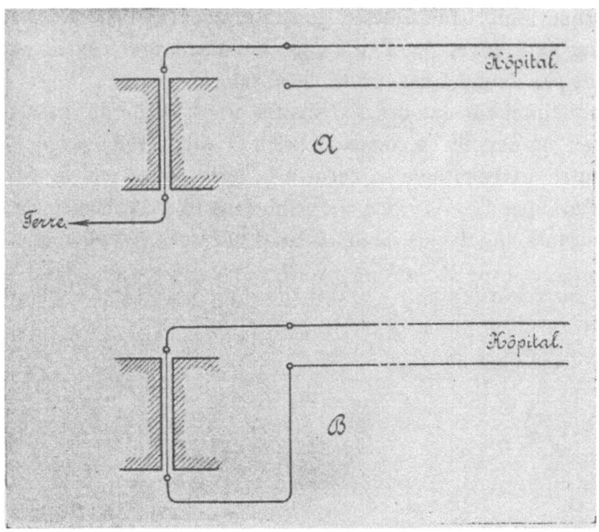

FIG. 11.

(1) Les matériaux nécessaires pour cette installation nous ont été fournis aussi, à notre entière satisfaction, par la maison FELTEN ET GUILLEAUME.

qu'un abonné reçoit un signal d'appel, des courants assez intenses se produisent dans le réseau, et, quand les divers fils ne sont pas parfaitement isolés les uns des autres, ces courants passent d'un fil à un autre, ce qui rend encore une fois incertaines les indications du galvanomètre.

Nous avons eu beaucoup de peine à isoler d'une façon aussi parfaite que possible les fils du galvanomètre. Le remplacement des fils terminaux, nus, tendus dans l'air, présentant nécessairement une isolation imparfaite aux points d'appui, par les câbles de plomb dont nous venons de parler, constituait déjà une amélioration considérable. D'ailleurs, l'emploi de ces câbles de plomb nous a permis de laisser de côté, sans danger, les parafoudres ordinaires, qui constituent toujours une source d'erreurs; il suffisait maintenant de mettre le manchon en plomb en communication avec le sol. L'isolement des câbles de plomb n'a jamais laissé à désirer, mais les endroits où s'établit le raccordement de la conduite souterraine aux fils aériens constituent, maintenant encore, des points faibles. Par un temps sec la résistance y atteint, il est vrai, 2000 à 3000 mégohms, mais en temps de pluie elle peut s'abaisser jusqu'à 10 mégohms et moins encore.

L'induction réciproque, surtout gênante aux extrémités des fils conducteurs, tendus sans enveloppe l'un à côté de l'autre, a été également diminuée notablement par l'emploi des câbles de plomb.

Mettons maintenant une des extrémités de la corde du galvanomètre en contact avec un des fils de communication du laboratoire avec l'hôpital, et relions l'autre extrémité de la corde à la terre, ainsi que le représente la figure schématique 11 𝔞. Dans ces conditions le galvanomètre est traversé par des courants vagabonds, produits dans le réseau téléphonique au moment

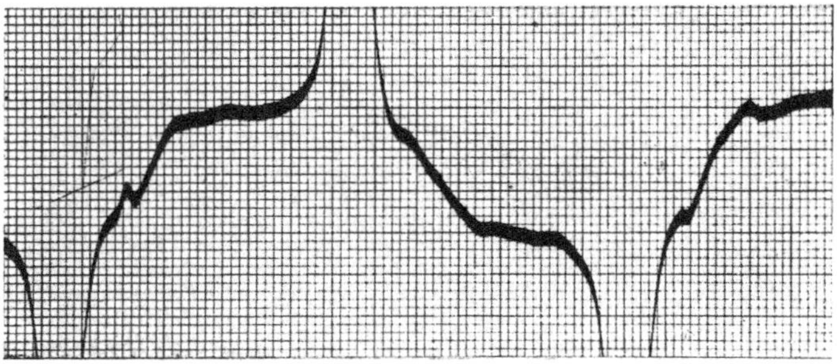

FIG. 12.

Absc. 1 mm. = 0.001 sec.; ordon. 1 mm. = 10^{-7} amp. 10

où une sonnerie électrique est mise en action pour avertir un abonné. Ces courants vagabonds sont causés par l'imperfection des isolations et par l'induction réciproque qui subsiste encore; ils sont assez puissants pour lancer entièrement hors du champs l'image de la corde. On peut cependant les affaiblir considérablement en laissant de côté la communication avec la terre, ainsi qu'on le voit sur le schéma fig. 11 𝔅, où les deux extrémités du galvanomètre sont reliées chacune à un des fils de communication du laboratoire avec l'hôpital. Mais même dans ces conditions on observe encore des vibrations de la corde, aussi longtemps qu'à l'hôpital même le circuit est interrompu, ou fermé par une très grande résistance. Elles ne cessent que quand on y ferme le circuit, soit directement, soit par intercalation d'une résistance relativement faible, comme celle du corps humain (variant de 1000 à 2000 ohms dans nos expériences). Or, ce sont là précisément les circonstances pratiques dans lesquelles nous opérons.

On voit dans la fig. 12 un photogramme obtenu en reliant avec intention une des extrémités de la corde du galvanomètre à la terre. Le galvanomètre avait une sensibilité à peu près 5 fois plus petite que celle que nous lui donnons dans le tracé des électrocardiogrammes ordinaires. Et cependant on constate que l'image de la corde est lancée complètement hors du champs par l'appel d'un abonné au téléphone. La vitesse du mouvement de la plaque était de 1 m. par sec., ce qui fait que 1 mm. en abscisse correspond à 0.001 sec., tandis que 1 mm. en ordonnée représente un courant de 10^{-7} amp.

La fig. 13, au contraire, représente un photogramme obtenu dans les mêmes conditions avantageuses que celles dans lesquelles nous enregistrons

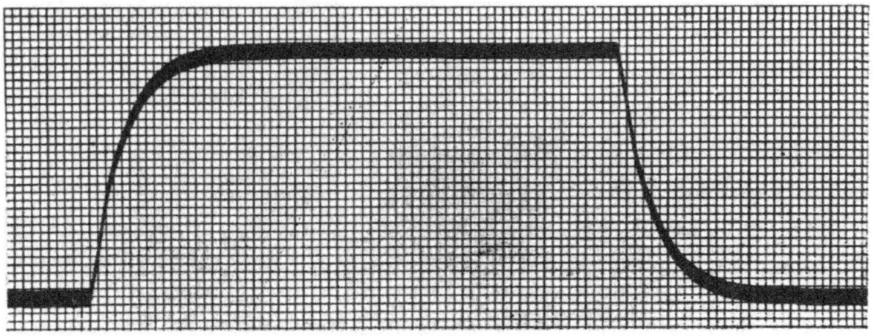

Fig. 13.

Absc. 1 mm. = 0.001 sec.; ordon. 1 mm. = 10^{-4} volts.

d'ordinaire les électrocardiogrammes de l'hôpital : sans fil de terre et en reliant les fils à l'hôpital par l'intermédiaire d'une résistance de 1500 ohms. On voit qu'il n'y a pas la moindre vibration; la corde reste absolument tranquille [1]. A un certain endroit du circuit nous avons intercalé subitement une différence de potentiel constante de 3 millivolts, sous l'influence de laquelle la corde a manifesté un écart de 30 mm.; 1 mm. correspond donc à 10^{-4} volts, ce qui est la sensibilité que nous appliquons régulièrement dans l'enregistrement des électrocardiogrammes.

Pendant le tracé, la plaque photographique se déplaçait avec une vitesse de 1 m. par sec. Un mm. en direction horizontale correspond donc de nouveau à 0.001 sec. Nous constatons sur le tracé que l'écart est achevé pour la plus grande partie au bout de 10 à 12 mm., c'est-à-dire en 1 à 1.2 centièmes de seconde. Cette durée de l'écart diffère à peine, tout au plus de quelques dix-millièmes de seconde, de celle que l'on obtient quand on n'emploie pas les fils de l'hôpital ; la différence est d'ailleurs si petite qu'elle peut être négligée dans toutes les expériences suivantes. Il y a néanmoins lieu de se demander quelle serait la durée qu'exigerait l'écart, si la distance du laboratoire à l'hôpital devenait beaucoup plus grande.

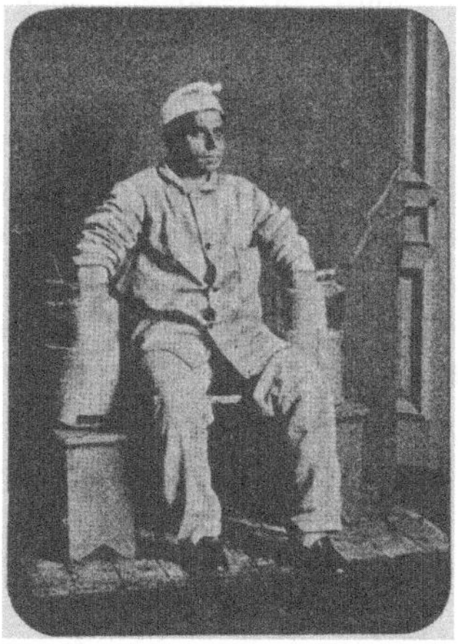

Fig. 14.

A mesure qu'augmente la longueur des fils de communication, leur self-induction, leur résistance et leur capacité augmentent également, et par là il est mis un terme à la distance des endroits que l'on peut relier avec succès. La conduite établie entre le laboratoire et l'hôpital a une longueur d'environ 1.5 km. Sa self-induction peut être négligée, tandis que sa résistance est de 106 ohms et sa capacité de 0.075 μf. Un calcul apprend

(1) Quand on applique la disposition 𝔅 de la fig. 11, ainsi que cela a eu lieu dans le cas de la fig. 13, les fils étant reliés à l'hôpital par une résistance médiocre (1500 ohms), l'immobilité de la corde est ordinairement assurée, même quand la pluie ou la neige ont réduit à moins de dix mégohms la résistance de l'isolation des fils de raccord.

qu'on pourrait se servir avec succès de conduites bien plus longues encore, et que l'on pourra raccorder avec succès Leyde à la Haye ou Harlem; je crois même que l'on pourrait établir une communication pratiquement assez bien utilisable entre Leyde et Rotterdam ou entre Leyde et Amsterdam.

Rendons-nous maintenant à l'hôpital et regardons-y un malade dont on est en train d'enregistrer l'électrocardiogramme. Il est commodément assis sur une chaise et plonge chaque main dans un grand vase, où aboutit un des fils de communication avec le laboratoire (fig. 14); ou bien il tient une main dans un des vases, et un pied dans l'autre (fig. 15). L'électrocardiogramme, dans ce cas un véritable *télécardiogramme*, est tracé au laboratoire. De cette manière l'opération est pratique et simple, et elle a sur le procédé de photographie ordinaire, où le sujet doit se trouver dans le voisinage du galvanomètre, l'avantage d'une plus grande rapidité. En effet, les soins que demande l'expérience sont partagés maintenant entre deux groupes de personnes, chaque groupe pouvant se mouvoir dans son propre local, sans courir le risque de gêner l'autre.

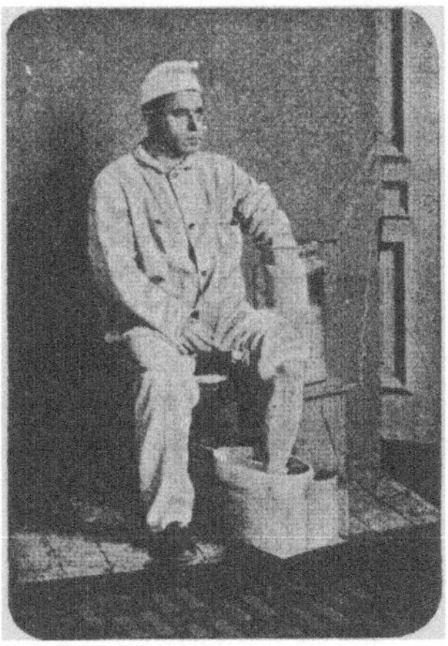

FIG. 15.

La fig. 16 est la reproduction du premier télécardiogramme que nous avons enregistré; c'est celui d'un homme sain et vigoureux; le courant provenait des deux mains (1). Il ne diffère en rien de celui que le même sujet fournit quand il se trouve au laboratoire, dans le voisinage même du galvanomètre. Les cinq sommets, dont le premier P est fourni par la systole des oreillettes et les quatres autres Q, R, S et T par celle des ventricules, présentent dans les deux cas la même

(1) Ce télécardiogramme a été tracé le 22 mars 1905. Grâce à la façon soigneuse dont elle fut préparée, cette première épreuve réussit immédiatement. Jusqu'a ce jour, 24 février 1906, donc au bout d'un an, pendant lequel nous avons enregistré une centaine d'électrocardiogrammes, et plus d'une fois des bruits et des souffles cardiaques de malades de l'hôpital, nous n'avons pas encore éprouvé le moindre accroc dans nos opérations. Les appareils du laboratoire, c'est-à-dire le galvanomètre et l'installation pour l'enregistrement, ainsi que les fils de communication avec l'hôpital sont invariablement restés en parfait état.

forme et la même grandeur. Chez ce sujet le sommet R est particulièrement élevé (1) et correspond à une différence de potentiel de deux millivolts.

Nous allons examiner maintenant quelques cardiogrammes de malades de l'hôpital, atteints de diverses affections cardiaques. En examinant ces malades nous sommes évidemment animés du désir de les guérir de leur mal. Tel est en effet le but du médecin. Malheureusement, nous devons être bien modestes, car la guérison n'est pas obtenue de si tôt. Nous devons en premier lieu tâcher de connaître dans tous ses détails le fonctionnement du cœur et les

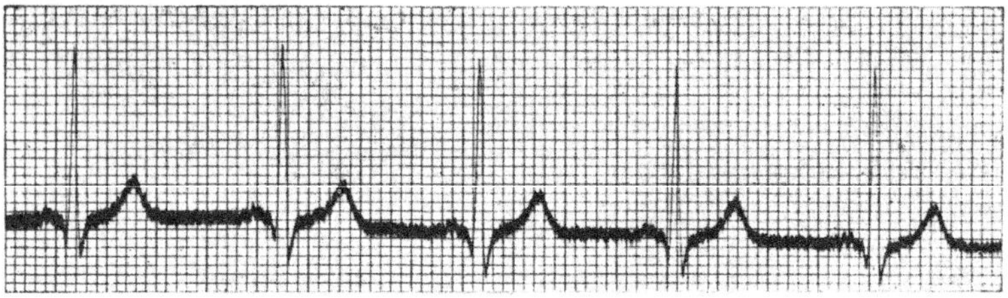

FIG. 16.

D. J. — Dérivation de la main droite à la main gauche.

causes de ses nombreux troubles; et nous basant ensuite sur la connaissance ainsi acquise et sur des vues plus claires, il est possible que dans un avenir encore éloigné nous soyons en état de soulager la souffrance des malades et de leur rendre la santé.

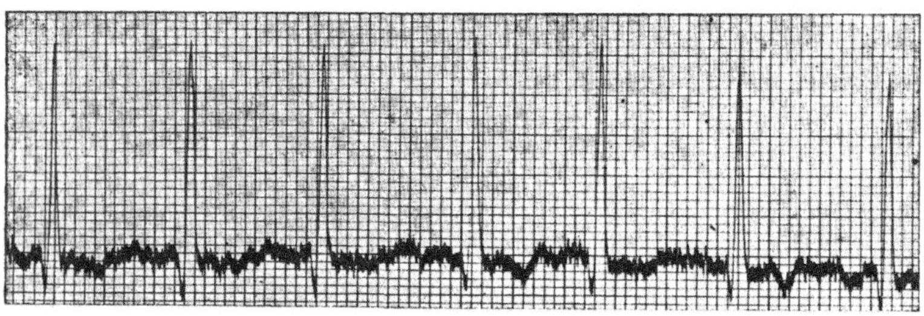

FIG. 17.

A. B. — *Insuff. mitralis.* — Dérivation de la main gauche au pied gauche.

Voici (fig. 17) l'électrocardiogramme obtenu en reliant la main gauche au

(1) La hauteur considérable du sommet R était occasionnée en partie par l'exercice corporel que le sujet venait de faire, peu de temps avant l'expérience. Il s'était notamment rendu à bicyclette du laboratoire à l'hôpital.

pied gauche d'une malade chez laquelle avait été constatée une affection de la valvule mitrale, consistant principalement en une insuffisance de cette valvule. On y remarque surtout un sommet dirigé vers le haut, d'une hauteur colossale, atteignant presque 30 mm., ce qui correspond à une différence de potentiel de 3 millivolts.

Je ne possède pas d'autre électrocardiogramme du même genre, obtenu en prenant le courant à la main gauche et au pied gauche. On aurait pourtant tort de considérer cette forme comme caractéristique pour une affection mitrale. On fera bien de ne pas se baser sur la forme de l'électrocardiogramme, du moins pas exclusivement, pour diagnostiquer un défaut de la valvule, puisque l'électrocardiogramme ne rend pas les mouvements de cette membrane. Le tracé est l'expression de la contraction du muscle cardiaque, et ce tracé n'est modifié que pour autant qu'un défaut dans le fonctionnement de la valvule a de l'influence sur cette contraction.

On ne doit pas oublier que la manière dont le cœur se contracte dépend à

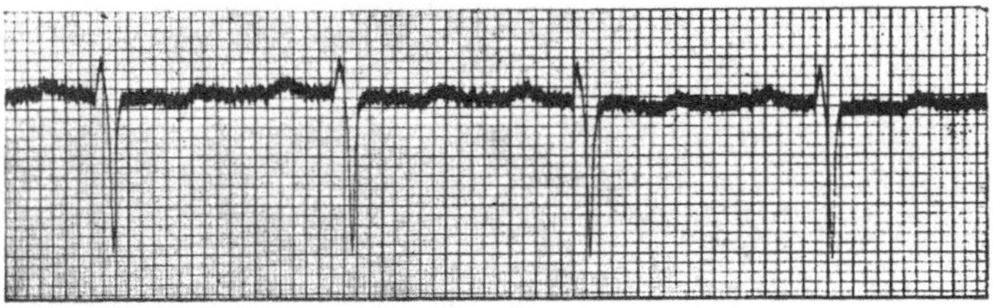

FIG. 18.

B. H. S. — *Insuff. aortae.* — Dérivation de la main gauche au pied gauche.

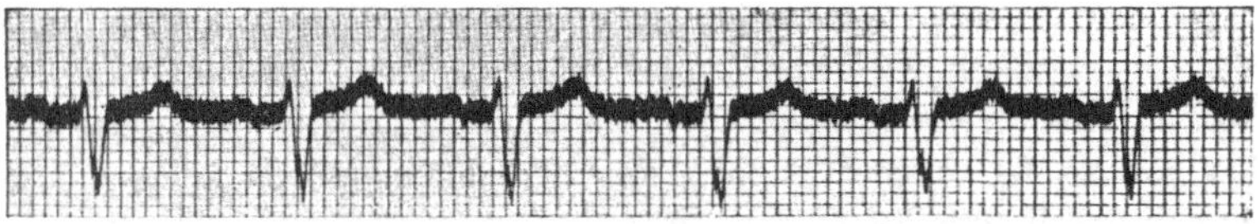

FIG. 19.

C. D. G. — *Insuff. aortae.* — Dérivation de la main gauche au pied gauche.

un haut degré de la nature et de l'intensité de la compensation qui s'établit, ainsi que de l'état plus ou moins maladif du muscle cardiaque lui-même. Dans ce cas particulier, on doit d'ailleurs comparer encore le degré de l'insuffisance avec la grandeur des autres défauts que présente la valvule mitrale. Ce n'est que par des recherches étendues que l'on pourra mettre en lumière la pleine signification de l'électrocardiogramme.

Comme pendant à l'insuffisance mitrale de la fig. 17, les fig. 18 et 19 montrent les télécardiogrammes de deux malades atteints d'insuffisance des valvules de l'aorte. Le courant provenait de nouveau de la main gauche et du pied gauche, et les courbes sont à un certain point de vue l'inverse de celle fournie par la malade à insuffisance mitrale : la grande pointe au commencement de la systole ventriculaire est tournée vers le bas.

Comme une insuffisance mitrale provoque surtout une hypertrophie du cœur droit, et une insuffisance aortique une hypertrophie du cœur gauche, il est naturel de présumer que l'hypertrophie de première espèce est accompagnée du développement d'une pointe *R* dirigée vers le haut, tandis que l'hypertrophie de deuxième espèce pourrait être la cause de la formation d'une pointe *R* dirigée vers le bas. J'ajouterai toutefois expressément que dans ces

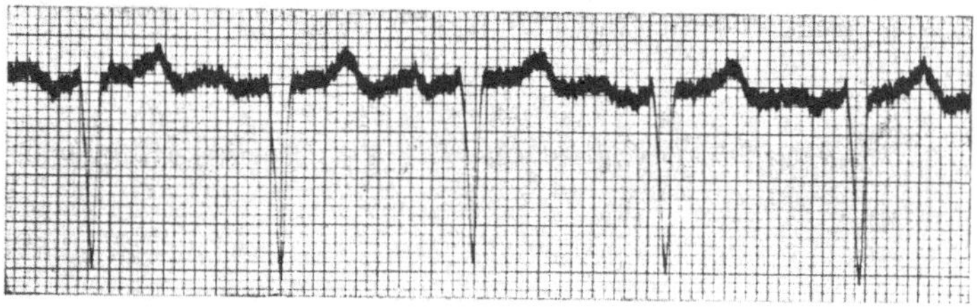

FIG. 20.

J. v. V. — *Hypertr. cord. sin.* — Dérivation de la main gauche au pied gauche.

considérations j'ai uniquement en vue les électrocardiogrammes obtenus par un raccordement de la main gauche et du pied gauche.

Or, cette prévision est confirmée par la fig. 20, obtenue chez un malade atteint d'artériosclérose et présentant une très forte hypertrophie du cœur gauche. Ici encore la communication a été établie entre la main gauche et le pied gauche. Le sommet *R*, dirigé vers le bas, correspond à une différence de potentiel de 2 millivolts environ.

La fig. 21 reproduit le télécardiogramme d'un malade souffrant d'une sténose mitrale, mais sans insuffisance ; le courant a été pris de la même façon que chez les quatre sujets précédents, c'est-à-dire à la main et au pied gauches. J'attire spécialement l'attention sur la forme tout à fait caractéristique de la systole des oreillettes, nettement renforcée et séparée en trois ou quatre temps bien distincts.

Ce renforcement et cette prolongation de la systole auriculaire est évidemment liée étroitement à l'existence de la sténose mitrale. L'entrave mise au courant sanguin par cette sténose a une influence compensatrice sur la contraction des oreillettes. On n'a jamais pu, à ma connaissance, indiquer d'aucune manière jusqu'ici cette modification dans l'oreillette gauche, la seule qui vienne en ligne de compte ; la méthode d'enregistrement des pulsations veineuses, qui peut rendre de si grands services dans l'examen de l'oreillette

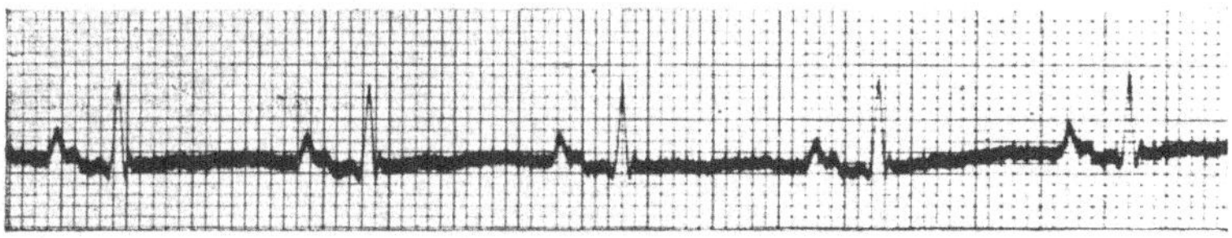

FIG. 21.

V. D. A. — *Stenosis mitralis.* — Dérivation de la main gauche au pied gauche.

droite, n'est absolument d'aucun usage pour les veines pulmonaires de l'homme, par suite d'obstacles anatomiques insurmontables.

Chez une deuxième malade atteinte de sténose mitrale, que nous avons eu l'occasion d'examiner, le sommet P correspondant à la contraction des oreillettes était moins allongé, il est vrai, mais était énormément surélevé, ainsi qu'on peut le voir dans la fig. 22. Ici le courant a été conduit de la main

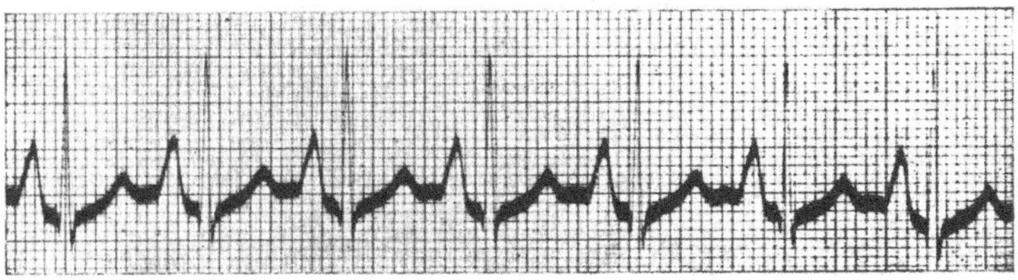

FIG. 22.

G. D. R. — *Stenosis mitralis.* — Dérivation de la main droite au pied gauche.

droite au pied gauche. En comparant ce sommet avec un sommet normal, tel que le représentent par exemple les fig. 7 et 8, l'anomalie due à la sténose mitrale saute aux yeux.

J'ai reproduit dans la fig. 23 un télécardiogramme fort remarquable, obtenu chez un malade atteint d'une dégénérescence du cœur (myodegeneratio cordis); le courant est dérivé de la main droite au pied gauche. On y constate qu'au sommet T, qui est le dernier dans tous les autres électrocardiogrammes, il en succède encore un autre. Ce sommet, que nous indiquerons par U, n'est égalisé que 0.5 sec. à peu près après le commencement de la systole ; ce qui prouve que dans ce cas pathologique la systole elle-même dure au moins 0.5 sec., et est donc caractérisée non seulement par une contraction irrégulière, mais encore par une durée extraordinairement longue.

La fig. 24 (dérivation de la main gauche au pied gauche) reproduit le télé-

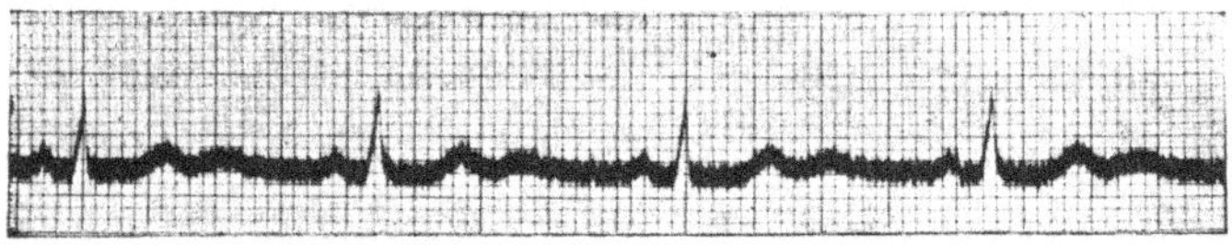

FIG. 23.

A. v. Y. — *Myodegeneratio cordis.* — Dérivation de la main droite au pied gauche.

cardiogramme d'un malade présentant une affection cardiaque congénitale, difficile à analyser dans tous ses détails. Dans le sommet dirigé vers le haut, on constate un crochet que l'on n'observe pas dans un électrocardiogramme normal.

On observe des modifications remarquables de la forme de la courbe dans les troubles du fonctionnement du cœur résultant d'un sport immodéré ; et un grand nombre d'autres circonstances pathologiques encore, qu'il serait trop long de mentionner ici, font sentir leur influence.

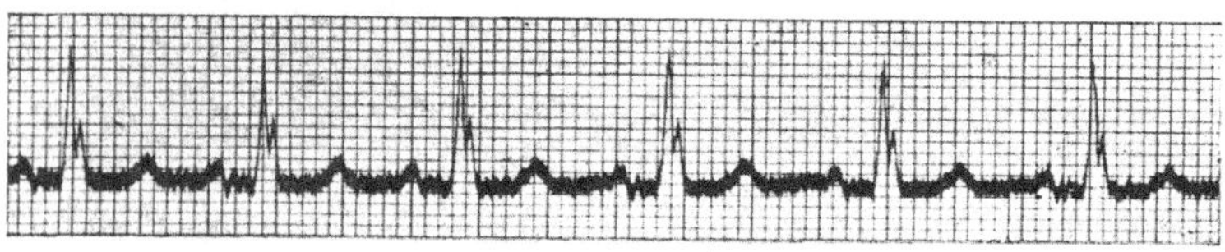

FIG. 24.

CH. N. — *Vitium cordis congenitale.* — Dérivation de la main gauche au pied gauche.

Dans ces recherches nous ne devons pas oublier qu'il peut se présenter des anomalies dans la situation du cœur, qui peuvent modifier la forme de l'électrocardiogramme sans que pour cela le fonctionnement du cœur soit lui-même anormal. Or, comme c'est précisément le mode de fonctionnement de cet organe que nous voulons déduire de l'électrocardiogramme, il est nécessaire que notre jugement soit rendu indépendant de l'influence que sa situation exerce sur la courbe. Voilà pourquoi il est nécessaire d'examiner pour chaque sujet les courbes obtenues par différents modes de dérivation. En pratique nous avons toujours appliqué les trois modes dont il a été question plus haut.

Qu'il me soit permis maintenant d'attirer l'attention sur un phénomène que nous avons observé dans le cours de nos recherches et qui a causé quelque surprise.

C'est un fait bien connu que, chez une personne présentant un pouls régulier, le rhythme des pulsations peut être soudainement interrompu, en ce sens que de temps en temps une pulsation manque dans la série régulière des

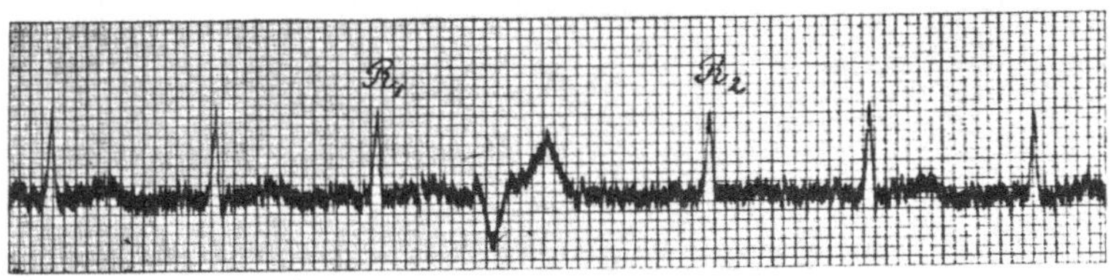

FIG. 25.

D. H. — *Convalescent du typhus.* — Dérivation de la main droite à la main gauche.

pulsations. Ces intermittences du pouls s'observent surtout chez des personnes qui ont été atteintes d'une maladie épuisant les forces du malade, comme le typhus. On s'attendrait à observer qu'au moment d'une intermittence du pouls l'électrocardiogramme est fortement affaibli ou fait même complètement défaut. Il est donc bien remarquable qu'au moment d'une intermittence il se développe précisément un courant relativement fort, souvent plus intense encore que celui de l'électrocardiogramme ordinaire.

La fig. 25 reproduit le télécardiogramme d'une personne en convalescence du typhus. La courbe enregistrée est un peu tremblotante, mais pour le reste le pouls peut être regardé comme normal. D'ailleurs ce tremblement ne provient pas des courants électriques du cœur, mais de ceux des muscles du squelette, ainsi que je le prouverai à une autre occasion. A un certain endroit entre les pulsations $\mathfrak{R}_1$ et $\mathfrak{R}_2$, le rhythme est soudainement interrompu par l'apparition d'un électrogramme atypique. Si le cœur s'était contracté normalement entre les battements $\mathfrak{R}_1$ et $\mathfrak{R}_2$, rien n'aurait manqué à la régularité du fonctionnement du cœur. Mais la pulsation normale entre $\mathfrak{R}_1$ et $\mathfrak{R}_2$ fait défaut et à sa place nous voyons apparaître la courbe atypique.

Dans notre laboratoire nous avons enregistré simultanément le pouls et l'électrocardiogramme d'une personne qui avait eu le typhus deux années auparavant. On constate sur le photogramme de la fig. 26 que le pouls, assez régulier au demeurant, est subitement absent, peu après que s'est manifesté un électrogramme atypique.

Il est bien remarquable que ce dernier se présente un peu avant l'instant où l'on s'attendrait à observer l'électrocardiogramme normal; il y a donc

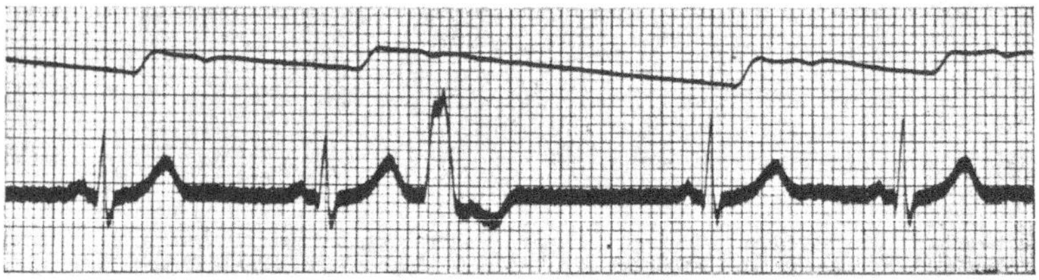

FIG. 26.

R. — *Intermittences.* — Dérivation de la main droite à la main gauche.

lieu de considérer le processus, qui accompagne le phénomène électrique atypique, comme la cause de l'absence de la contraction normale du cœur. Le fonctionnement atypique du cœur consiste ici en une extra-systole, suivie d'une pause compensatrice.

Avec le convalescent de l'hôpital nous avons pu faire une observation frappante. En même temps que nous observions au laboratoire les écarts du galvanomètre, le clinicien, M. le Prof. NOLEN, observait à l'hôpital le pouls du sujet. Chaque fois que nous constations au laboratoire un écart atypique, nous en avertissions par un court signal téléphonique le clinicien, qui constatait après chaque avertissement une intermittence du pouls.

Comme à l'examen attentif du pouls on ne peut constater l'intermittence qu'à la fin de l'instant où la pulsation aurait dû se produire, tandis que l'écart atypique du galvanomètre apparaît déjà dans une phase antérieure, comme on s'en aperçoit en inspectant le photogramme, le galvanomètre permet de prédire les intermittences du pouls. Aussi pouvions-nous, à la grande surprise de M. NOLEN, l'avertir téléphoniquement un instant d'avance quand il allait constater une intermittence du pouls.

Il arrive parfois qu'il se manifeste avec un électogramme atypique un pouls négatif, comme on peut le voir dans le photogramme 27 suivant. Ce fait ne doit pas nous étonner, puisque l'électrogramme atypique est l'expression d'une contraction atypique du cœur et qu'en général une telle contraction pourrait bien produire une pareille irrégularité dans l'onde artérielle.

Nous devons toutefois faire remarquer que le sphygmogramme de la fig. 27 a été obtenu en appliquant un tambour explorateur sur le cou du sujet dans la région de la carotide. Bien que cela me paraisse peu probable, il n'est pas impossible pourtant qu'une modification du courant sanguin dans la veine jugulaire ait eu une influence sur la forme de la courbe.

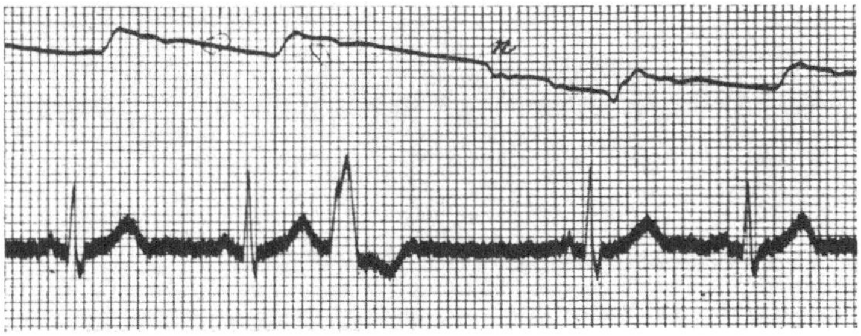

Fig. 27.

R. — *Intermittences.* — Dérivation de la main droite à la main gauche.

En ce moment, nos observations ne sont pas encore suffisantes pour permettre de donner, déjà dès à présent, une explication satisfaisante du phénomène; mais le phénomène lui-même est tellement frappant, que j'ai cru bien faire en ne le passant pas sous silence. La dépression que l'on observe en *n* n'est pas, du reste, produite par un mouvement fortuit et sans importance du style enregistreur; cela est prouvé par le fait qu'on l'observe à ce seul endroit dans toute une série de pulsations, tandis que dans une autre série on observe une dépression analogue, à peu près au même instant après la fin d'un autre électrogramme atypique. La différence de temps entre la fin de l'électrogramme et l'apparition du pouls négatif est de 0.32 sec. dans la fig. 27, tandis qu'elle est de 0.28 sec. dans le deuxième cas, figuré fig. 29. Ces intervalles, qui me paraissent très grands, semblent prouver qu'une contraction cardiaque atypique continue à exercer une influence pendant un temps relativement long.

Il arrive parfois qu'un électrogramme atypique ne se manifeste que fort tard, et alors on observe ce fait remarquable, que le rhythme du pouls n'est pour ainsi dire pas interrompu, voyez p. ex. fig. 28.

On sait depuis longtemps qu'il peut se présenter des contractions cardiaques sans pouls. On les a décrites sous le nom d'extra-systoles, c'est-à-dire de systoles inopportunes, et on en a distingué qui avaient leur origine dans les oreillettes, dans le faisceau de His et dans les ventricules. On a parlé

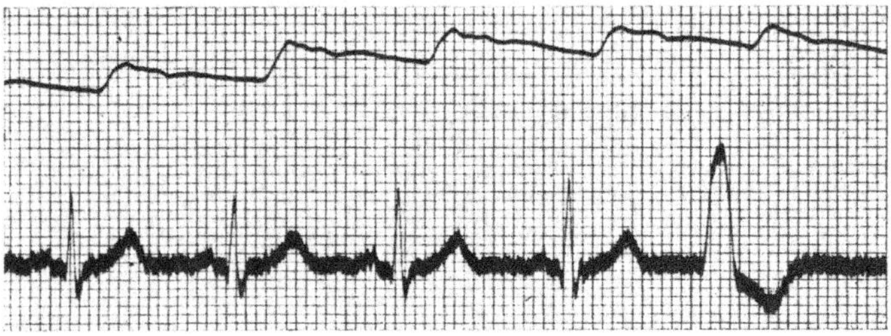

Fig. 28.

R. — *Intermittences.* — Dérivation de la main droite à la main gauche.

aussi de contractions frustranées, non accompagnées de pouls, parce que la systole serait incomplète et ne serait pas assez forte pour vaincre la pression dans l'aorte.

Mais dans toutes ces explications on a méconnu l'essence même du phénomène. Dans le cas de la fig. 28 on ne peut pas parler d'une extra-systole, pas plus que d'une systole frustranée, puisque la systole ne se manifeste pas à contre-temps et que le pouls qu'elle produit est fortement accusé.

La cause du phénomène doit être cherchée dans la façon dont le cœur se contracte. L'onde de contraction est atypique, de sorte que nous avons le droit de parler d'une contraction cardiaque ou d'une systole atypiques. Celle-ci peut se produire à un moment indu, et alors on peut l'appeler évidemment une extra-systole; ou bien elle peut se produire sans être accompagnée d'un pouls, et alors on peut parler naturellement de contraction frustranée, mais on ne doit pas attacher à ces mots une signification plus grande. En décrivant les extra-systoles on s'est probablement laissé induire en erreur par les phénomènes d'auscultation et par l'intensité du pouls, et on a cru que les contractions cardiaques devaient *toujours* être d'autant plus faibles qu'elles succédaient plus tôt à une systole antérieure.

Pourtant on constate qu'en réalité les contractions cardiaques atypiques qui se manifestent immédiatement après une systole diffèrent relativement peu de celles qui viennent après une pause normale ou à peu près. C'est ce que l'on reconnaît nettement quand on compare les fig. 26 et 27 d'une part avec la fig. 28 d'autre part. L'intervalle de temps entre la systole précédente, normale, et la contraction cardiaque atypique est d'environ 0.04 sec. dans les deux premières figures, tandis qu'il atteint 0.24 sec. dans la dernière, soit

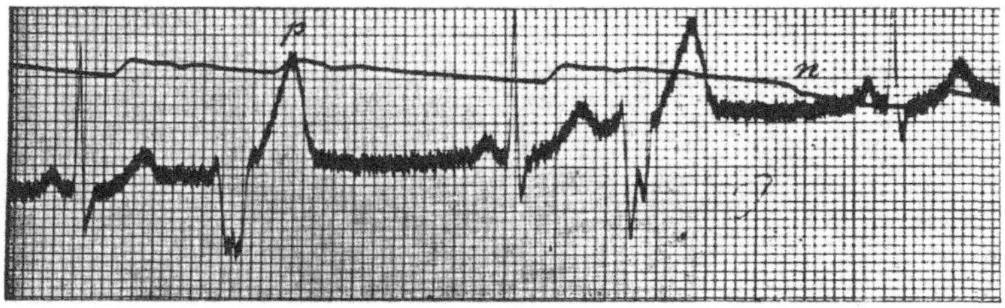

FIG. 29.

R. — *Intermittences.* — Dérivation de la main droite au pied gauche.

une valeur six fois plus grande, et cependant dans ce dernier cas les sommets de l'électrogramme ne sont pas beaucoup plus élevés.

Notre manière de voir est confirmée d'ailleurs par la fig. 29, qui fait voir l'électrogramme du même sujet, mais pour une dérivation du courant de la main droite vers le pied gauche. La première contraction atypique vient après un repos assez long, et développe une pulsation intense *p*, tandis que la deuxième contraction atypique succède presque immédiatement à une systole normale et est accompagnée d'un pouls négatif *n*.

Et cependant il n'y a qu'une différence insignifiante entre les deux électrogrammes atypiques.

J'ai à peine besoin de dire qu'il résulte de tout ceci que le cœur est déjà en état de se contracter fortement bientôt après la fin de la période réfractaire, et que ce phénomène est tout à fait en contradiction avec quelques-unes des idées courantes au sujet du fonctionnement du cœur.

Il est plus que probable que nos contractions cardiaques atypiques donnent aussi l'explication des phénomènes que l'on a décrits sous les noms de bigéminie du cœur, hémisystolie et systolie alternante, et dont les explications plus ou moins subtiles que l'on en a données jusqu'ici doivent être rejetées pour la plupart (1).

On voit dans la fig. 30 le télécardiogramme d'un individu chez lequel

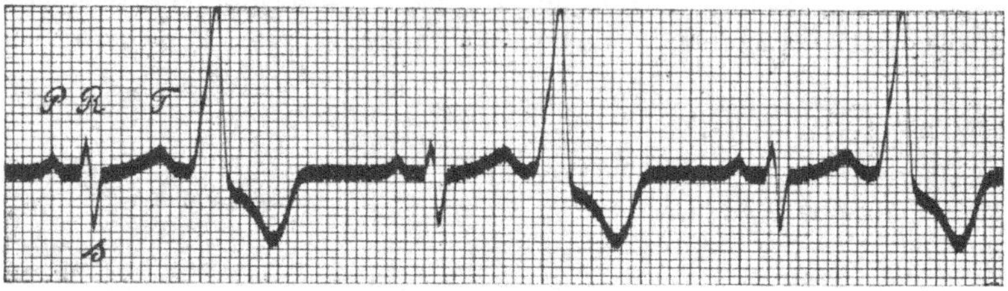

FIG. 30.

S. K. — *Bigéminie du cœur.* — Dérivation de la main droite au pied gauche.
Absc. 1 mm. = 0,04 sec. ; ord. 1 mm. = 2×10^{-4} volts.

on a constaté une bigéminie du cœur; il a d'ailleurs le "pouls lent permanent" typique. On a constaté chez lui 80 battements du cœur et seulement 40 pulsations par minute. Le photogramme a été obtenu en dérivant le courant de la main droite au pied gauche; 1 mm. en abscisse correspond, comme d'habitude, à 0.04 sec.; mais, avec la sensibilité ordinaire du galvanomètre, les mouvements de l'image de la corde avaient une telle amplitude, que cette image quittait les bords de la plaque photographique. Voilà pourquoi nous avons, par exception, donné à la corde une tension plus forte, de telle sorte que 1 mm. en ordonnée correspond à 2×10^{-4} volts, c'est-à-dire au double de la valeur ordinaire.

(1) Que surtout on ne croie pas, à la suite des considérations précédentes, que je veuille méconnaître en aucune façon les mérites d'un grand nombre de cliniciens, qui ont entrepris avant moi l'étude des mêmes questions en se servant de la méthode d'enregistrement mécanique. Puisque je parle à présent du télécardiogramme, ce n'est pas le moment de parler de la bibliographie, fort étendue, relative au mécanisme et à l'innervation du fonctionnement du cœur dans son ensemble. Qu'il me soit permis cependant de faire une exception en faveur des études remarquables : « The study of the pulse » etc., Edinburgh 1902, d'un anglais, M. JAMES MACKENZIE, et de notre clinicien de Groningue, M. le Prof. WENCKEBACH : « Die Arhytmie als Ausdruck » etc. Leipzig 1903.

Qu'il me soit permis aussi d'exprimer comme mon opinion personnelle qu'à l'aide des méthodes d'investigation mécaniques on n'a pas été capable, même avec la plus grande perspicacité, d'établir avec certitude la nature et l'essence des contractions cardiaques atypiques. Et en ce sens les méthodes d'investigation électriques nous ont réellement permis de faire un pas en avant.

Avec la dérivation employée ici, l'électrocardiogramme normal ne donne lieu à aucune remarque particulière. On voit un sommet bien net P, provenant de la contraction des oreillettes; des sommets ventriculaires le premier Q est absent et le troisième S est fortement développé. Or à chaque courbe normale succède immédiatement un électrogramme atypique, avec un sommet très élevé, dirigé vers le haut, qui correspond à une différence de potentiel d'environ 4 millivolts (1).

Parfois on constatait chez le sujet une série de systoles normales, interrompues de temps en temps par une contraction atypique du cœur. Une autre fois nous avons pu constater une série de trois contractions atypiques successives, absolument identiques; enfin nous avons pu reconnaître aussi deux formes différentes de contractions atypiques.

Je craindrais d'entrer dans trop de détails si je m'attardais à la considération de ces phénomènes. Cependant, avant de quitter les contractions cardiaques atypiques, je désirerais faire à leur propos deux remarques.

D'abord, leur existence est beaucoup plus générale qu'on ne serait tenté de l'admettre. Le plus souvent on ne songera à l'existence de contractions cardiaques atypiques chez un malade que quand on aura observé chez lui des intermittences du pouls. Mais, dans les cas où les contractions du cœur sont inégales et irrégulières, il est difficile de distinguer les diverses causes de cette irrégularité et il est presque impossible de constater au toucher une intermittence du pouls.

C'est ainsi qu'il put arriver que chez un sujet dont le pouls, inégal et irrégulier, donnait 150 pulsations par minute, on ne crut pas à l'existence de contractions cardiaques atypiques, et que le galvanomètre donna la preuve du contraire; la fig. 31 peut servir d'exemple.

La deuxième remarque que je voudrais faire concerne le rapport entre la façon dont le cœur se contracte et la forme du pouls artériel. Quelques physiologistes ont prétendu que certains sommets du sphygmogramme artériel provenaient d'irrégularités dans la contraction du muscle cardiaque au moment de la systole, et quelques cliniciens ont, de leur côté, défendu une

(1) Dans la dissertation de M. le Dr GOTELING VINNIS, Leyde 1905, on trouve le cardiogramme mécanique du même sujet. On voit par les courbes publiées par M. VINNIS que la pulsation du cœur est redoublée. La seconde partie, régulièrement répétée, d'une courbe est tantôt de même grandeur, tantôt un peu plus petite que la première.

pareille manière de voir dans l'explication d'un pouls lent anacrote. Or, l'exactitude de ces assertions ne saurait être mieux contrôlée qu'au moyen

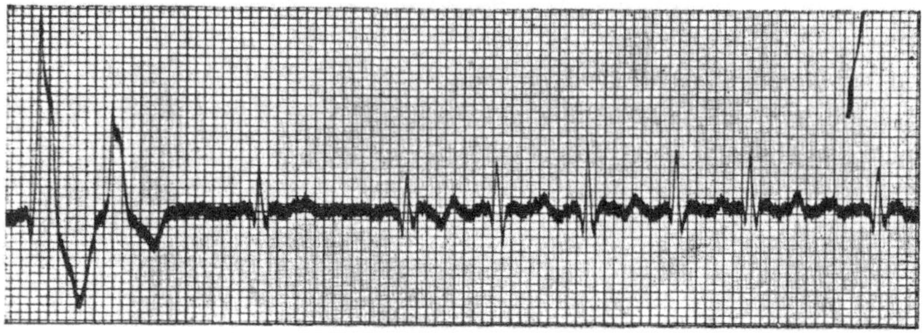

FIG. 31.
H. v. W. — *Pulsus inaequalis et irregularis.* — Dérivation de la main gauche au pied gauche.

de l'électrocardiogramme; mais les observations que nous avons faites dans ce but sont encore trop peu nombreuses pour que la question puisse être considérée comme définitivement résolue.

Pour finir cet examen des télécardiogrammes, je donnerai encore quelques considérations sur le rapport qui existe entre les systoles des oreillettes et des ventricules. Nous savons que dans la plupart des cas ce rapport est très intime, de sorte que normalement toute systole ventriculaire est précédée d'une systole auriculaire et qu'inversement cette dernière est toujours suivie d'une systole des ventricules. Dans ces conditions il n'est pas sans importance de mesurer exactement l'intervalle entre l'action des oreillettes et celle des ventricules.

Si l'on se propose de faire cette détermination par enregistrement mécanique, on doit tracer simultanément le pouls d'une artère et celui d'une veine, ce qui donne souvent des difficultés; l'électrocardiogramme, au contraire, nous permet d'atteindre aisément le but avec toute la précision désirable. Je n'ai qu'à renvoyer à la fig. 9, où 1 mm. en abscisse représente 0.01 sec. On y constate qu'il s'écoule 0.175 sec. entre le commencement de la systole des oreillettes et le commencement de la systole des ventricules, tandis qu'il y a un intervalle de 0.055 sec. entre la fin de la systole des oreillettes et le commencement de la systole des ventricules. L'électrocardiogramme d'une autre personne, enregistré dans les mêmes conditions et représenté fig. 10, fournit des intervalles beaucoup plus petits, respectivement de 0.13 et 0.035 sec.

D'après M. Mackenzie on peut dire qu'il y a retard dans le rapport entre les deux sections du cœur, du moment que l'intervalle A_s— V_s dépasse 0.2 sec., et dans ces conditions certains médicaments, tels que la digitale très renommée et souvent employée, sont dangereux. Il ne serait pas difficile de se servir de l'électrocardiogramme pour poursuivre pas à pas l'influence de divers médicaments sur la grandeur de l'intervalle en question. Et ce que je dis ici d'un examen de l'intervalle A_s— V_s, s'applique aussi, en général, à tout examen quantitatif de la fonction cardiaque. Le système de coordonnées dans lequel nos courbes sont tracées facilite singulièrement de pareilles mesures.

Quand le pouls est fréquent, il peut arriver que la contraction des oreillettes, dans chaque nouvelle révolution du cœur, succède si rapidement à la systole ventriculaire de la révolution précédente, que la pause cardiaque disparaît presque. Il se peut même que la systole ventriculaire et celle des oreillettes qui lui succède, aient lieu en partie en même temps. Alors les tracés représentatifs de l'action de ces deux sections du cœur se recouvrent partiellement. Il y a chevauchement des systoles. Et quand la contraction de l'oreillette est tellement prématurée, que le muscle du ventricule est encore dans l'état latent de la systole précédente quand il est atteint par une nouvelle excitation, la succession régulière des actions des deux parties du cœur est troublée.

Ces considérations sont confirmées par les télécardiogrammes des fig. 31 et 32. Cette dernière figure a été obtenue chez un malade présentant une dextérocardie, produite par une exsudation pleurétique du côté gauche. Le pouls est assez régulier, tandis que sa fréquence est grande : environ 126 pulsations par minute. La pause du cœur fait complètement défaut. Tandis que partout ailleurs dans la figure on n'observe que deux petites élévations entre deux sommets R successifs, il importe d'attirer l'attention sur la présence de *trois* élévations pareilles entre les sommets que j'ai indiqués par R_1 et R_2. L'élévation moyenne correspondant, selon toute probabilité, à une contraction des oreillettes qui n'a pas été suivie d'une contraction ventriculaire.

Remarquons encore que l'on trouve dans la fig. 31 une particularité analogue et que dans les deux figures 31 et 32 les contractions des ventricules présentent toutes espèces de petites irrégularités variables, qui n'existent pas chez les cœurs normaux.

La succession régulière des actions des oreillettes et des ventricules est également troublée quand il y a un obstacle à la transmission des excitations

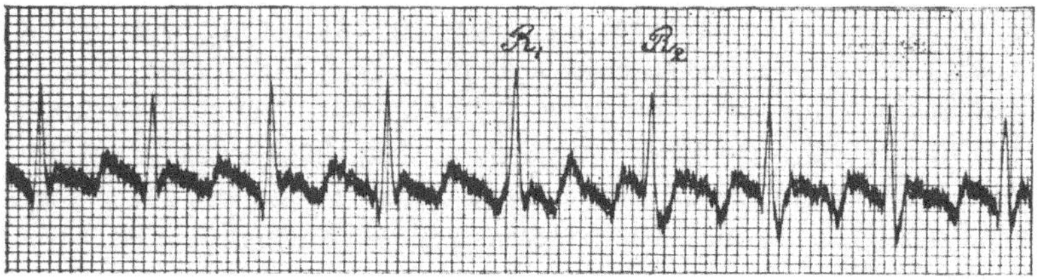

FIG. 32.

L. — *Dextérocardie par suite d'une pleurésie.* — Dérivation de la main gauche au pied gauche.

entre les deux parties du cœur ; il faut alors plus d'une contraction auriculaire pour provoquer une systole des ventricules (Herzblock).

Il se peut d'ailleurs que tout rapport entre la fonction des oreillettes et celle des ventricules ait cessé ; alors les deux parties du cœur travaillent indépendamment l'une de l'autre, chacune avec son rhythme propre. Un tel état peut être provoqué dans le cœur des mammifères, quand on sectionne le faisceau de communication entre les oreillettes et les ventricules, qui a été découvert par W. His jun. et qui porte son nom ; on doit avoir soin toutefois de ne pas mutiler le cœur assez profondément pour qu'il s'arrête. Cette expérience, qui a été décrite pour la première fois par His lui-même, a été répétée après lui avec succès par d'autres expérimentateurs, entre autres Léon Fredericq et Max Humblet à Liége et H. E. Hering à Prague. Après la section dont il s'agit, — ou encore après l'écrasement du faisceau —, un cœur de mammifère présente le phénomène remarquable d'une entière indépendance des systoles auriculaires et ventriculaires, ce qu'on nomme une *allorhythmie.*

Au moyen de l'électrocardiogramme on peut parfaitement bien faire voir l'état d'un cœur blocké et l'allorhythmie. La figure 33 reproduit l'électrocardiogramme d'un chien, dans un état de narcose profonde par le chloroforme. Le courant a été conduit de la patte antérieure droite vers la patte postérieure gauche, et dans sa forme générale le tracé présente, comme on le reconnaît à la figure, une grande analogie avec celle d'un électrocardiogramme humain. J'ai indiqué par a_1, a_2 etc. les sommets des oreillettes et nous remarquons que le dernier sommet des ventricules *T*, qui est dirigé vers le haut dans la plupart des électrocardiogrammes humains, est dirigé ici vers le bas.

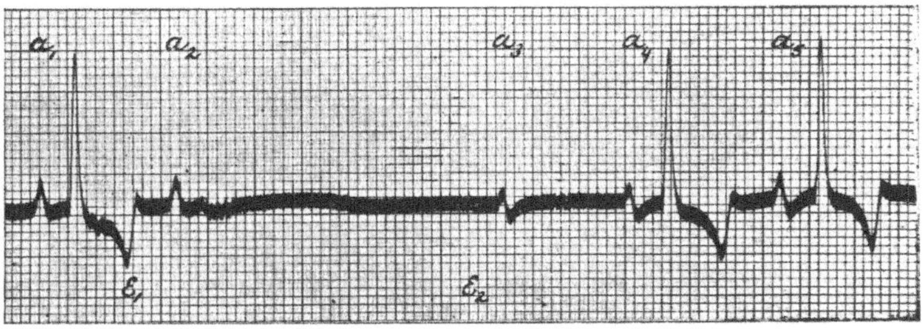

Fig. 33.

Chien. — *Excitation du nerf vague. Block du cœur.* — Dérivation de la patte antérieure droite à la patte postérieure gauche

Entre $\mathcal{E}_1$ et $\mathcal{E}_2$ le bout périphérique du nerf vague droit a été excité. Après le commencement de cette excitation, la systole du cœur, déjà commencée, s'est achevée, puis il est venu encore une systole des oreillettes en a_2, après quoi le cœur est resté en repos jusqu'à la fin de l'excitation.

Quand l'excitation a pris fin, il s'est manifesté en a_3 la première contraction auriculaire à laquelle ne succède pas de systole ventriculaire : à ce moment donc se présente un “ block „. Ce n'est qu'en a_4 que ce “ block „ est levé et que le rapport entre la systole des oreillettes et celle des ventricules se rétablit complètement.

Quand la narcose est plus profonde encore, et que l'excitation du nerf vague est encore plus forte, le “ block „ du cœur s'accentue encore. On observe alors, après une longue pause produite par l'excitation du nerf vague, un certain nombre de contractions auriculaires successives, précédant la première systole ventriculaire qui se développe. C'est ce que montre la fig. 34 suivante, obtenue avec un autre chien, profondément narcotisé ; le courant est également dirigé de la patte droite de devant vers la patte postérieure gauche.

On voit sur la figure les oscillations des courants électriques, qui commencent à se manifester après que l'excitation du nerf vague a occasionné un état de repos de 3 sec. Ce n'est que la cinquième contraction des oreillettes qui est suivie d'une systole ventriculaire.

Les deux dernières figures prouvent que la nature de la contraction auriculaire est modifiée par l'excitation du nerf vague, tandis qu'il n'y a pour ainsi dire aucune différence entre les systoles ventriculaires (fig. 33) avant et après l'excitation.

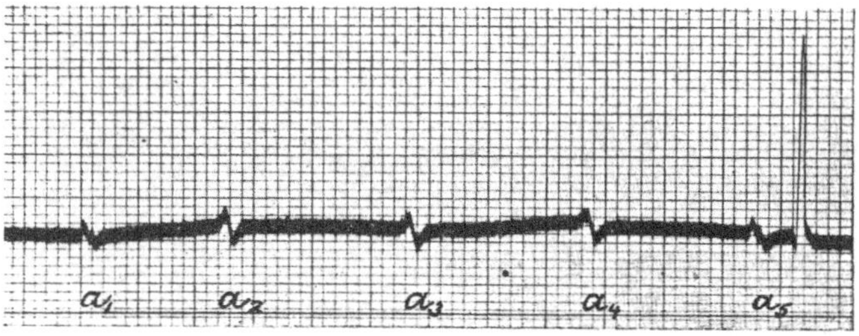

Fig. 34.
Chien. — *Excitation du nerf vague.* — Dérivation de la patte antérieure droite à la patte postérieure gauche.

La fig. 1 de la planche 3 représente les électrocardiogrammes d'un troisième chien, chez lequel il n'y a plus aucun rapport entre les contractions des oreillettes et des ventricules, de sorte que le fonctionnement du cœur est absolument allorhythmique. Ici encore le courant a été pris à la patte antérieure droite et à la patte postérieure gauche. Les sommets auriculaires, que j'ai indiqués par les lettres a_1, a_2 etc., s'observent à des distances régulières, et il en est de même des sommets qui se rapportent aux systoles des ventricules; mais, tandis que la fréquence des systoles auriculaires est d'environ 55, celle des systoles des ventricules est d'environ 35 par minute.

Je compte traiter à une autre occasion, avec plus de détails, les phénomènes provoqués par l'excitation du nerf vague, et les circonstances dans lesquelles on peut produire chez le chien le " block „ et l'allorhythmie du cœur. Revenons maintenant à l'électrocardiogramme de l'homme.

Dans quelques cas bien rares on peut observer chez des malades une allorhythmie complète du cœur. Nous avons eu l'occasion d'enregistrer le télécardiogramme d'une femme qui présentait ce phénomène ; on le trouve dans les fig. 2 et 3 de la planche 3 ; le courant était dirigé de la main droite vers le pied gauche.

La malade avait 29 pulsations par minute seulement. On voit que le rhythme des contractions auriculaires, indiquées par a_1, a_2 etc., est absolument indépendant du rhythme des contractions ventriculaires. Il y a environ

10 à 11 contractions auriculaires sur 4 ventriculaires, et, comme ce rapport ne peut être représenté par celui de deux nombres assez petits, les élévations provenant des oreillettes sont inégalement distribuées parmi celles dues aux ventricules, ou bien elles se confondent avec ces dernières en des points différents du tracé.

Il est généralement aisé de reconnaître une superposition des tracés auriculaires et ventriculaires. C'est ainsi qu'en a_5 et a_{10} (pl. 3, fig. 2) on voit un sommet d'oreillettes entre les sommets S et T de la systole ventriculaire, tandis qu'aux points a_3 et a_8 de la même figure le sommet des oreillettes tombe sur la branche descendante du sommet T.

Dans le premier et le dernier électrocardiogramme de la fig. 3, pl. 3, les superpositions sont remarquables. Dans le dernier électrocardiogramme de cette figure, le sommet des oreillettes coïncide exactement, en a_{10}, avec la pointe du sommet T, et de cette superposition résulte évidemment une élévation plus haute et plus aiguë que le sommet T des autres électrocardiogrammes.

Dans la première systole ventriculaire de la figure, en a_1, le maximum de l'élévation auriculaire vient à peu près 0.04 sec. après la pointe du sommet T. Alors que l'élévation ventriculaire a déjà atteint son plus haut point et que commence sa période de descente, par laquelle l'image de la corde reviendrait vers la position d'équilibre, surgit la branche ascendante du sommet des oreillettes, qui tend à écarter de nouveau vers le haut l'image de la corde. Les deux effets se combinent, avec ce résultat, qu'il se forme un plateau horizontal au lieu d'une pointe.

Il est à peine nécessaire de dire qu'à l'aide des télécardiogrammes le diagnostic du mal est très facile et ne laisse pas le moindre doute.

Mais quoique dans les fig. 2 et 3 de la planche 3 les contractions ventriculaires atypiques fassent complètement défaut, je ne puis pas passer sous silence que j'ai pu les observer chez le même sujet, dans une autre série de télécardiogrammes, de sorte que l'écart que présente le fonctionnement de son cœur est plus compliqué qu'on ne serait peut-être tenté de l'admettre.

Dans une très intéressante leçon de clinique, publiée dans le *Nederlandsch Tijdschrift voor Geneeskunde,* M. Pel présente un malade du même genre et insiste avec raison sur les difficultés de l'enregistrement simultané du mouvement du cœur et du pouls veineux. Et pourtant on ne pouvait pas encore se passer jusqu'ici de cette méthode d'investigation, quand il s'agissait d'établir le rapport entre les contractions des oreillettes et des ventricules. M. PEL dit que c'est " une opération qui demande beaucoup de temps et qui est fort subtile et délicate; elle soumet à une rude épreuve la patience des auditeurs „, quand on la fait dans une leçon de clinique, " et son résultat est fort incertain „.

Quand on essaie de remplacer le procédé de l'enregistrement mécanique par l'examen aux rayons de RÖNTGEN, il me semble qu'on ne saurait obtenir des résultats satisfaisants, aussi longtemps que l'on ne réussit pas à fixer sous forme d'images graphiques les mouvements passagers du cœur.

A propos des tracés obtenus par enregistrement mécanique, M. PEL dit que leur mesure et leur analyse sont une source d'interprétations fausses, et il avance cette prédiction, quelque peu imprudente, " que nous ne serons jamais en état de nier, chez les malades, l'existence de contractions ventriculaires excessivement faibles. „

Ces difficultés, tracées par M. PEL en des couleurs aussi vives, ne se présentent pas dans l'enregistrement des télécardiogrammes ; presque toutes les épreuves réussissent, sont obtenues en quelques minutes et fournissent un résultat absolument certain ; la méthode n'exige pas une habileté particulière de la part de l'observateur, et elle unit, à une précision qui laisse peu à désirer, le grand avantage qu'elle permet de faire usage de mesures absolues. Cependant, si tels sont les arguments que l'on peut fournir en faveur des télécardiogrammes, nous ne devons pas méconnaître les inconvénients de la méthode.

Les appareils avec lesquels on opère demandent une installation particulière et prennent beaucoup de place ; comparés avec les cardiographes et sphygmographes ordinaires, ils sont coûteux et compliqués ; ils ne peuvent être maniés que par des assistants qui ont appris à s'en servir. Or, il ne serait peut-être pas raisonnable d'exiger des assistants pour les cours de clinique, dont les études sont déjà si lourdes, des études techniques encore plus fortes qu'elles ne le sont en ce moment.

C'est donc dans un laboratoire de physiologie où les appareils sont à leur place, que ce genre de travaux doit être effectué. Et là où il y a un lien, tant réel que figuré, entre ce laboratoire et l'hôpital, là où les circonstances sont favorables à la collaboration du physiologiste et du clinicien, — l'un et l'autre restant le maître sur son propre terrain, — là on pourra se servir avec succès, comme j'espère vous l'avoir prouvé, à côté des méthodes mécaniques ordinaires, des nouvelles méthodes de recherche par l'électricité.

VI
L'enregistrement des bruits du cœur de l'homme à l'aide du galvanomètre à corde

When Einthoven published phonocardiograms for the first time (I), he used the capillary electrometer. Although his tracings sufficed for studying time relations, as he intended, Einthoven was well aware of their shortcomings. These were in fact evident, as one can see by comparing the tracings from the present paper to those of the earlier one. A new feature is the inclusion of phonocardiograms from patients in the hospital, in particular from patients with mitral stenosis and insufficiency. They ware obtained in the same way as the electrocardiograms in "Le Télécardiogramme". It is understable that for this technical reason no pulse tracings or apex cardiograms could be added as reference. On the other hand, Einthoven stresses the fact that in this way phonocardiography can be used for clinical diagnosis just like electrocardiography.

At that time only a guess could be made as to the identity of the murmurs under the guidance of the silent diastolic period, which in this patient appeared much shorter in the phonocardiogram than at auscultation. Einthoven diagnosed in this case a presystolic murmur, a three-phasic systolic murmur and a diastolic murmur.

An air leak (stopcock) was introduced between the funnel on the thorax and the microphone to avoid mechanical disturbances of low frequency.

In the same year 1907 Einthoven discovered the third heart sound (85, 86), as cited in chapter 1. In this case the person (a healthy young man) was examined in the laboratory; the carotid pulse and jugular venous pulse were taken as reference tracings. 8 years later Einthoven's assistant Battaerd published a new series of phonocardiograms in Heart (cited in chapter 1) in which he used two string galvanometers whose movements, displaying phonocardiogram and electrocardiogram respectively, were recorded on the same photographic plate.

L'ENREGISTREMENT DES BRUITS DU CŒUR DE L'HOMME À L'AIDE DU GALVANOMÈTRE À CORDE,

PAR

W. EINTHOVEN.

AVEC LA COLLABORATION DE

A. FLOHIL et P. J. T. A. BATTAERD.

Il y a déjà quelques années que nous avons élaboré au laboratoire de physiologie de Leyden une méthode pour enregistrer les bruits du cœur [1]); comme instrument enregistreur on se servait dans cette méthode de l'électromètre capillaire. Les courbes que j'ai publiées à cette époque ne faisaient pas seulement connaître l'instant auquel un bruit cardiaque commençait ou cessait [2]), mais elles apprenaient aussi les différences de qualité de ces bruits.

Pourtant les tracés ne donnaient par eux-mêmes qu'une représentation graphique inexacte des bruits examinés. Pour en déduire la représentation graphique exacte il eût fallu les soumettre à des mesures de longue durée et à de nombreux calculs, qui n'ont pas été effectués alors. En 1894 on s'est contenté des images photographiques elles-mêmes, parce qu'elles donnaient déjà des formes très typiques pour le premier bruit et le deuxième, tels qu'on les obtient chez le lapin et en divers endroits de la région précordiale chez l'homme.

---

[1]) W. EINTHOVEN et M. A. J. GELUK, Die Registrirung der Herztöne, PFLÜGER's *Arch. f. d. gesammte Physiol.*, 57, 617, 1894.

[2]) La méthode de HÜRTHLE (*Deutsche mediz. Wochenschr.*, 1893, n°. 4) avait en particulier pour but d'indiquer nettement le moment précis du commencement d'un bruit cardiaque. Il en est de même de la méthode de HOLOWINSKI, *Arch. de physiol. norm. et path.*, (5), 8, 893, 1896.

Et cependant on conçoit que des images précises sont préférables aux courbes directement enregistrées par l'électromètre capillaire [1]); or, on obtient déjà un degré de précision suffisant en remplaçant simplement l'électromètre capillaire par un galvanomètre à corde, beaucoup plus sensible et réagissant beaucoup plus rapidement.

J'ai déjà montré [2]) jusqu'à quel point le galvanomètre à corde est capable de reproduire exactement des vibrations rapides. Parmi ma collection de fils de quartz argentés, c'est le n°. 20 qui est le plus léger. Il a 2,5 cm. de longueur et 1 μ d'épaisseur, et ne pèse que $1{,}5 \times 10^{-7}$ g. environ, un poids si petit qu'aucune balance ne l'accuse. Ce fil peut être tendu comme une corde de violon, et exécute alors des vibrations dont la période propre est de 0,31 σ. Cette période correspond à celle d'un son de 3230 vibrations par sec., ce qui est environ le *sol*^{4} dièze (*gis*^{4}), ou presque le son le plus haut d'un piano ordinaire.

Mais la tension du fil peut encore être augmentée sans danger de rupture. On pourrait d'ailleurs prendre un fil plus court, de sorte qu'on peut disposer si l'on veut de périodes de vibration plus petites encore.

Mais il est inutile de profiter de ces avantages pour enregistrer les bruits du cœur. On sait en effet que la hauteur des sons produits par l'activité cardiaque est beaucoup plus basse que celle des sons dont je viens de parler, de sorte que les vibrations amorties de la corde choisie doivent être la reproduction presque irréprochable du mouvement périodique qui lui est communiqué par les bruits du cœur.

Mais bien que l'on puisse prétendre que le fil de quartz du galvanomètre à corde est capable de suivre exactement les vibrations aériennes produites par les bruits, il n'est pas encore dit par là que toutes les difficultés qui se présentent dans l'enregistrement soient résolues. Dans la méthode que nous avons appliquée, les vibrations de l'air produites par le son à enregistrer doivent d'abord mettre en mouvement la plaque

[1]) Tout récemment encore M. Otto Frank a insisté sur ce point; voir *Münch. mediz. Wochenschrift*, 51e Jahrg., n°. 22, 1904.

M. Frank a réussi à enregister les bruits cardiaques directement, par voie mécanique, mais je n'ai jamais vu de reproductions des courbes qu'il a obtenues. Elles ne figurent pas dans sa note susmentionnée. Au sujet d'une tentative d'enregistrement mécanique de bruits cardiaques, voir aussi Hürthle, *Zentralbl. f. Physiol.*, 18, 617, 1904.

[2]) Voir plusieurs publications dans ces *Archives*, depuis 1903.

d'un microphone, traversé par un courant continu que fournit une source de courant constant. Les vibrations de la plaque font naître des variations d'intensité dans le courant du microphone, et ce sont ces variations qui, par l'intermédiaire d'un transformateur, mettent en mouvement le fil de quartz du galvanomètre à corde. On aura donc à tenir compte non seulement des propriétés du fil de quartz, mais encore de celles du microphone et du transformateur.

Il est vrai qu'au point de vue de la reproduction de vibrations de haute fréquence les microphones du commerce ne satisfont pas à d'aussi hautes exigences que le galvanomètre à corde, mais pour notre but, qui est d'enregistrer les bruits cardiaques, nous pouvions sans difficulté faire usage d'un appareil BERLINER, adopté par mainte société téléphonique. La construction d'un transformateur convenable ne présente pas de difficultés non plus. J'ai fait construire dans ce but un transformateur réglable, sans fer et sur bobines d'ébonite; mais nous pouvions faire usage, sans grand préjudice, d'un appareil d'induction ordinaire de DU BOIS-REYMOND ou de HELMHOLTZ, pourvu que nous enlevions le fer de la bobine primaire. Je laisserai de côté ici les calculs qui ont été faits pour arriver au transformateur le mieux approprié à notre but; je les communiquerai à une autre occasion, lorsque je parlerai de l'enregistrement de sons très élevés.

La figure ci-contre fait voir comment le son d'un bruit du cœur est amené au microphone.

Le microphone M est assujetti au milieu d'un anneau en fer assez lourd, non représenté dans la figure, qui est suspendu en trois points pour être à l'abri des trépidations, de la façon recommandée par M. JULIUS. Les trois fils d'acier auxquels l'anneau est suspendu sont munis de ressorts d'acier à leur extrémité inférieure, de manière à amortir des secousses verticales aussi bien que horizontales.

B est un tube métallique courbé, muni d'un tube latéral Z qui porte un robinet K. Le tube B même est solidement fixé à un pilier ou à une table murale, et l'une de ses extrémités est reliée au microphone par un tube en caoutchouc c_1, l'autre à l'entonnoir T d'un stéthoscope par l'intermédiaire d'un tube en caoutchouc c_2. Ce dernier tube a environ 75 cm. de longueur. On peut prendre l'entonnoir en main et l'agiter sans que le microphone présente la moindre trace de trépidation. On peut s'en assurer au moyen d'un miroir de mercure, dont les rides constituent un réactif très sensible aux secousses, et au moyen duquel on peut vérifier aisément, et à chaque instant, la perfection de la méthode de Julius.

Le robinet K est toujours laissé largement ouvert, de sorte que la pression de l'air dans le système des tubes $c_1 B c_2$ reste toujours égale à la pression de l'air extérieur. De cette façon on exclut absolument la transmission de secousses ou de chocs du stéthoscope au microphone,

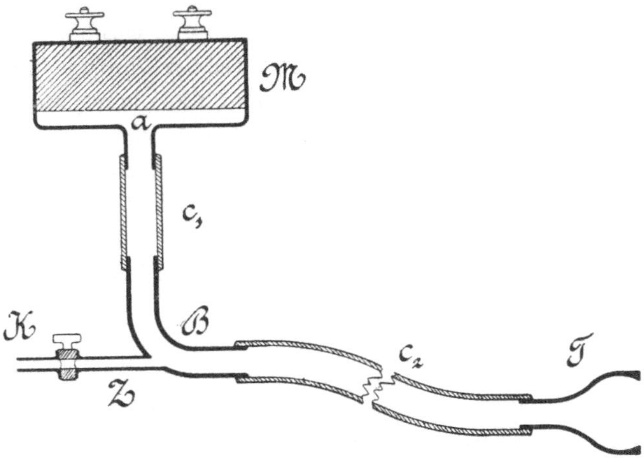

qui ne peut donc être frappé que par des ondes provenant de vibrations de l'air.

Sur les planches XII et XIII sont reproduits un certain nombre de photogrammes de bruits du cœur, obtenus à l'aide du galvanomètre à corde [1]). Le fil de quartz dont nous avons fait usage, le n°. 15, n'était pas aussi léger que le n°. 20, mais il était toujours fortement tendu et satisfaisait suffisamment aux conditions exigées. Comme d'ordinaire nous projetions, pendant l'enregistrement des courbes fournies par le galvanomètre à corde, suivant la méthode de Garten [2]) un réseau de milli-

---

[1]) Nous sommes tout disposés à envoyer des reproductions de nos négatifs à tous ceux qui nous en exprimeront le désir.

[2]) Dr. Siegfried Garten, *Abhandl. der K. Sächs. Gesellsch. d. Wissensch. zu Leipzig*, Mathem.-phys. Kl., 26, n°. 5, 1901.

mètres carrés sur la plaque sensible, ce qui facilitait considérablement, dans la suite, la mesure des bruits enregistrés.

La vitesse de rotation du disque à rayons était fort constante et correspondait toujours exactement à la valeur fixée d'avance. Les écarts étaient inférieurs à 1 : 1000, de sorte que les distances entre les ordonnées fournissent une bonne mesure du temps, sauf à certains endroits, régulièrement espacés, qui correspondent à des rayons qui ont été déplacés fortuitement.

Mais la vitesse de déplacement de la plaque sensible a été le plus souvent trop grande pendant les expériences, ce qui fait que les distances entre les ordonnées sont plus grandes que 1 mm. Bien que cette circonstance soit sans influence sur la précision des mesures de temps, les appareils ont été modifiés depuis, en vue de nouvelles expériences, de telle sorte que la vitesse de déplacement de la plaque sensible pût être mieux réglée.

En faisant les photogrammes reproduits à la suite de ce travail, nous avons donné à la plaque deux vitesses:

Dans les figures 1 et 2 de la plauche XII et 8 et 9 de la planche XIII 1 mm. en abscisse correspond à 0,04 sec., tandis que dans les autres figures 1 mm. en abscisse a une valeur de 0,02 sec.

On aurait pu donner à la plaque sensible des vitesses plus grandes encore, p. ex. jusqu'à 1000 mm. p. sec. [1]. Mais, si l'on applique ces grandes vitesses à l'étude de la forme des ondes sonores, on perd l'avantage de reproduire un grand nombre de bruits du cœur sur une petite étendue.

Les différences entre les courbes reproduites dans ce travail et celles obtenues auparavant à l'aide de l'électromètre capillaire sautent aux yeux. Nous n'avons pas à y insister et il suffit que nous fassions remarquer la symétrie presque parfaite par rapport à la ligne zéro, qui caractérise les courbes actuelles.

Les figures 1, 2, 3 et 4 représentent les bruits de la pointe du cœur chez quatre personnes différentes. On reconnaît aisément quelles sont les vibrations de la corde qui correspondent au bruit systolique et quelles autres correspondent au bruit diastolique Je les ai d'ailleurs distinguées par les chiffres 1 et 2, et j'ai indiqué la durée de la systole

---

[1]) Voir p. ex. les figg. 12 et 13 dans ces *Archives*, (2), 11, 249 et 250, 1906.

par une accolade qui s'étend du commencement du premier bruit jusqu'au commencement du second.

Si l'on examine les photogrammes de plus près, on remarque en premier lieu quelques particularités communes aux divers tracés. On voit que chez tous les sujets le premier bruit est plus intense et de plus longue durée que le deuxième. Il est impossible d'attribuer une hauteur à ces bruits, parce qu'ils sont irréguliers, et sont comparables à de courtes secousses plutôt qu'à des sons musicaux. Mais, quelque irréguliers que soient ces bruits, ils sont caractéristiques pour chaque personne. Si l'on compare p. ex. les premiers bruits des diverses révolutions cardiaques de la fig. 1, on constate une identité tellement grande, qu'on dirait que ce sont toutes copies d'un seul et même modèle. Il en est de même des bruits diastoliques, et, bien qu'il y ait des différences entre les figures relatives à diverses personnes, à chaque figure en particulier s'applique la même remarque qu'à la fig. 1.

Pour bien juger des différences présentées par les quatre figures entr'elles, on doit tenir compte de deux circonstances. En premier lieu j'ai déjà dit que la vitesse de la plaque sensible était deux fois plus grande pendant l'obtention des épreuves 3 et 4 que pour les épreuves 1 et 2. En second lieu les courants électriques qui sont conduits vers le galvanomètre n'ont pas été affaiblis au même degré pour les quatre photogrammes. Il s'ensuit que de la différence d'amplitude des vibrations de la corde dans ces quatre photogrammes on ne peut pas conclure à une différence d'intensité des bruits du cœur. L'installation galvanométrique était tellement sensible, que l'image de la corde aurait été lancée hors du champ si l'on avait voulu enregistrer les bruits du cœur avec leur intensité propre. Dans tous les photogrammes il a donc fallu réduire plus ou moins l'amplitude des mouvements de la corde. C'est surtout chez des sujets jeunes et maigres, dont la paroi thoracique est mince, de sorte que les bruits sont forts, comme dans le cas *Mo* fig. 3, et puis encore dans certains cas pathologiques, que l'on est obligé de réduire notablement les mouvements de la corde.

Cette réduction peut s'effectuer de plusieurs manières et il ne serait pas difficile d'employer dans cette réduction des mesures déterminées, de manière à pouvoir déduire des dimensions des courbes obtenues et du degré de réduction les intensités réelles. Mais pour le moment nous n'avons pas encore fait de pareils calculs et nous nous sommes contentés de diminuer le courant dans le microphone de manière à obtenir des écarts convenables dans les mouvements de la corde.

Mais *un même photogramme* permet de déduire immédiatement les rapports d'intensité des divers sons de la fréquence et de l'amplitude des vibrations de la corde; l'intensité de chaque son est notamment proportionnelle au produit du carré de la fréquenee et du carré de l'amplitude.

Pour pénétrer plus loin dans l'étude des différences entre les bruits de la pointe du cœur chez les quatre sujets examinés, il faudra porter son attention, non seulement sur la fréquence et la forme générale des vibrations sonores, mais encore sur le rapport des amplitudes des vibrations du premier et du deuxième bruit, sur la durée de chacun des deux bruits en particulier, et sur la durée de la systole et de la diastole.

Les figures 5 (pl. XII) et 6 (pl. XIII) reproduisent les bruits de l'artère pulmonaire de deux personnes, tels qu'on les observe près du sternum dans le deuxième espace intercostal de gauche. On remarque nettement la différence avec les bruits de la pointe. Le premier bruit a une durée plus courte, tant pour ce qui regarde la valeur absolue qu'en comparaison avec la durée du 2e bruit. C'est surtout cette dernière circonstance qui saute immédiatement aux yeux.

Dans la fig. 5 la phase entre le premier et le deuxième bruit n'est pas absolument tranquille, bien que l'auscultation n'eût révélé chez le sujet *Ba*, un jeune homme sain et dont le cœur fonctionnait normalement, aucun souffle systolique à l'orifice de l'artère pulmonaire. Les vibrations entre le premier bruit et le deuxième sont d'autant plus remarquables que le fil de quartz revient presque complètement au repos à chaque grand silence.

Dans la fig. 6 appartenant au sujet *Ou* on voit, contrairement à ce que présentait la fig. 5, que le deuxième bruit est nettement plus fort que le premier, et que dans l'intervalle entre le 1er et le 2e bruit il y a tout aussi peu de vibrations que pendant le grand silence.

Je finirai cette note en indiquant simplement les figg. 7, 8, 9 et 10 de la planche XIII. Elles représentent les bruits et les souffles du cœur de trois malades de l'hôpital de l'université de Leyden. Pendant que les malades restaient à l'hôpital, leurs bruits cardiaques étaient enregistrés, à l'aide du galvanomètre à corde, au laboratoire de physiologie, distant d'à peu près 1,5 km. J'ai décrit dernièrement, dans une note sur le télécardiogramme [1]), la façon dont les deux établissements sont reliés à l'aide de fils électriques, jusqu'à quel point la précision des images graphiques est influencée par l'emploi des câbles de raccordement, et jusqu'à combien de kilomètres on peut porter la distance du malade à l'appareil enregistreur, avant que les résultats soient notablement contrariés. Nous n'y reviendrons plus maintenant et nous passerons directement à l'examen des photogrammes.

La fig. 7 nous donne à voir les bruits de l'artère pulmonaire d'un malade dont le cœur fait nettement entendre un souffle systolique. Dans le photogramme le premier bruit passe graduellement à un souffle; il n'y a pas de limite bien marquée entre le premier ton et le souffle, tandis que le deuxième ton, plus fort que le premier, est nettement séparé du souffle, de sorte que l'instant où la diastole commence peut être indiqué avec une assez grande précision. Remarquons encore que pendant le grand silence on ne constate presque pas la moindre vibration de la corde.

La fig. 8 représente les bruits que l'on entend à la pointe du cœur d'une malade atteinte de sténose et d'insuffisance mitrale. Chez cette malade la main ressent à la pointe du cœur un frémissement présystolique, et le stéthoscope révèle un souffle présystolique et un souffle systolique. Sur le photogramme, où ces deux bruits de souffle sont nettement accusés, le premier est indiqué par *a*.

La fig. 9 reproduit les bruits de l'artère pulmonaire de la même malade. On voit qu'ici les souffles présystolique et systolique n'existent plus, ou sont à peine sensibles; de plus on constate que le deuxième bruit est faible par rapport au premier. La question de savoir si le deuxième ton de l'artère pulmonaire, — qui est important au point de vue clinique —, est renforcé ne se résout souvent que difficilement par l'examen au stéthoscope, et dans le cas spécial dont il s'agit la réponse était restée douteuse. Il va de soi que, vu les rapports anatomiques variables du thorax, on ne prendra pas la peine de déterminer l'intensité absolue du son, mais qu'on se contentera de comparer les intensités relatives des bruits, et d'estimer p. ex. le rapport d'intensité du 2e bruit de l'artère pulmonaire et du 1er bruit de la même artère ou du 2e bruit de l'artère pulmonaire et du 2e bruit de l'orifice aortique. Mais même ces comparaisons-là

---

[1]) Ces *Archives*, (2), 11, 239, 1906.

ne sont pas sans difficulté pour l'oreille, surtout parce qu'on a affaire à des bruits dont la durée et le caractère sont différents [1]).

Dans ces circonstances il est permis d'attendre de bons résultats de l'enregistrement des bruits cardiaques. Si l'on met la fig. 9 de notre malade à côté des figg. 5 et 6, qui reproduisent les bruits de l'artère pulmonaire de deux jeunes gens bien sains, dont le cœur fonctionne normalement, on est en droit de conclure sans réserve que le deuxième ton de l'artère pulmonaire de la malade n'est pas renforcé, du moins en comparaison du premier bruit de la même artère.

Pour les figures dont nous nous sommes occupés jusqu'ici il était aisé de mettre les tracés en rapport avec les observations d'auscultation à l'aide du stéthoscope; mais l'explication de la fig. 10, dont nous allons nous occuper pour finir, présente de grandes difficultés. Cette figure donne les bruits que l'on entend à la pointe du cœur d'un jeune homme atteint d'insuffisance de la valvule mitrale, accompagnée d'une forte dilatation et hypertrophie des deux moitiés du cœur. Au stéthoscope on perçoit à la pointe un souffle systolique prolongé, assez égal, dont il n'est pas bien possible de saisir le commencement, mais qui finit brusquement en passant au bruit diastolique, un peu étouffé il est vrai, mais pas faible. Entre le bruit diastolique et le commencement du souffle systolique consécutif il y a nettement un silence.

Cette description ne s'accorde pas avec la forme de la courbe reproduite fig. 10. Cette figure accuse pour chaque révolution cardiaque, en dehors du grand silence, cinq bruits parfaitement distincts, qui ont été indiqués par a, s_1, s_2 et s_3 et 2. Quelle est la signification de ces bruits et quel est leur ordre de succession dans la révolution, voilà ce que nous n'avons pas pu déterminer avec certitude. Pour cela notre expérience est encore insuffisante, mais nous ne doutons pas qu'un examen poursuivi nous permettra bientôt d'expliquer d'une façon satisfaisante les „cardiophonogrammes", comme on peut appeler nos tracés.

---

[1]) Selon M. Max Wien, Pflüger's *Arch.*, 97, 1, 1903, des sons bas de 50 vibrations par seconde doivent être objectivement plusieurs millions de fois plus forts que des sons élevés de 2000 vibrations p. sec., pour produire une sensative auditive également intense. Dans Engelmann's *Arch. f. Physiol.* 1904, p. 25, MM. H. Zwaardemaker et F. H. Quix font connaître des différences qui s'accordent en principe avec les précédentes quant à la forme, mais dont la valeur est d'un autre ordre de grandeur.

Pour le moment nous ne faisons qu'avancer provisoirement l'hypothèse explicative suivante:

a = souffle présystolique;

s_1, s_2, s_3 = trois phases du souffle systolique;

2 = bruit diastolique;

p = grand silence;

et l'accolade dans la figure est supposée limiter une révolution cardiaque.

Une des difficultés de l'explication de la figure réside dans la durée du grand silence. A l'examen au stéthoscope ce temps paraît être assez long, tandis que sur le photogramme il apparaît avec une très courte durée. Si l'on voulait attribuer le défaut de concordance entre les deux méthodes d'observation à des erreurs d'enregistrement, il faudrait admettre qu'un bruit fortuit a mis en mouvement la corde enregistrante précisément dans le temps silencieux du fonctionnement du cœur. Mais une pareille supposition est fort peu probable, puisqu'il y a plus de 7 révolutions consécutives qui ont été tracées sur le photogramme, et que ces révolutions ne laissent à désirer que fort peu au point de vue de la similitude.

A notre avis c'est l'imperfection de notre oreille qui en est la cause. La raison pour laquelle on entend aussi régulièrement un silence est probablement celle-ci, que notre oreille qui vient d'être frappée par le bruit relativement fort du ton diastolique est temporairement fatiguée. Le calme que l'on observe serait donc comparable au silence qui semble se produire après une forte détonation, bien qu'il y ait encore de faibles bruits.

J'ai déjà fait remarquer que l'oreille est un guide peu sûr, quand il s'agit d'estimer l'intensité d'un son, et il n'est pas nécessaire de rappeler d'autres défauts encore de cet organe pour être persuadé qu'un observateur pourra tirer profit de la méthode d'enregistrement des bruits du cœur. Nous ne voulons pas dire par là que l'auscultation ordinaire d'un malade doive être remplacée par la méthode d'enregistrement, mais uniquement ceci, que la dernière méthode peut être appliquée avec succès pour compléter ce qui manque à la première.

L'enregistrement des bruits cardiaques deviendra-t-elle jamais une méthode clinique, ou bien est-il déjà permis maintenant de la considérer comme telle? Cela dépend des exigences que l'on croit devoir poser à une méthode clinique. Ici s'appliquent les mêmes considérations que celles que j'ai faites à la fin de l'article sur le télécardiogramme.

Le galvanomètre à corde est un instrument assez compliqué et très coûteux, il exige une installation particulière et ne peut être employé que moyennant le concours d'assistants exercés, de sorte que pour le moment le clinicien, assis au chevet du malade, ne s'en servira pas encore. Mais on peut opposer à cela qu'on ne doit demander à l'observateur que la connaissance de l'instrument dont il se sert, et qu'il n'a pas besoin de posséder une habileté particulière; de plus, on peut dire que presque chaque épreuve photographique réussit et est faite en quelques minutes.

Les instruments nécessaires pour l'enregistrement ne sauraient trouver place dans la chambre des malades, mais un raccordement convenable par des fils électriques lève cette difficulté. Bien que la communication entre le laboratoire de physiologie et l'hôpital de l'université de Leyden fonctionne depuis plus de deux ans, il ne s'est jamais présenté le moindre accroc, et là où il sera possible d'obtenir la collaboration du physiologiste et du clinicien, rien ne s'oppose à l'application clinique de l'enregistrement des bruits du cœur.

VII
Weiteres über das Elektrokardiogramm

Together with the "Le Télécardiogramme" (V) the following paper marks the beginning of electrocardiography as a science and a clinical diagnostic method. Their fundamental importance for the interpretation of the electrocardiogram was stressed by Johansson in his appreciation of Einthoven's work on behalf of the Nobel Prize Committee.

In the introduction to the present paper Einthoven presents electrocardiography as a diagnostic tool and points out the objective and quantitatively measurable character, in contrast to mechanical (apical) cardiography. That his own technique for this method was inferior to that of Marey, has been mentioned in chapter 1. It becomes clear in this introduction that his esteem for this type of examination was very low; characteristically he abhors the idea that many physiologists only accept curves of a predetermined and dictated shape. (condensed translation by H.A.S.) This may refer to the influence of Marey (see ch. 1) who undoubtedly was right in stating, that a cardiogram taken near, but not exactly at the point of contact of the heart with the thoracic wall, provides a negative (downwards) image of the normal tracing.

Einthoven starts to discuss the electrocardiogram from the isolated frog heart and the intact dog. In doing this he develops a series of practical arrangements concerning such matters as: the speed of registration, the calibration and adjustment of sensitivity, the choice of positive and negative direction of electrocardiographic waves in relation to the deflections of the string, that is to the direction of the heart's action current. All these arrangements, which are essential for the mutual comparison of electrocardiograms were settled by Einthoven in such a way that they have been automatically followed by all clinicians ever since. Surely numerous difficulties have been avoided in this way and progress in electrocardiography has been fostered.

In comparing the direct leads from the isolated frog's heart and the extremity leads from the dog it is pointed out that the current, taken in direct leads from a small region, is influenced by variable factors – such as humidity – whereas in the leads from the intact body the current stems, as it were, from all points of the heart together ("gleichsam von samtlichen Punkten des Herzens zugleich abgeleitet"). In reprint IX this thought has been worked out, as we shall see.

The experiments in the dog are mainly concerned with section and stimulation of the vagus nerve. Th effect on the height of the individual waves is studied and found conspicuous in the P and T waves; also the effect on time relations (slight changes of the systolic period, pronounced changes in heart rate). Strong vagus stimulation is seen to be followed by cardiac arrest and heart block*. Gaskell's experiment in the tortoise heart according to which vagus stimulation increased an existing injury current, is repeated in the dog, but not confirmed. Because of its theoretical importance the "Gaskell effect" was generally interpreted as an anabolic effect of vagus stimulation. Einthoven and Rademaker repeated later Gaskell's experiment in the tortoise (113, see also reprint XI) and established its misleading character.

In dealing with the human electrocardiogram it is stated that in analogy to the experiments in the dog, it is now obvious that the small irregular vibrations, noted in the initial tracings are due to muscular tremor. The influence of leads and the importance of a consistent choice and denomination are again discussed. In this connection the rule of the relation between the leads (lead II - Lead I = lead III) is now clearly formulated as a means of checking both the reliability of the registration and identification of the individual waves. That waves from different leads, bearing the same name, often do not occur at identical instants of the heart cycle, is proven by measuring distances between the waves.

The changes in the electrocardiogram, induced by the respiratory movements are pointed out. Here it is thought likely, that this might be due to changes in the negative interpleural pressure. In continuation of II, the influence of exercise on heart rate, P and T waves is discussed. As far as the T waves are concerned various factors are enumerated which in experiments or human pathology modify the T waves, such as withdrawal of blood and hypertrophy respectively. Electrocardiograms from patients are demonstrated, e.g. with left ventricular hypertrophy and adhesive pericarditis. Clinical heart block is shown in electrocardiograms with the jugular venous and carotic pulses as reference tracings. From the general conclusions regarding the mechanism of the electrocardiogram the following can be noted:

1) The function of the conducting system, described by Tawara a little earlier, is appraised and the conclusion is drawn that contraction must occur almost simultaneously at many points in the ventricles. Nevertheless an attempt is made to follow the path of the spread of

* A more extensive study of the effect of electrical stimulation and sectioning of the vagus nerve, as well as the effect of vagotropic drugs (morphine, atropine) was made by Einthoven and Wieringa (96, 97, 100).

excitation (base to apex, to the right and to the left) from the presence and height of the individual waves in the electrocardiogram. (In later publications Einthoven largely refrained from such attempts).

2) The height of the waves changes in some circumstances in the same way as the force of the heart.
3) The "atypical" contractions (i.e. ventricular premature beats) are discussed in terms of a widened complex, which is ascribed to a longer pathway, and also to variability of the following pulse. The latter is shown to be dependent on the timing of the extrasystole within the cardiac cycle. The eventuality of automatic ventricular beats with a normal profile, however, is shown in a case of clinical heart block.

Finally it should be noted, that the electrocardiographic signs of left and right ventricular hypertrophy were described for the first time by Einthoven, i.e. in V (Le Télécardiogramme) and in the paper which follows here. Lewis confirmed this in his book*, adding: From time to time further evidence to support this view has accumulated and it now sufficiently establishes the signs as the most reliable we possess of *preponderance* of one or other ventricle in hypertrophy."

* THOMAS LEWIS: The mechanism and graphic registration of the heart beat 3rd Ed 1925.

(Aus dem physiologischen Laboratorium in Leiden.)

Weiteres über das Elektrokardiogramm.

Nach gemeinschaftlich mit
Dr. B. Vaandrager angestellten Versuchen mitgeteilt
von
W. Einthoven.

(Mit 41 Textfiguren und Tafeln XI und XII.)

Inhaltsübersicht.

1. Einleitung.

Mit dem Worte „Kardiogramm" wird bald die Kurve, welche den Herzstoss wiedergibt, bald die Figur gemeint durch welche die Druckvariationen in einer Kammerhöhle angegeben werden. In letzterer Bedeutung hat das Kardiogramm bei dem Studium der Herzwirkung vortreffliche Dienste geleistet, aber in dem zuerst genannten Sinne hat es nur geringen Wert.

Durch eine gegen die Regio cordis gedrückte und mit einer Registriertrommel verbundene Aufnahmekapsel wird man bei derselben Person bald diese, bald jene Linie erhalten: eine geringe Verschiebung der Kapsel, ein schwächeres oder kräftigeres Anlegen an die Brustwand hat grössere Veränderungen in der Form des Kardiogrammes zur Folge als die ausgeprägtesten anatomischen Abweichungen des Herzens. Viele Physiologen meinen sogar, das Registrieren des Ictus cordis habe nur dann Wert, wenn man die Aufnahmekapsel auf der Brustwand so lange verschiebe, dass endlich der Hebel der mit der Kapsel verbundenen Registriertrommel eine Kurve von einer vorher bestimmten, vorgeschriebenen Form schreibe.

Die Untersuchung des „Elektrokardiogrammes" ist nicht mit obigen Schwierigkeiten verbunden und darf als eine erwünschte Ergänzung der Herzuntersuchungsmethoden betrachtet werden. Während die rhythmischen Stromesschwankungen des schlagenden Froschherzens schon 1856 den Forschern A. Kölliker und M. Müller bekannt waren, gelang es Aug. D. Waller erst 33 Jahre später, 1889, die Ströme des menschlichen Herzens nachzuweisen.

Behufs einer kritischen Übersicht der älteren einschlägigen Literatur können wir auf die Dissertationen von W. T. de Vogel[1]) und K. de Lint[2]) verweisen. Für unseren Zweck genügt die Bemerkung, dass die Untersuchung der elektrischen Erscheinungen des Herzens durch die Anwendung des Saitengalvonometers[3]) in eine neue Phase eingetreten ist[4]). Dieses Instrument kann in vielen Fällen das früher so häufig gebrauchte Kapillar-Elektrometer mit Vorteil ersetzen.

Es sei uns vergönnt, an dieser Stelle mit wenigen Worten des Telekardiogrammes Erwähnung zu tun[5]). Der Name Telekardiogramm rührt von der grossen Entfernung her, in welcher sich das zu untersuchende Individuum von dem Registrierapparat befindet. Das physiologische Laboratorium in Leiden ist mittels elektrischer Leitungsdrähte mit dem dortigen Universitäts-Krankenhause verbunden, wodurch es möglich ist, die Kranken in dem Spitale mit dem im Laboratorium fest aufgestellten elektrischen Messinstrument zu untersuchen.

Die Kurven, die man auf diese Weise von den Aktionsströmen des menschlichen Herzens erhält, und welche man mit Recht „Tele-

1) W. T. de Vogel, Bijdrage tot de kennis der electrische verschijnselen van het hart. Academisch proefschrift. Leiden 1893. Siehe auch Onderzoekingen Physiol. Laborat. Leiden 2. R. I.

2) K. de Lint, Bijdrage tot de kennis van het normale electrocardiogram van den mensch. Academisch proefschrift. Leiden 1896. Siehe auch Onderzoekingen Physiol. Laborat. Leiden 2. R. III.

3) Siehe: Ein neues Galvanometer. Annalen der Physik, 4. Folge, Bd. 12 S. 1059. 1903. Über einige Anwendungen des Saitengalvanometers. Ibidem Bd. 14 S. 182. 1904. Weitere Mitteilungen über das Saitengalvanometer. Ibidem Bd. 21 S. 483. 1906.

4) Siehe: Die galvanometrische Registrierung des menschlichen Elektrokardiogramms, zugleich eine Beurteilung der Anwendung des Kapillar-Elektrometers in der Physiologie. Pflüger's Arch. f. d. ges. Physiol. Bd. 99 S. 472. 1903.

5) Siehe: „Le Télécardiogramme". Arch. intern. de Physiol. t. 4 p. 132. 1906.

kardiogramme“ nennen darf, lassen verschiedene Abweichungen von der normalen Herzwirkung erkennen, wodurch auch diese selbst besser beleuchtet wird. Typische Formen von Elektrokardiogrammen zeigen sich bei Hypertrophie des rechten Herzens durch Mitralis-Insuffizienz, Hypertrophie des linken Herzens durch Aorta-Insuffizienz, Hypertrophie der linken Vorkammer durch Mitralis-Stenosis und ferner noch bei vielen anderen Abweichungen, von denen wir nur noch die Myodegeneratio cordis und die kongenitalen Herzfehler nennen.

Da der Aktionsstrom der Vorkammern im Elektrokardiogramm fast immer sehr deutlich von dem Aktionsstrom der Kammern unterschieden werden kann, lassen die Kurven das Verhältnis zwischen Vorkammer- und Kammerkontraktion in einer Weise erkennen, welche an Bestimmtheit und Genauigkeit die gewöhnlichen mechanischen Registriermethoden weit übertrifft. Herzblock- und Allorhythmiezustände werden im Telekardiogramm mit sehr befriedigender Schärfe und Entschiedenheit wiedergegeben.

Sehr merkwürdig sind auch die elektrischen Erscheinungen, die bei einer sogenannten Extrasystole eintreten. Der Aktionsstrom bekommt dabei eine Form, die stark von dem gewöhnlichen Elektrokardiogramm abweicht, was darauf hinweist, dass der Ursprung und die Fortpflanzung der Kontraktionswelle in den Kammern während einer Extrasystole nicht mit denen einer normalen Herzkontraktion übereinstimmen. Ferner hat der Augenblick, in welchem die Extrasystole sich entwickelt, im Zusammenhang mit der Form und der Grösse des arteriellen Pulses auf die Bedeutung dieser unzeitigen Herzwirkung neues Licht geworfen.

Vor kurzem ist eine Mitteilung erschienen von F. Kraus und G. F. Nicolai, die sich auch des Saitengalvanometers bedient und besonders die klinische Bedeutung des Elektrokardiogrammes des näheren untersucht haben [1]). Da sie versprechen, bald eine ausführliche Abhandlung über ihre Arbeit veröffentlichen zu wollen, brauchen wir hier keine eingehende Beschreibung ihrer Resultate zu geben. Wir können aber schon jetzt mitteilen, dass sie imstande waren, unsere

1) F. Kraus und G. F. Nicolai, Über das Elektrokardiogramm unter normalen und pathologischen Verhältnissen. Berliner klin. Wochenschr. 44. Jahrg. S. 765 und 811. 1907. — Später sind noch zwei kurze Mitteilungen von Kraus und Nicolai erschienen (vgl. Zentralbl. f. Physiol. vom 28. Dez. 1907 und Deutsche medizin. Wochenschr. vom 2. Januar 1908).

35 *

Ergebnisse der Hauptsache nach zu bestätigen. Es besteht ein guter Grund für die Erwartung, dass bald die Anwendung des Saitengalvanometers überhaupt und namentlich das Registrieren des Elektrokardiogrammes in der Klinik allgemeiner üblich wird.

Die saitengalvanometrische Untersuchung des Elektrokardiogrammes ist auch noch von Max Cremer[1]) und von J. de Meyer[2]) angewendet worden. Für eine kurze Beschreibung ihrer Arbeit verweisen wir auf die Dissertation von Dr. B. Vaandrager[3]).

2. Die Drahtverbindungen und das Elektrokardiogramm des Frosches.

In der untenstehenden Fig. 1 ist die Drahtverbindung abgebildet. Von dem Akkumulator A geht der Hauptstrom durch den Kommutator C, den Schlüssel S und zwei Widerstände R_1 und R_2. Der Weg des Hauptstromes ist durch eine dicke gezogene Linie angegeben.

Von R_2 wird ein Nebenstrom abgezweigt, welcher in der Figur durch eine dünne gezogene Linie abgebildet ist, und in welchem sich die Wippen P_1 und P_2, der Graphitrheostat K und das Galvanometer G befinden.

Die Wippe P_1 ermöglicht, den Nebenstrom entweder durch einen Widerstandskasten R_3 oder nach den mit dem Froschherzen verbundenen Elektroden zu leiten. Da die elektromotorische Kraft des Akkumulators auf 2 Volt gerechnet werden darf, und in den Widerstandskasten R_1 20000 Ohm eingeschaltet sind, wird man mit jedem Ohm des Kastens R_2 einen Potentialunterschied von 0,1 Millivolt in den Nebenschluss einschalten. Diese absichtliche Herstellung eines Potentialunterschiedes im Kreise, in welchem sich das Herz und das Galvanometer befinden, ist nötig, um eine bleibende elektrische Spannung, die oft zwischen den Ableitungsstellen des Herzens vorkommt, kompensieren zu können.

---

1) Max Cremer, Über die direkte Ableitung der Aktionsströme des menschlichen Herzens vom Ösophagus und über das Elektrokardiogramm des Fötus. Münchener medizin. Wochenschr. 1906 Nr. 17. Vgl. auch Verhandl. des Kongresses für innere Medizin 1906.

2) J. de Meyer, Sur de nouveaux courants d'action du cœur et sur les variations de l'oscillation négative. Communication préliminaire (Travail du Hallerianum de Berne). Arch. internat. de Physiol. t. 5 p. 76. 1907.

3) B. Vaandrager, Verdere onderzoekingen over het electrocardiogram. Inauguraldissertation. Leiden 1907. Siehe auch Onderzoekingen Physiol. Laborat. Leiden, 2. R. VII.

Der Kommutator *C* ermöglicht es uns, die Richtung des kompensierenden Stromes nach Bedürfnis zu verändern.

Zuweilen ist die durch das ruhende Herz entwickelte elektromotorische Kraft so gross, dass bei den gewöhnlichen Verbindungen und ohne die Anwendung eines Kompensationsstromes das Saitenbild des Galvanometers aus dem Gesichtsfelde geschlagen wird. Unter diesen Verhältnissen ist es erwünscht, einen Augenblick den Graphitrheostat *K*, in welchen 100 000 oder 1 000 000 Ohm eingeschaltet werden können, zu benutzen. Die Ausweichung der Saite

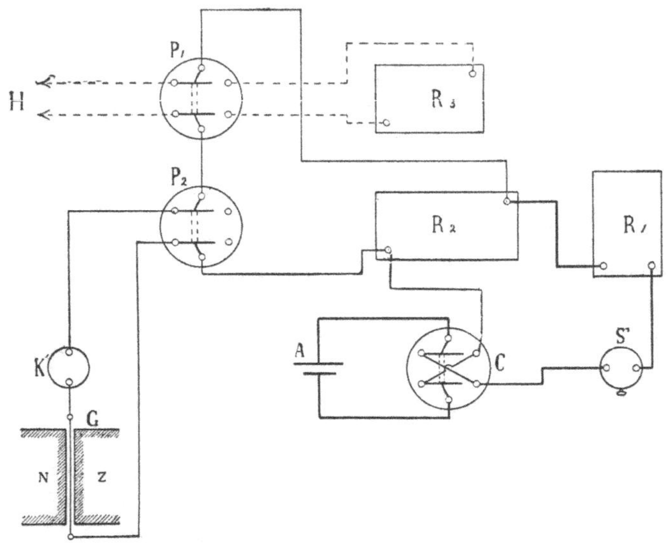

Fig. 1. Schema der Drahtverbindungen.

bleibt dabei innerhalb bestimmter Grenzen, welche die Kompensation des Herzstromes erleichtern. Nachdem der Strom durch die Anwendung des Graphitrheostats ungefähr kompensiert ist, wird dieser wieder ausgeschaltet, während darauf die Kompensation mit aller erwünschten Genauigkeit weiter vollendet wird.

Die Empfindlichkeit des Galvanometers wird durch Veränderung der Quarzdrahtspannung immer so geregelt, dass das Verhältnis der Anzahl von Millivolts Spannung, die in den Galvanometerkreis angebracht wird, zu der Anzahl von Zentimetern Verschiebung des Saitenbildes durch eine kleine ganze Zahl ausgedrückt wird. Bei der Registrierung der Elektrokardiogramme des Menschen und des

Hundes, wobei der Strom von verhältnismässig weit vom Herzen liegenden Körperteilen abgeleitet wurde, war dieses Verhältnis in der Regel = 1, so dass mithin jedem Zentimeter Verschiebung des Saitenbildes 1 Millivolt entsprach. Bei der Registrierung der elektromotorischen Schwankungen des isolierten Froschherzens konnte jedoch diese empfindliche Einstellung des Galvanometers nicht erhalten bleiben. Die Ausschläge wurden dabei oft unzweckmässig gross, so dass es erwünscht war, die Empfindlichkeit des Galvanometers um einige Male zu verringern.

Die richtige Einstellung der Galvanometerempfindlichkeit kann, obgleich die Saite unter dem Einfluss der Herztätigkeit rhythmische Schwankungen aufweist, mit ziemlich grosser Genauigkeit zustande gebracht werden. Während das Herz in den Kreis eingeschaltet ist, bringt man mit Hilfe des Widerstandskastens R_2 einen Spannungsunterschied von einer gewissen Anzahl von Millivolts in den Kreis an. Der Quarzfaden muss dann so gespannt werden, dass das Saitenbild um die vorher bestimmte Anzahl von Zentimetern verschoben wird, was an dem Stande während der Herzpausen, bei denen die Saite in Ruhe ist, leicht kontrolliert werden kann.

Der Widerstand des Herzens wird, zusammen mit dem der Elektroden, nach der Substitutionsmethode gemessen. Durch das Umschlagen der Wippe P_1 wird an der Stelle des Herzens der Widerstandskasten R_3 eingeschaltet, und in diesem ein solcher Widerstand angebracht, dass die Herstellung desselben Spannungsunterschiedes in den Kreis wieder einen gleich grossen Ausschlag des Saitenbildes verursacht. Der in dieser Weise gefundene Widerstand ist dann dem gesuchten gleich.

Um Irrthümern bei der Beurteilung der Form der Elektrokardiogramme vorzubeugen, beobachteten wir bei der Herstellung der Verbindungen einige bestimmte Regeln. Der Erregungsstrom des Elektromagneten wird immer in solcher Richtung durchgeleitet, dass in dem den Quarzfaden enthaltenden Felde die magnetischen Kraftlinien, die nach der Konstruktion des Galvanometers der optischen Achse parallel laufen müssen, dieselbe Richtung haben wie die Lichtstrahlen. Unter diesen Verhältnissen schlägt das Saitenbild, das mittels eines Prismas um 90° um die Achse gedreht ist, nach oben aus, wenn der Quarzfaden von unten nach oben durchströmt wird.

Nun wird bei der Registrierung aller Elektrokardiogramme der proximale Teil des Herzens oder was dem zunächst liegt mit dem oberen, der distale Teil des Herzens mit dem unteren Ende des Quarzfadens verbunden. Eine Negativität der Herzbasis in Beziehung zur Herzspitze wird in unseren Elektrokardiogrammen folglich immer durch einen aufwärts gerichteten Ausschlag des Saitenbildes angegeben. Ebenso sorgten wir dafür, dass das Saitenbild nach oben ausschlug, jedesmal wenn bei Stromableitung von rechts nach links das rechte Herz negativ wurde in Beziehung zum linken.

Wir haben die elektromotorischen Schwankungen des isolierten Froschherzens hauptsächlich in der Absicht untersucht, die Kontraktionswelle, die über den Herzmuskel fortschreitet, von Punkt zu Punkt verfolgen zu können. Selbstverständlich ist bei einer solchen Untersuchung eine unerlässliche Bedingung, dass das Herz durch die Manipulationen der Isolierung und durch das Anlegen der Elektroden nicht verletzt wird.

Wir verwendeten Elektroden, die nach dem Prinzip von E. du Bois-Reymond konstruiert waren: einen amalgamierten Zinkstab in einer mit gesättigter $ZnSO_4$-Lösung gefüllten Röhre. Die Röhre ist am unteren Ende mit Zinksulfat-Ton geschlossen. Gegen diesen ist Ringer-Ton geklebt, in welchen ein in Ringer-Lösung getränkter Lampendocht gepflanzt wird. Der Lampendocht, den man mit dem Herzen in Berührung bringt, ist sehr weich und biegsam und macht alle Bewegungen des Herzens leicht mit, so dass er das Herz nicht beschädigen kann.

Auch beim Präparieren des Herzens haben wir grosse Sorgfalt beobachtet, allein ungeachtet aller von uns getroffenen Maassnahmen, haben wir unseren Zweck nicht erreicht. Die Formen der von uns erhaltenen Elektrokardiogramme sind in hohem Grade voneinander verschieden, und es war uns nicht möglich, den Weg, den die Kontraktionswelle im Herzmuskel nimmt, in dieser Weise mit genügender Bestimmtheit kennen zu lernen. Auch die Versuche, die wir angestellt haben, den Strom von dem blossgelegten Herzen in situ abzuleiten, blieben ohne befriedigenden Erfolg. Dagegen konnten wir wohl konstante Elektrokardiogramme erhalten, wenn die Elektroden an die Vorder- und Hinterpfoten des Frosches angelegt wurden; aber weil bei einer solchen Ableitung verschiedene höhere Tiere und namentlich der Mensch selbst bequemere Beobachtungsobjekte lieferten, haben wir auf die weitere Untersuchung des Froschherzens verzichtet. Nur sei hier noch bemerkt, dass die auf diese Weise erhaltenen Elektrokardiogramme des Frosches im allgemeinen eine grosse Ähnlichkeit mit denen des Hundes und des Menschen aufweisen.

Verfolgt man einen anderen Zweck als wir, so reicht ein weniger empfindliches und weniger schnell arbeitendes Messinstrument als das Saitengalvanometer aus, während dann doch noch das Studium der elektromotorischen Erscheinungen des isolierten Froschherzens zu einer Anzahl merkwürdiger Ergebnisse führen kann. Dies hat besonders Samojloff[1]) gezeigt, der bei seiner Untersuchung von dem Kapillarelektrometer Gebrauch machte.

Unsere Bemerkung, dass die Formen der Elektrokardiogramme des isolierten Froschherzens in hohem Grade wechseln, hat früher schon Waller[2]) für das isolierte Säugetierherz gemacht, und auch Samojloff weist auf die Schwierigkeiten hin, die durch den fortwährenden Formenwechsel der so erhaltenen Kurven dem Beobachter geboten werden. Er schreibt nämlich[3]): „Will man aber die Form des Elektrokardiogrammes näher charakterisieren, so stösst man auf Schwierigkeiten; letztere bestehen darin, dass das Elektrokardiogramm ein ungemein wechselndes Bild darstellt. Vergleicht man Bilder von Elektrometerkurven verschiedener Herzen, so ist das Auffälligste dabei die Mannigfaltigkeit der Kurvenformen. Beobachtet man die Tätigkeit eines und desselben Froschherzens längere Zeit, z. B. ein paar Stunden oder noch länger, unter gleichen Bedingungen, so kann man schon aus dem Spiel der projizierten Hg-Kuppe oder noch besser auf Grund einer Reihe photographischer Kurven erkennen, dass wir es mit einer Erscheinung zu tun haben, die sehr allmählich aber ununterbrochen wechselt."

Weshalb diese Formen in so hohem Grade wechseln im Gegensatz zu der grossen Konstanz der Form des menschlichen Elektrokardiogrammes und desjenigen von Tieren, bei denen die Strom-

---

1) A. Samojloff, Beiträge zur Elektrophysiologie des Herzens. Engelmann's Arch. f. Physiol. 1906 Suppl. S. 207.

2) A. D. Waller, On the elektromotive changes connected with the beat of the mammalian heart, and of the human heart in particular. Philosophical Transactions of the Royal Society of London vol. 180 (B.) p. 169. 1889.

3) A. a. O. S. 209.

ableitung von unlädierten Körperteilen stattfindet, wird von Samojloff auf eine in jeder Hinsicht befriedigende Weise erklärt. Im isolierten Froschherzen beeinflussen die Temperatur die Feuchtigkeitsverhältnisse und die unvermeidlichen Verletzungen den Weg, den die Kontraktionswelle von Punkt zu Punkt durch den Herzmuskel nimmt. Die beiden Punkte, von denen der Strom abgeleitet wird, weisen darum ihren Potentialunterschied zu stark wechselnden Zeiten auf, während beim Anlegen der Elektroden an die Hände oder an eine Hand und einen Fuss eines Menschen der Strom gleichsam von sämtlichen Punkten des Herzens zugleich abgeleitet wird. Wir haben es dann mit einer Resultante der Herzströme zu tun, einer Art von Durchschnittsstrom, der wohl konstanter sein muss als die an zwei gesonderten Punkten der Herzoberfläche zum Vorschein kommende Potentialschwankung.

Auch die gewöhnliche mechanische Kontraktionskurve des Herzens ist eine Resultante der spezifischen Kontraktionskurven aller Muskelfasern.

Samojloff zeigt weiter, dass das Elektrokardiogramm ebenso deutlich wie die mechanische Kontraktionskurve des Herzens eine Extrasystole, eine refraktäre Periode und eine kompensatorische Pause aufweist. Die gedehnte und verstärkte Post-Extrasystole und die polyrhythmische Herztätigkeit werden durch die elektrischen Erscheinungen sogar schon verraten, wenn sie sich noch so wenig herausgebildet haben, dass sie kaum oder noch gar nicht durch die mechanische Kontraktionskurve angegeben werden.

3. Das Elektrokardiogramm des Hundes.

Bei der Registrierung des Elektrokardiogrammes des Hundes haben wir verschiedene Stromableitungsmethoden angewendet. An erster Stelle wurden dieselben Elektroden gebraucht, die bei früheren Untersuchungen im Laboratorium schon wiederholt bei der Registrierung menschlicher Elektrokardiogramme benutzt wurden. Sie werden im folgenden Abschnitt eingehender besprochen werden. Es genügt hier mitzuteilen, dass der Hund mit einer Vorder- und einer Hinterpfote in je einer der beiden Elektroden stand.

Auf diese Weise konnten wir zwar sehr brauchbare Elektrokardiogramme erhalten, und waren wir zugleich sicher, dass die Hunde durch die Untersuchung nicht in abnormale Zustände gerieten; allein die Methode wurde doch bald aufgegeben, da es sich als nicht leicht erwies, die Tiere während der Registrierung vollkommen ruhig zu erhalten. Die Hunde zitterten meistens sichtlich, wodurch der Stand der Saite unruhig wurde. Vielleicht genügt auch schon die beim Aufrechtstehen erforderliche Muskelanstrengung, wechselnde elektrische Ströme von merklicher Stärke hervorzurufen.

Wird der Hund niedergelegt und chloroformiert, so hören die kleinen frequenten Saitenschwingungen auf, und man erhält ein reineres Elektrokardiogramm. Ausserdem kann man bei einem ruhig liegenden, schlafenden Hunde leichter den Blutdruck registrieren, die Erfolge der Vagusreizung untersuchen und die verschiedenen übrigen Manipulationen vornehmen, welche für die weitere Untersuchung erforderlich sind. Die meisten der von uns registrierten Elektrokardiogramme von Hunden sind deshalb bei liegender Körperhaltung des Tieres hergestellt worden.

Einen Versuch, das Galvanometer mit dem Tiere mittels als Haarseile unter die Haut gebrachter Lampendochte zu verbinden, gaben wir bald auf. Den ausserhalb der Haut befindlichen Teil des Dochtes konnten wir nicht gleichmässig genug feucht erhalten, der Widerstand der Elektroden war sehr gross und schon die geringsten Bewegungen des Tieres waren imstande, einen Ausschlag des Saitenbildes herbeizuführen.

All diese Schwierigkeiten wurden beseitigt, als wir von zwei ziemlich breiten flanellenen Binden Gebrauch machten, welche jede um eine sorgfältig von Haaren entblösste Hautfalte geklemmt wurden. Die Binden wurden mit NaCl-Lösung feucht gehalten und mit ihren freien Enden jede in eine mit derselben Lösung gefüllte Tonzelle eingetaucht. Diese Tonzelle stand in einem Glaszylinder, in welchem sich eine gesättigte $ZnSO_4$-Lösung und eine amalgamierte Zinkplatte befanden. Letztere war mittels eines Leitungsdrahtes mit dem Galvanometer verbunden.

Diese Elektroden befriedigten in jeder Hinsicht. Kleine Bewegungen des Hundes hatten keine Ortsveränderung des Saitenbildes zur Folge, und der Widerstand war verhältnismässig gering, da der Gesamtwiderstand des Tieres und der Elektroden von 2000 bis 4000 Ohm betrug.

Das Elektrokardiogramm des Hundes, obgleich in der Form nicht ganz mit dem des Menschen übereinstimmend, weist doch keine prinzipiellen Unterschiede von demselben auf. Die fünf Spitzen

P, *Q*, *R*, *S* und *T* des menschlichen Elektrokardiogrammes, die schon früher beschrieben worden sind [1]), und die wir im folgenden Abschnitt des näheren werden besprechen müssen, sind in der Regel auch im Elektrokardiogramm des Hundes vorhanden.

Der Einfluss der Stellen, von denen der Strom abgeleitet wird, auf die Form der Kurve weist beim Hunde sehr viel Übereinstimmung auf mit dem Einfluss, den die Ableitungsstellen auf die Form der menschlichen Kurve ausüben. Von den vielen Aufnahmen, die uns zur Verfügung stehen, mögen einige wenige zum Beispiel dienen.

In den Figuren 2, 3 und 4 sind die Elektrokardiogramme wiedergegeben [2]), die wir erhielten, indem der Strom in drei verschiedenen Weisen abgeleitet wurde. In Fig. 2 wurde der Strom

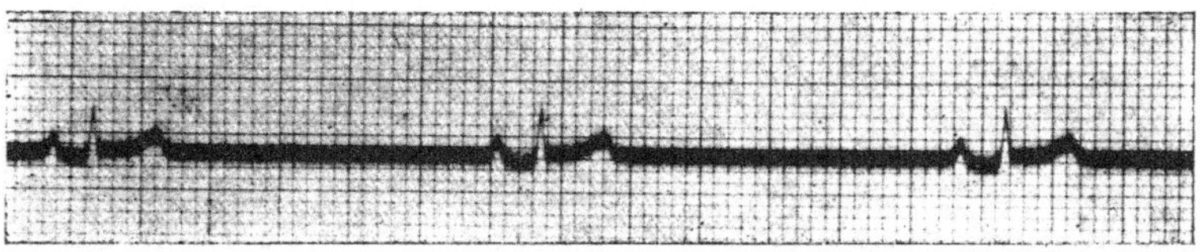

Fig. 2. Hund. Stromableitung von rechter und linker Vorderpfote. Absz. 1 mm = 0,04 Sek. Ordin. 1 mm = 10^{-4} Volt.

von den beiden Vorderpfoten abgeleitet (Ableitung I), in der folgenden Figur von der rechten Vorder- und der linken Hinterpfote (Ableitung II) und in Fig. 4 von der linken Vorder- und der linken Hinterpfote (Ableitung III).

Wie wir schon im vorigen Abschnitt erwähnt haben, sind die Verbindungen immer so gewählt worden, dass beim Negativwerden des proximalen Teiles oder des rechten Teiles des Herzens das Saitenbild nach oben ausschlägt. Während der Registrierung der Elektrokardiogramme wurde, ebenso wie bei den schon früher im Laboratorium angestellten Untersuchungen, ein Netz von Quadratmillimetern auf der empfindlichen Platte entworfen.

1) Siehe mehrere Aufsätze in Pflüger's Arch. f. d. ges. Physiol. und in Onderzoekingen physiol. Laborat. Leiden.

2) Wir sind gern bereit, Kopien unserer ursprünglichen Negative, die ungleich deutlicher und schärfer sind als die Textfiguren und die Tafeln, auf Anfrage den Fachgenossen zu übersenden.

Die Bewegungsgeschwindigkeit der Platte betrug in den drei oben genannten Figuren 25 mm pro Sekunde, so dass 1 mm Abszissenlänge 0,04 Sekunden entspricht, während die Empfindlichkeit des Galvanometers dergestalt geregelt war, dass 1 mm Ordinatlänge einem Potentialunterschiede von 0,1 Millivolt entspricht.

Die Figuren geben zu verschiedenen Bemerkungen Anlass. Erstens ist es auffällig, dass bei Ableitung I von den beiden Vorderpfoten im Gegensatz zur Darstellung Waller's ein deutliches Elektrokardiogramm mit ziemlich grossen Potentialunterschieden erhalten wird. Waller[1]) teilt den Körper des Hundes in einen vorderen und einen hinteren Teil ein. Stromableitung von dem vorderen

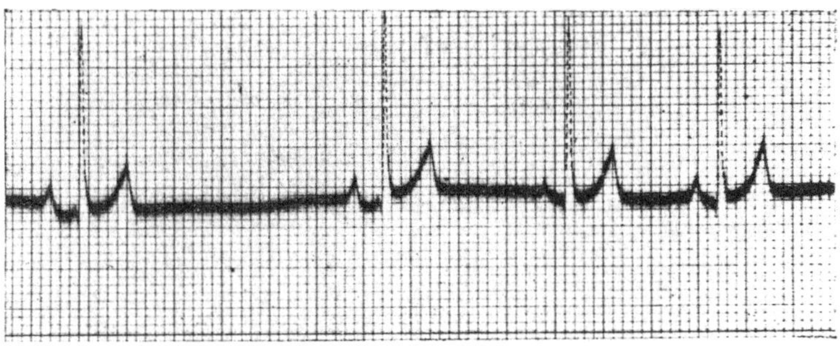

Fig. 3. Hund. Stromableitung von rechter Vorderpfote und linker Hinterpfote. Absz. 1 mm = 0,04 Sek. Ordin. 1 mm = 10^{-4} Volt.

nach dem hinteren Teile, z. B. von einer Vorderpfote nach einer Hinterpfote sollte eine günstige Kombination bilden und mithin deutliche rhythmische Schwankungen im elektrischen Messapparat hervorrufen, während bei Ableitung von der einen Vorderpfote nach der anderen oder von einer Hinterpfote nach der anderen eine ungünstige Kombination gebildet werden sollte, wobei keine oder so gut wie keine wechselnden Potentialunterschiede zum Vorschein kommen sollten.

Tatsächlich sind bei Ableitung von den beiden Hinterpfoten die durch die Herzwirkung verursachten Potentialunterschiede gering, obgleich doch noch sichtbar, aber wir sehen an Fig. 2, dass die Behauptung Waller's für Ableitung I von den beiden Vorderpfoten nicht ganz zutrifft.

---

1) A. a. O. S. 192.

Wie bei den durch Anwendung verschiedener Stromableitung erhaltenen Kurven des Menschen, wechselt in den drei obenerwähnten Elektrokardiogrammen des Hundes das gegenseitige Verhältnis der Höhen der verschiedenen Spitzen.

Namentlich Spitze *R* ist bei Ableitung II gross (siehe Fig. 3) im Vergleich mit den meisten übrigen Spitzen, während bei Ableitung I (siehe Fig. 2) die drei wichtigsten Spitzen *P*, *R* und *T* weniger voneinander verschieden sind.

Die Spitze *Q* ist bei Ableitung I nicht oder kaum vorhanden, während sie bei Ableitung II und III sehr scharf ist und eine Höhe von 1—2 mm erreicht. Keine einzige dieser drei Kurven weist eine Spitze *S* auf.

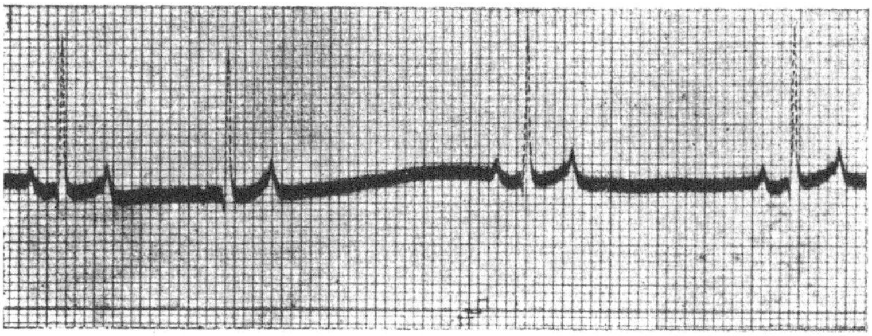

Fig. 4. Hund. Stromableitung von linker Vorderpfote und linker Hinterpfote. Absz. 1 mm = 0,04 Sek. Ordin. 1 mm = 10^{-4} Volt.

Bei Ableitung III erweisen zufälligerweise in der photographischen Aufnahme (von welcher in Fig. 4 nur ein Teil reproduziert ist) einige Spitzen sich als sehr inkonstant. So variiert die Höhe der Vorkammerspitze *P* zwischen — 0,4 und + 1,2 $\times$ 10^{-4} Volt, während die Höhe der Spitze *T* zwischen 3 und 4 $\times$ 10^{-4} Volt schwankt.

Die Frage, wie die Entstehung der verschiedenen Spitzen erklärt werden muss, und zu welchen Bemerkungen sie in bezug auf die Fortschreitung der Kontraktionswelle im Herzmuskel Anlass geben, wird besser bei der Besprechung der Formen des menschlichen Elektrokardiogrammes im folgenden Abschnitt erörtert. Wir beschränken uns hier auf die Wiedergabe einer Tabelle, in der die Höhen der Spitzen der letzten drei Figuren in Millimetern, d. h. in Zehntausendsteln eines Volts, angegeben sind.

Vergleicht man die drei abgebildeten Kurven mit menschlichen Elektrokardiogrammen, wie sie z. B. in „Le Télécardiogramme“

abgebildet sind und im folgenden Abschnitt näher zur Sprache kommen werden, so fällt es vor allem auf, dass die grosse Spitze *R* von kurzer Dauer ist. Ist sie dabei zugleich hoch, wie bei Ableitung II (siehe Fig. 3), so wird sie viel schärfer und spitzer als der gleichnamige Gipfel beim Menschen.

Tabelle I.

	P	*Q*	*R*	*S*	*T*
Ableitung I . . .	1,3	—	4	—	1,8
Ableitung II . . .	2,2	— 1,2	22	—	6,0
Ableitung III . .	variierend zwischen — 0,4 und + 1,2	— 1,2	10	—	variierend zwischen 3 und 4

Die grosse Geschwindigkeit, mit der das Saitenbild sich auf- und abwärts bewegt, veranlasst, dass die Schattenlinien, welche den Umriss der Spitze bezeichnen, äusserst fein werden, so dass sie, obgleich auf den ursprünglichen Negativen noch gut sichtbar, bei der Reproduktion oft verloren gehen. Deutlichkeitshalber haben wir darum in einigen Figuren längs den Umrissen der Spitze *R* mit Tinte eine gestrichelte Linie gezogen. Diese Retouche ist besonders deshalb gestattet, weil sie als solche deutlich genug auffällt und unmöglich dafür angesehen werden kann, dass sie den übrigen auf rein photographischem Wege erhaltenen Teilen der Figuren gleichwertig sei.

Wünscht man die Form der Spitze *R* besser zu beurteilen, so kann man die Kurve bei grösserer Geschwindigkeit der empfindlichen Platte registrieren. In Fig. 5 ist das Elektrokardiogramm eines anderen Hundes bei Ableitung II von der rechten Vorder- und der linken Hinterpfote abgebildet. Die Empfindlichkeit des Galvanometers war wiederum so geregelt, dass 1 mm einer Ordinat einer Spannung von 10^{-4} Volt entsprach, aber die Geschwindigkeit der empfindlichen Platte ist viermal grösser als früher, so dass 1 mm einer Abszisse jetzt 0,01 Sekunde entspricht.

Durch die grosse Geschwindigkeit der empfindlichen Platte sind die Umrisse der Spitze *R* im Photogramm breit genug geworden, um auch in der Reproduktion zu ihrem Rechte zu kommen. Man sieht jetzt deutlich, dass die Spitze *R* nur 3 mm, d. h. 0,03 Sekunden, anhält, während die gleichnamige Spitze beim Menschen, so wie dieselbe z. B. in Fig. 9 und 10 von „Le Télécardiogramme“ und auch in den Figuren von Abschnitt 4 dieser Abhandlung abgebildet ist, eine Dauer von 0,04—0,05 Sekunden besitzt.

Auch die Vorkammerspitze *P* ist, wie sich bei einer Vergleichung der verschiedenen Kurven leicht herausstellt, in der Regel schärfer, d. h. von kürzerer Dauer, und höher beim Hunde als beim Menschen. In Fig. 5 finden wir für die Dauer ungefähr 0,05 oder 0,06 Sekunden, während die Höhe 5×10^{-4} Volt beträgt. Im Photogramm (von dem in Fig. 5 nur ein Teil reproduziert ist) sind wieder grössere Höhen- und Dauerunterschiede der Vorkammerspitzen vorhanden, als wir bei menschlichen Elektrokardiogrammen beobachtet haben.

Es braucht kaum bemerkt zu werden, dass nicht alle Hunde gleiche Elektrokardiogramme aufweisen. Viele unterschieden sich von den beiden oben untersuchten darin, dass sie, was freilich auch

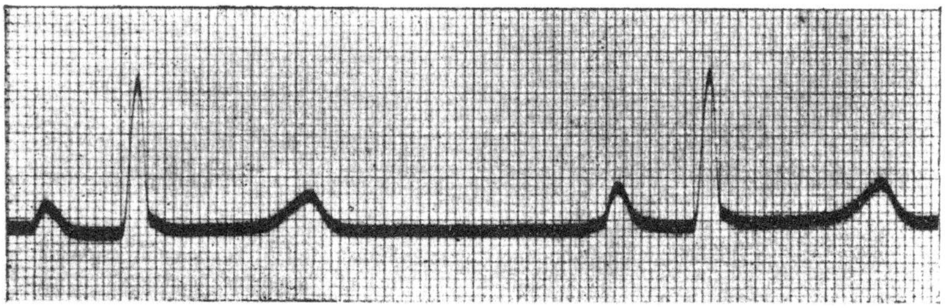

Fig. 5. Hund. Stromableitung von rechter Vorderpfote und linker Hinterpfote Absz. 1 mm = 0,01 Sek. Ordin. 1 mm = 10^{-4} Volt.

bei Menschen vorkommt, eine sehr kleine oder eine negative Spitze *T* besitzen. Bei Menschen wird diese Erscheinung hauptsächlich bei Ableitung III, bei Hunden dagegen sowohl bei Ableitung II als bei bei Ableitung III konstatiert.

Wir finden es nicht nötig, in dieser Abhandlung alle Verschiedenheiten der von uns registrierten Elektrokardiogramme des Hundes zu reproduzieren. Nur diene Fig. 6 als Beispiel einer Kurve mit einer negativen Spitze *T*. Die Stromableitung hat hier von einer rechten Vorder- und einer linken Hinterpfote stattgefunden, während die Abszissen und Ordinaten die gewöhnlichen, in Fig. 2, 3 und 4 schon erwähnten Werte haben. Die scharfen Spitzen *P* und *R* und die negative, eigentümlich geformte, ziemlich scharfe Spitze *T* stellen zusammen ein Bild dar, wie in manchen Elektrokardiogrammen des Hundes wahrgenommen wird.

Weil bei Abteilung II die grössten Potentialschwankungen zum Vorschein kommen, haben wir meistens diese Ableitung benutzt. Wo wir nicht ausdrücklich das Gegenteil bemerken, ist bei allen in diesem Abschnitt noch zu besprechenden Elektrokardiogrammen die Ableitung II von der rechten Vorder- und der linken Hinterpfote angewendet worden.

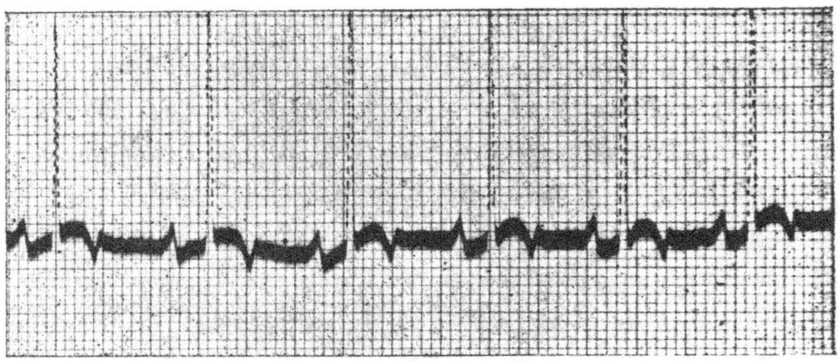

Fig. 6. Hund. Stromableitung von rechter Vorderpfote und linker Hinterpfote. Absz. 1 mm = 0,04 Sek. Ordin. 1 mm = 10^{-4} Volt.

Vagusreizung.

Die elektrischen Erscheinungen, welche die Herztätigkeit begleiten, können namentlich einiges Licht auf die Frage nach dem Einfluss von Vagusreizung werfen. Es existiert eine ausgebreitete Literatur über den Einfluss des Nervus vagus auf den Mechanismus der Herzwirkung [1]), woraus hervorgeht, dass mancher Punkt dieser Nervenfunktion unaufgeklärt geblieben ist, während eine Anzahl von Forschern, die bei verschiedenen, zuweilen sehr nahe verwandten Tierarten experimentiert haben, zu ganz verschiedenen Resultaten gelangt sind.

Wir dürfen z. B. an die Frage erinnern, ob der Nervus vagus ausser auf die Frequenz auch Einfluss auf die Kraft der Herzwirkung ausübt, und weiter an die Frage, ob dieser Nerv auf die Vorkammern oder aber auf die Kammern wirkt. Ohne behaupten zu wollen, dass diese Fragen durch direkte mechanische Untersuchung nicht gelöst werden können, bemerken wir doch, dass die ge-

1) Siehe z. B. R. Tigerstedt, Lehrbuch der Physiologie des Kreislaufs. Leipzig 1893, und E. A. Schäfer, Textbook of Physiology vol. 2. Edinburgh and London. 1900.

bräuchlichste Methode, den Mechanismus der Herztätigkeit nach dem Puls zu beurteilen — wobei das Herz selbst nicht blossgelegt zu werden braucht und folglich auch keinen schädlichen Einflüssen ausgesetzt ist —, uns hierbei im Stich lässt.

Vaguswirkung bei einem isolierten Säugetierherzen ist unter anderem von H. E. Hering[1]) und von J. Rihl[2]), bei einem blossgelegten Säugetierherzen besonders von Rehfisch[3]), der unter Engelmann's Leitung arbeitete, näher untersucht worden.

Die elektrische Untersuchung, die hier aushelfen könnte, ist von Gaskell[4]), Gotch[5]), Burdon Sanderson[6]), Fano[7]) und Boruttau[8]) vorgenommen worden. Bei den Versuchen Gaskell's, die vieles Aufsehen erregten, wurde der Strom von der stillstehenden rechten Vorkammer der Schildkröte abgeleitet, wobei eine Elektrode auf der lädierten Spitze, die andere auf der unlädierten Basis der genannten Vorkammer angelegt wurde. Merkwürdigerweise zeigte es sich, dass der Demarkationsstrom, der mit Hilfe eines empfindlichen Galvanometers beobachtet wurde, bei Vagusreizung verstärkt wurde.

Es sind weitgehende Betrachtungen an die Ergebnisse dieses Versuchs geknüpft worden: die Vagusreizung sollte einen assimila-

---

1) H. E. Hering, Über die unmittelbare Wirkung des Accelerans und Vagus auf automatisch schlagende Abschnitte des Säugetierherzens. Pflüger's Arch. Bd. 108 S. 281. 1905.

2) J. Rihl, Über Vaguswirkung auf die automatisch schlagenden Kammern des Säugetierherzens. Ibidem Bd. 114 S. 545. 1906. Man findet bei Rihl auch eine Besprechung der einschlägigen Literatur.

3) E. Rehfisch, Über die Reizung des Herzvagus bei Warmblütern mit Einzelinduktionsschlägen. Engelmann's Arch. f. Physiol. Supplbd. S. 152. 1906.

4) W. H. Gaskell, On the action of muscarin upon the heart, and on the electrical changes in the non-beating cardiac muscle brought about by stimulation of the inhibitory and augmentor nerves. The Journal of Physiology vol. 8 p. 404. 1887.

5) Gotch, Inhibition of tortoise heart. Proceedings of the physiolog. society. July 2, 1887, p. 26.

6) Burdon Sanderson, Ibidem p. 27.

7) Fano et Fayod, De quelques rapports entre les propriétés contractiles et les propriétés électriques des oreillettes du cœur. Arch. ital. de Biologie t. 9 p. 143. 1888.

8) Boruttau, Über die elektrischen Erscheinungen am Herzen bei Vagusreizung. Zentralbl. f. Physiol. Bd. 19 S. 301. 1905.

torischen Prozess im Herzmuskel hervorrufen, wobei dann eine elektropositive Stelle im Herzen noch stärker positiv werden sollte.

Wir halten es nicht für wünschenswert, hier auch die Arbeit der anderen erwähnten Forscher eingehend zu besprechen, zumal die von ihnen angewendeten Methoden nicht ganz einwandfrei sind. Sie haben alle die elektrischen Erscheinungen bei direkter Stromableitung von verschiedenenen Stellen des blossgelegten oder isolierten Herzens studiert. Im vorigen Abschnitt haben wir aber schon darauf hingewiesen, dass, wenn die Elektroden unmittelbar auf das blossgelegte Herz angelegt werden, die Form des Elektrokardiogrammes unsicher und schwankend bleibt, mag das Organ auch noch so sorgfältig präpariert sein, und mag man auch noch so weiche und biegsame, den Bewegungen der verschiedenen Herzteile leicht folgenden Elektroden anwenden. Man entbehrt eine bestimmte Basis für die Beurteilung der Veränderungen, welche die Potentialschwankungen erleiden, und die in einem bestimmten Moment durch einen willkürlichen Reiz hervorgerufen werden.

Dasselbe Bedenken können auch die Versuche Gaskell's erregen. Diese werden wegen der weitgehenden Schlüsse, die man daraus ziehen kann, in den Lehr- und Handbüchern der Physiologie als sehr wichtig dargestellt; sie werden zu den klassischen Versuchen gerechnet. Aber wir halten es für nicht unmöglich dass die technischen Schwierigkeiten der von Gaskell angewendeten Methode seine Folgerungen unsicher machen, und meinen, dass einiger Zweifel an der Richtigkeit seiner Resultate noch wohl berechtigt heissen darf.

Merkwürdig ist es gewiss, dass niemand weniger als Gotch[1]), indem er mit einem empfindlichen Kapillarelektrometer ein Gaskellpräparat untersuchte, keine Differenz im Potentialunterschied bemerken konnte, wenn in einem Falle Stillstand durch Vagusreizung verursacht wurde, während im anderen Falle ein vorübergehender Stillstand durch die gewöhnliche Diastole des Herzens vorhanden war.

Burdon Sanderson[2]) macht die Annahme, das Kapillarelektrometer von Gotch sei nicht empfindlich genug gewesen. Er meint, der Versuch sei sehr schwierig und könne nur mit Hilfe eines empfindlichen Galvanometers ausgeführt werden, während er den Potentialunterschied, der durch Vagusreizung entsteht, für noch

---

1) A. a. O.

2) A. a. O.

nicht 0,0005 Volt grösser hält als den Potentialunterschied, der bei einer gewöhnlichen Diastole gefunden wird.

Das Saitengalvanometer kann unseres Erachtens hier sehr nützlich sein, da das Instrument empfindlich genug ist, um eine Isolierung oder Blosslegung des Herzens im Körper des Tieres überflüssig zu machen. Im Hinblick auf die Versuche Gaskell's würde es gewiss nicht unwichtig sein, das saitengalvanometrische Elektrokardiogramm der lebenden Schildkröte aufzunehmen und die Veränderungen zu studieren, die darin durch Vagusreizung hervorgerufen werden können. Wir haben uns aber auf die Untersuchung des Hundeherzens beschränkt.

Während bei einem ruhig schlafenden Hunde der Strom von zwei Pfoten abgeleitet wird, kann der Vagus gereizt werden. Das Herz gibt zuvor das Elektrokardiogramm in seiner vollkommen zuverlässigen, bestimmten Form. Sieht man diese Form sich zeitweilig ändern, um darauf wieder normal zu werden, so darf man sich auf ein in dieser Weise erhaltenes Resultat mehr verlassen als auf Ergebnisse, die bei der Untersuchung eines isolierten Herzens erhalten werden.

Schon in dem mehr erwähnten Aufsatz über „Le Télécardiogramme" werden einige Elektrokardiogramme von Hunden abgebildet, bei denen der Einfluss von Vagusreizung nachgewiesen werden konnte. Wir vervollständigen hier die erwähnten Beobachtungen.

In Fig. 7 ist das Elektrokardiogramm eines Hundes reproduziert, der mit unversehrten Vagis untersucht wird. Nach der Aufnahme werden beide Vagi durchschnitten, und unmittelbar darauf wird eine neue Kurve, Fig. 8, registriert. Beide Figuren sind bei Stromableitung von der rechten Vorder- und der linken Hinterpfote erhalten worden, während zugleich der Blutdruck registriert wurde [1]).

Der auffälligste Unterschied, den beide Figuren aufweisen, ist die grössere Frequenz der Herzschläge nach dem Durchschneiden der Vagi. In Fig. 7 beträgt die Frequenz 103 Schläge in der Minute, in Fig. 8 ist dieselbe $2^1/_4$ mal grösser und beträgt 226 Schläge in der Minute. Diese starke Vermehrung beweist, dass die unversehrten

---

1) Für eine Beschreibung der Methode, nach welcher der Blutdruck registriert wurde, verweisen wir auf die Dissertation von Dr. Vaandrager. Hier sei nur erwähnt, dass 1 mm einer Ordinate auf dem Photogramm einer Blutdruckvariation von 10 mm Hg entspricht.

Vagi einen kräftigen Tonus unterhielten. In Fig. 8 folgen die Herzschläge so rasch aufeinander, dass die Kammersystole der vorhergehenden Periode noch nicht abgelaufen ist, wenn schon die neue Vorkammerkontraktion der folgenden Periode wieder beginnt. Die beiden Kontraktionen werden superponiert, was sich im Elektrokardiogramm reiner und deutlicher zeigt als in mancher auf mechanischem Wege erhaltenen Kurve.

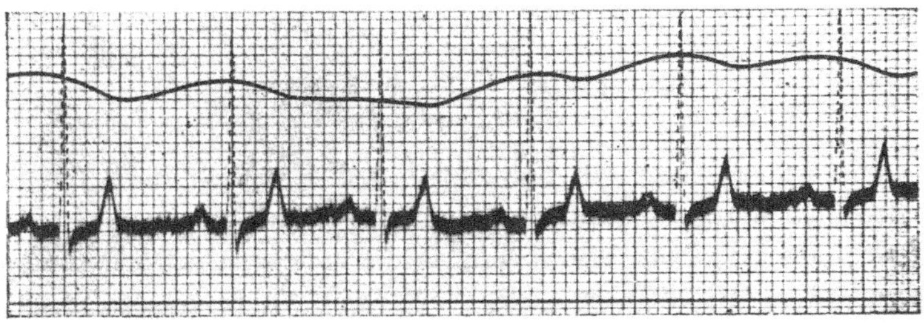

Fig. 7. Hund. Beide Vagi unversehrt. Blutdruck und Elektrokardiogramm. Stromableitung von rechter Vorderpfote und linker Hinterpfote. Absz. 1 mm = 0,04 Sek. Ordin. 1 mm = 10^{-4} Volt.

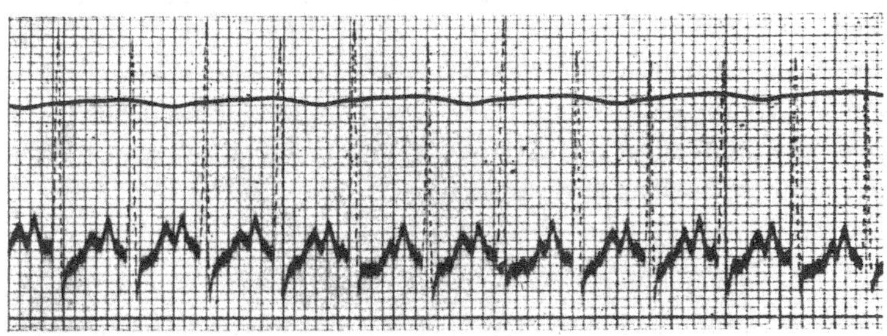

Fig. 8. Hund. Beide Vagi durchschnitten. Unmittelbar nach Fig. 8 aufgenommen. Die Stromableitung und der Wert der Koordinaten sind unverändert.

Die Superposition der elektrischen Schwankungen erschwert das Finden des richtigen Nullpunktes der Diastole. Man kann dafür die kurze horizontale Strecke nehmen, welche da und dort zwischen den Spitzen S und T der Kammersystole vorhanden ist, und deren Niveau nur wenig von dem Niveau der zwischen der Vorkammerspitze P und der ersten Kammerspitze Q befindlichen Phase abweicht.

Gehen wir von einem Durchschnittswerte dieser beiden Saitenstände als einer Basis aus, so können wir die Höhe der verschiedenen Spitzen in Fig. 8 leicht messen und mit jener der Spitzen von Fig. 7 vergleichen.

In der folgenden Tabelle sind die Messungsresultate in Millimetern oder Spannungsbeträgen von 10^{-4} Volt wiedergegeben. Die Ziffern geben die Durchschnittswerte an, die mit Benutzung der zur Verfügung stehenden langen Reihen von Elektrokardiogrammen berechnet sind, von denen Fig. 7 und 8 nur kurze Stücke reproduzieren.

	P	*Q*	*R*	*S*	*T*
Fig. 7	1,5	0,5	23	2	5
Fig. 8	4	0,5	23	3	4,5

Wir sehen, dass die Spitzen *Q* und *R* gleich hoch bleiben; *T* wird bei durchgeschnittenen Vagis ein wenig kleiner, *S* etwas grösser, aber weitaus die wichtigste Veränderung erfährt die Vorkammerspitze *P*, die bei durchschnittenen Vagis nahezu dreimal so hoch ist als bei unversehrten.

Wir müssen uns auch fragen, wie es mit den Zeitverhältnissen der Herztätigkeit steht. Selbstverständlich wird beim Wegfall des Vagustonus und der dadurch verursachten starken Zunahme der Pulsfrequenz die Herzpause verkürzt, und wir sahen schon oben, dass hierdurch eine Superposition von Kammer- und Vorkammerkontraktion entsteht. Aber unsere Frage nach den Zeitverhältnissen betrifft besonders die Zeitdauer der Systole. Wir finden durchschnittlich für die Dauer der Vorkammerkontraktion:

bei unversehrten Vagis 1,5 mm = 0,06 Sekunden,
„ durchschnittenen „ 1,2 „ = 0,05 „

Der Zeitraum zwischen dem Beginn der Vorkammerkontraktion und dem Beginn der Kammerkontraktion ist durchschnittlich:

bei unversehrten Vagis 3,3 mm = 0,13 Sekunden,
„ durchschnittenen „ 2,2 „ = 0,09 „

Die Dauer der Kammerkontraktion darf proportional angenommen werden dem in beiden Figuren leicht messbaren Abstand zwischen den Gipfeln der Spitzen *R* und *T*. Dieser Abstand beträgt:

bei unversehrten Vagis 4 mm = 0.16 Sekunden,
„ durchschnittenen „ 3,2 „ = 0,13 „

Die drei gemessenen Zeitwerte werden also durch den Wegfall des Vagustonus sämtlich verkürzt.

Wir lassen es vorläufig dahingestellt, ob die Veränderungen, welche die Höhe und die Dauer der Spitzen des Elektrogrammes beim Wegfall des Vagustonus erfahren, in direktem oder aber in indirektem Zusammenhang mit der Vaguswirkung stehen, aber in beiden abgebildeten Figuren sind sie leicht zu konstatieren, so dass an ihrem Vorhandensein nicht gezweifelt werden kann.

Obgleich wir aus der Höhe der Spitzen *P* und *R* nicht mit Bestimmtheit auf die Kraft schliessen können, mit welcher die Vorkammern und die Kammern sich zusammenziehen, so haben wir doch allen Grund, anzunehmen, dass bei den ziemlich gleichförmigen Figuren, womit wir in unserem Falle zu tun haben, die Höhe der Spitzen auch ungefähr einen Maassstab für die Kraft der Kontraktion an die Hand gibt. Dies voraussetzend folgern wir, dass beim Wegfall des Vagustonus die Vorkammerkontraktion wohl, die Kammerkontraktion nicht verstärkt wird. Zugleich werden, wie die Zeitmessungen lehren, sowohl die Dauer der Kammer- als die der Vorkammerkontraktion verkürzt, während der Übergang von der Vorkammer- zur Kammersystole erleichtert wird.

Im folgenden Abschnitt kommen wir beim menschlichen Elektrokardiogramm noch auf die Veränderung, welche die Kraft und die Dauer der Herztätigkeit erleiden, wenn im allgemeinen die Frequenz gesteigert wird, zurück. Jetzt müssen wir untersuchen, ob die Erfolge direkter Vagusreizung die oben erwähnten Ergebnisse in bezug auf die Vaguswirkung bestätigen.

In Fig. 9 sieht man den Erfolg schwacher Vagusreizung bei einem fünften Hunde abgebildet. Der Strom wird wieder von der rechten Vorder- und der linken Hinterpfote abgeleitet, während die Signallinie den Moment angibt, wo der durchschnittene rechte N. vagus an seinem peripherischen Ende gereizt wird. Die reizenden Induktionsströme bleiben nicht ganz im Nerv lokalisiert. Es werden Stromzweige gebildet, welche auch das Galvanometer erreichen und dem Saitenbilde so deutliche Schwingungen mitteilen, dass wir dadurch Gelegenheit bekommen, die Anzahl der in der Sekunde angebrachten Induktionsschläge genau zu zählen: es finden 62 Unterbrechungen in der Sekunde statt.

Wir müssen hier ausdrücklich erwähnen, dass der Induktionsapparat sowohl wie der Hund und das Saitengalvanometer sorgfältig von der Erde isoliert waren. Dass trotzdem ein deutlich merkbarer Stromübergang erfolgt, mahnt wohl zur Vorsicht; aber weil hier der

Ort nicht ist, die Mittel zu besprechen, durch welche man diesem Stromübergang vorbeugen kann, und weil dessen Betrag so gering ist, dass das Ergebnis unserer Versuche dadurch wahrscheinlich nicht verändert wird, dürfen wir uns damit begnügen, dass wir darauf aufmerksam gemacht haben.

In Fig. 9 sind nur zwei Erscheinungen, welche als Folge der Vagusreizung sehr auffallen:

1. die Verlängerung der Herzpause mit der dadurch herbeigeführten Verminderung der Herzfrequenz und
2. die Verkleinerung der Vorkammerspitze *P*.

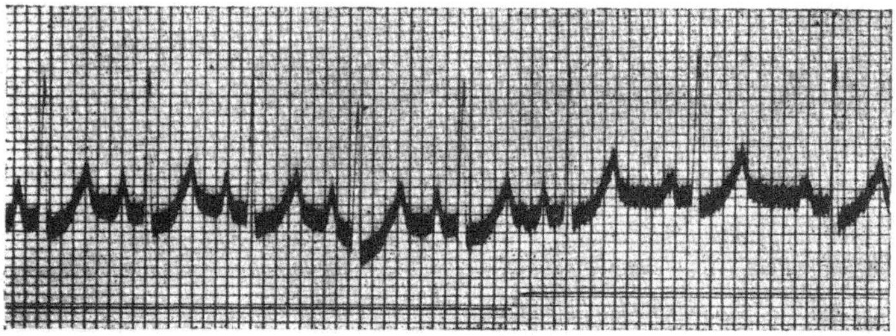

Fig. 9. Hund. Stromableitung von rechter Vorderpfote und linker Hinterpfote. Absz. 1 mm = 0,04 Sek. Ordin. 1 mm = 10^{-4} Volt. Schwache Vagusreizung.

Von den sonstigen Veränderungen, die weniger deutlich sind, kann mit Sicherheit nur noch eine kleine Verlängerung der Zeitdauer der Kammersystole erwähnt werden, die durch eine Vergrösserung des Abstandes zwischen den Gipfeln der Spitzen *R* und *T* zu erkennen ist. Vor der Vagusreizung beträgt dieser Abstand durchschnittlich 0,14 Sekunden, während der Vagusreizung 0,15 Sekunden. Der Einfluss der schwachen Vagusreizung, insofern man denselben konstatieren kann, stimmt also völlig überein mit dem, was die Durchschneidungsversuche erwarten liessen.

Reizt man den Vagus stärker, so dass das Herz zum Stillstehen gebracht wird, so erhält man Kurven, die, je nachdem die Bedingungen, unter denen der Versuch erfolgt, modifiziert werden, einige Unterschiede aufweisen. Es gibt jedoch einige Effekte, die konstant zum Vorschein kommen. So werden die ersten Kontraktionen, die nach dem Stillstande erfolgen, ausnahmslos von einer veränderten Vorkammerspitze begleitet.

Wir verfügen über 24 Reihen von Elektrokardiogrammen, bei denen durch starke Vagusreizung ein zeitweiliger Stillstand des Herzens erzielt wurde, und für welche bei sieben Hunden der Strom von der rechten Vorder- und der linken Hinterpfote abgeleitet worden war. Bei allen erhaltenen Kurven ist ein deutlicher Einfluss der Vagusreizung auf die Vorkammerkontraktion zu konstatieren[1]). Zuweilen wird die Vorkammerspitze bloss verkleinert, ohne dass ihre Form dabei eine deutliche Veränderung erleidet, wie unter anderem in der vorhergehenden, bei schwacher Vagusreizung erhaltenen Figur zu sehen ist. Aber oft wird auch die Form der Spitze modifiziert. Anstatt einer einzigen Erhebung über die Nullinie, der eine Senkung bis auf die ursprüngliche Höhe folgt, sieht man, dass die Kurve unmittelbar nach der Erhebung bis unter die Nullinie herabsinkt, um darauf allmählich wieder bis zu ihrem ursprünglichen Niveau zu steigen. In „Le Télécardiogramme" findet man diese Form der Vorkammerspitze als Folge von Vagusreizung beim Hunde in den Fig. 33 und 34 abgebildet.

Wir reproduzieren in Taf. XI, Fig. 1 noch ein anderes Beispiel, das an Deutlichkeit nichts zu wünschen übrig lässt. Zwischen den zwei, durch die Signallinie bezeichneten Augenblicken wird das peripherische Ende des durchgeschnittenen rechten Vagus mit Induktionsströmen gereizt. An den Schwingungen des Saitenbildes sieht man, dass, ebenso wie in der Textfigur 9, sich Zweige des reizenden Stromes durch das Galvanometer ausbreiten. Nachdem die Reizung schon eingesetzt hat, findet erst noch eine volle Periode der Herzwirkung statt, der alsdann ein Stillstand während der weiteren Reizung folgt. Sehr bald nach dem Aufhören der Reizung fängt das Herz wieder zu schlagen an. Die ersten Vorkammerspitzen weisen die oben beschriebenen Veränderungen auf, die allmählich geringer werden und beim sechsten Herzschlage etwa verschwinden. Von dem sechsten Herzschlag nach dem Stillstande ab ist keine oder so gut wie keine Veränderung der Vorkammerspitzen mehr merklich.

Ausser der oben beschriebenen Veränderung bemerken wir in der Figur noch als eine weitere Folge von Vagusreizung auf die

1) Vollständigkeitshalber sei hier mitgeteilt, dass wir ein Photogramm, das bei Stromableitung von den beiden Vorderpfoten erhalten wurde, und bei dem nur verhältnismässig kleine Spitzen zum Vorschein kamen, nicht mitrechnen. Bei peripherischer Vagusreizung erfolgte wohl ein vorübergehender Stillstand des Herzens, aber keine deutliche Veränderung in der Form der Vorkammerspitzen.

Wirkung der Vorkammern, dass die Dauer der Vorkammerkontraktion und auch das Intervall zwischen dem Beginn der Atriumsystole und dem Beginn der Ventrikelsystole ein wenig verlängert sind.

Alle hier beschriebenen Erscheinungen bestätigen die Ergebnisse der Versuche über den Vagustonus (siehe Fig. 7, 8 und 9) und müssen als konstante Folgen von Vagusreizung betrachtet werden.

Bevor wir den Einfluss des Vagus auf die Wirkung der Ventrikel näher beschreiben, erwähnen wir erst noch einige inkonstante auf die Vorkammern bezügliche Erscheinungen. Unter gewissen Umständen, besonders bei tiefer Chloroformnarkose, wird bei Vagusreizung die Leitung von den Vorkammern nach den Kammern dermaassen erschwert, dass auf die ersten schwachen, nach dem Stillstand des Herzens eintretenden Vorkammerkontraktionen keine Ventrikelsystolen folgen. In „Le Télécardiogramme“ sind in den Fig. 33 und 34 ein paar Beispiele dieses Zustandes von Herzblock gegeben. Wir reproduzieren in Taf. XI, Fig. 2 noch ein anderes Beispiel, bei welchem ausser dem Elektrokardiogramm noch der Blutdruck registriert ist. Das peripherische Ende des durchschnittenen rechten Vagus wird zwischen E und E_1 mit Induktionsströmen gereizt, wodurch der Blutdruck von 130 bis auf 32 mm Hg sinkt und ein Herzblock zum Vorschein kommt, der nach dem Obenerwähnten keiner weiteren Erklärung bedarf.

Die Veränderungen, welche sich bei Vagusreizung im Kammerelektrogramm zeigen, sind im allgemeinen weniger konstant als die der Vorkammerkurve. Als einzige konstante Veränderung, die wir in der Kammerkurve haben nachweisen können, nennen wir eine geringe Verlängerung der Dauer der Kammersystole. In Fig. 1, Taf. XI ist der Abstand zwischen den Gipfeln der Spitzen R und T vor der Reizung 0,14 Sek., während der entsprechende Abstand bei der ersten Systole nach der Reizung 0,02 Sek. mehr, also 0,16 Sek. beträgt. In Fig. 2, Taf. XI ist der gleichnamige Abstand vor der Reizung 0,185 Sek., nach der Reizung 0,20 Sek.

Die hier zum Vorschein kommenden Differenzen sind zwar gering, aber wir dürfen sie doch nicht übersehen, weil sie konstant vorzukommen scheinen und z. B. auch in den Fig. 7, 8 und 9 vorhanden sind, wo nur der normale Vagustonus resp. eine schwache Vagusreizung wirksam war.

Eine andere Frage ist natürlich, ob die nachgewiesene konstante Veränderung nun auch als ein Beweis für den direkten Einfluss des

Vagus auf die Herzkammern gelten darf. Wir glauben dies bezweifeln zu dürfen, nicht nur, weil die betreffende Veränderung uns dafür zu gering scheint, sondern namentlich auch deshalb, weil ihr Betrag in gar keinem Zusammenhang mit der Stärke der Vagusreizung steht.

Die Verlängerung des Abstandes zwischen den Gipfeln der Spitzen *R* und *T* muss vielleicht als eine Folge des veränderten Blutstroms von den Vorkammern nach den Kammern aufgefasst werden, während es auch möglich ist, dass eine Verengung der Aa. coronariae ihren Einfluss auf das Elektrogramm geltend macht.

Von den inkonstanten Veränderungen, die das Kammerelektrogramm aufweist, nennen wir an erster Stelle die Modifizierung der Spitze *T*. Ist diese Spitze vor der Vagusreizung aufwärts gerichtet, so kann sie nach der Vagusreizung verkleinert oder sogar nach unten gerichtet sein. Ist sie schon vor der Vagusreizung nach unten gerichtet, so kann sie nach der Reizung vertieft sein, wie z. B. in Fig. 2, Taf. XI ersichtlich ist.

Beide Veränderungsarten kommen vielfach vor, was durch eine Anzahl von Photogrammen, die zu unserer Verfügung stehen, aber hier nicht reproduziert werden, bewiesen wird. Ein einziges Mal sahen wir nach Vagusreizung eine atypische Herzkontraktion eintreten.

Die inkonstanten Veränderungen müssen verschiedenen Nebenumständen zugeschrieben werden, und es liegt noch weniger Grund vor, sie als Folgen direkter Vaguswirkung aufzufassen, als die zuerst genannten konstanten Veränderungen.

Wir weisen hier auch noch flüchtig auf den Reaktionsunterschied zwischen Vorkammern und Kammern hin. Erstere erholen sich nach einem durch starke Vagusreize verursachten Stillstand allmählich; sie fangen nach dem Stillstande zuweilen mit sehr schwachen, allmählich stärker werdenden Kontraktionen an und erreichen erst nach einiger Zeit ihre normale Kraft, eine Erscheinung, von der besonders in Fig. 34 von „Le Télécardiogramme" ein gutes Beispiel zu finden ist, die aber auch schon in Fig. 2, Taf. XI beobachtet werden kann.

Die Kammern verhalten sich ganz anders und folgen dem „Alles- oder Nichtsgesetz": wenn nach dem durch Vagusreizung verursachten Stillstande die Vorkammern schon wieder angefangen haben, sich rhythmisch zu kontrahieren, bleiben die Kammern oft noch einige Zeit in Ruhe. Sobald jedoch auch sie anfangen zu funktionieren, entwickeln sie gleich ihre volle Kraft[1]), und zwar meistens in einem Moment, wo die Vorkammern noch deutlich eine Nachwirkung der Vagusreizung aufweisen.

Schliesslich kommen wir kurz auf die positive Stromschwankung Gaskell's zurück. Die Schlüsse, welche Gaskell aus seinen Versuchen mit dem Schildkrötenherz zog, dürfen nicht auf das Hundeherz anwendbar erachtet werden. Wenigstens zeigt sich in unseren Elektrokardiogrammen des Hundes keine positive Stromschwankung als Folge von Vagusreizung.

Eine positive Stromesschwankung würde vermutlich im Gegensatz zu der aufwärts gerichteten normalen Vorkammerspitze eine Senkung des Saitenbildes zur Folge haben, aber man sieht, dass in den Fig. 1 und 2 der Taf. XI während der Vagusreizung das Saitenbild gerade höher steht als während der vorhergehenden und nachfolgenden diastolischen Phasen.

Diese Ortsveränderung, die übrigens gering ist und in Fig. 2, Taf. XI nur 1,2 Zehntausendstel eines Volts erreicht, wird wahrscheinlich durch andere Einflüsse als durch Wirkungen im Herzen verursacht. Wo das Galvanometer durch die Saitenschwingungen deutlich das Vorhandensein von Stromzweigen nachweist, die sich von dem reizenden Strome weit ausserhalb des gereizten Nerven ausbreiten, dort darf man voraussetzen, dass auch einige Körpermuskeln des Versuchstieres getroffen werden, welche alsdann ihren Aktionsstrom durch das Galvanometer schicken könnten.

Auch der direkte Stromübergang von dem Induktionsapparat nach dem Galvanometer könnte uns bei der Beurteilung des Nullstandes der Saite irreführen.

All diese Zweifel erwachsen aus dem Umstande, dass unsere Versuche nicht in der Absicht angestellt worden sind, zu untersuchen, ob die positive Stromesschwankung wohl oder nicht existiert. Wir sind davon überzeugt, dass das Problem mittels des durch das Saitengalvanometer registrierten Elektrokardiogrammes, — wenn nur die dafür nötigen technischen Vorbedingungen beachtet werden — mit aller wünschenswerten Sicherheit gelöst werden kann.

---

1) Siehe über den Zusammenhang zwischen dem Betrag der Potentialschwankungen und der Kraft der Herzkontraktion die einige Seiten früher in dieser Abhandlung darüber gemachte Bemerkung.

Verschiedene andere Einflüsse, welche die Form des Elektrokardiogrammes des Hundes modifizieren können.

Von den Umständen, welche die Form des Elektrokardiogramms des Hundes beeinflussen können, haben wir namentlich die Verblutung und die Chloroformnarkose untersucht.

Die deutlichste Veränderung, die nach Blutentziehung im Elektrokardiogramm erfolgt, ist das Tieferwerden der Spitze *T*. In der untenstehenden Fig. 10 ist das Elektrokardiogramm desselben Hundes abgebildet, von dem wir Fig. 2, Taf. XI erhalten haben, aber jetzt, nachdem dem Tiere aus der A. cruralis 100 ccm Blut entzogen worden sind.

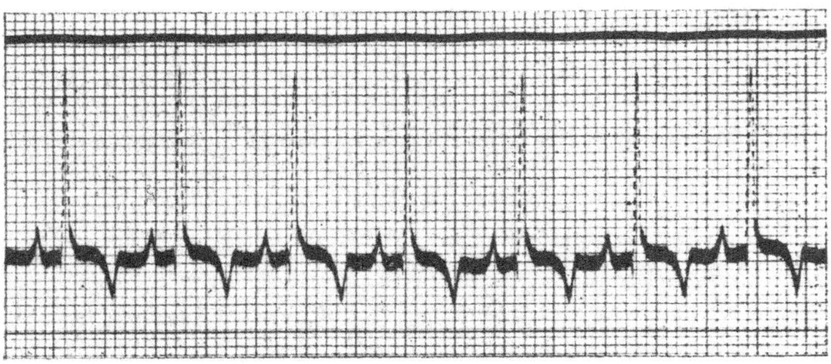

Fig. 10. Hund nach Blutentziehung.

Man sieht, dass die Spitze *R*, die in Fig. 2 der Tafel ungefähr 19×10^{-4} Volt erreicht, in Fig. 10 bis auf etwa 21×10^{-4} Volt vergrössert ist. Die Vorkammerspitzen sind in letzterer Figur auch deutlich höher geworden, aber am auffälligsten ist die Veränderung der Spitze *T*. Während einige Zeit nach der Registrierung von Fig. 2, Taf. XI das Elektrokardiogramm sich wieder ganz von den Folgen der Vagusreizung erholt und die Spitze *T* ihre ursprüngliche Grösse und Form zurückbekommen hatte, ist sie jetzt viel tiefer geworden. Nach der Blutentziehung hat die Spitze grosse Ähnlichkeit mit dem Bilde, das Fig. 2 der Tafel unmittelbar nach Vagusreizung von ihr aufweist. Der Blutdruck, der in Fig. 2 der Tafel vor der Vagusreizung 130 mm betrug, erreicht in Fig. 10 nur 110 mm.

Nun wird dem Tiere durch Öffnung der Bauchaorta noch mehr Blut entzogen. Das unter diesen Verhältnissen registrierte Elektrokardiogramm ist in Fig. 11 abgebildet.

Der Blutdruck beträgt am Beginn der Figur 21 mm, am Ende nur noch 13 mm Hg. Die Spitze *R* ist kleiner geworden und erreicht nur 14×10^{-4} Volt, während die Spitze *T* noch um $2{,}4 \times 10^{-4}$ Volt vertieft ist.

Der Einfluss der Blutentziehung auf die Form des Elektrokardiogrammes, der aus den beiden zuletzt abgebildeten Figuren hervorgeht, bestärkt uns in der Meinung, dass die Vertiefung der Spitze *T* nach Vagusreizung nicht die Folge direkter Vaguswirkung auf die Herzkammern ist, sondern Nebenumständen zugeschrieben werden muss. Nimmt doch bei Herzstillstand durch Vagusreizung der Blutdruck bedeutend ab, und die modifizierte Weise, in der das Herz sich zusammenzieht, könnte schon allein aus dieser Erniedrigung des Blutdruckes genügend erklärt werden.

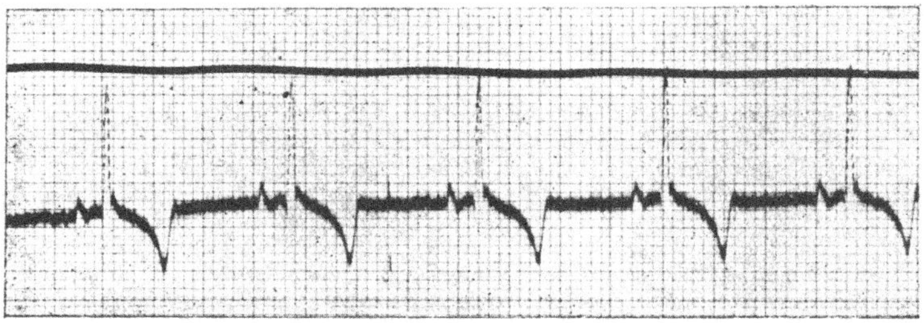

Fig. 11. Hund. Bauchaorta geöffnet.

Eine derartige Veränderung wie durch Blutentziehung wird im Elektrokardiogramm durch tiefe

Chloroformnarkose

hervorgerufen. In Fig. 12 sieht man die Kurve, die wir von einem Hunde bei oberflächlicher Chloroformnarkose erhielten, während unmittelbar darauf sehr viel Chloroform verabfolgt und Fig. 13 registriert wurde. Man sieht, wie beim Tieferwerden der Narkose die Spitze *T* eine Formveränderung erfährt und dabei $3{,}2 \times 10^{-4}$ Volt unter die Nullinie sinkt.

Es gibt noch eine Anzahl anderer Veränderungen, die durch eine tiefe Chloroformnarkose in den elektromotorischen Erscheinungen des Herzens, d. h. folglich auch in der Herztätigkeit selbst, hervorgerufen werden. Wir haben manchmal die Narkose so weit getrieben, dass die eigenen Atembewegungen des Hundes aufhörten, wodurch die Erscheinungen von O-Mangel und CO_2-Vergiftung sich mit denen der Chloroformnarkose vermischten und die Anwendung künstlicher Atmung nötig war, das Tier am Leben zu erhalten. Die Chloroformmenge bis zu einem Maximum steigern zu können, haben wir später den Atmungsapparat benutzt, der schon früher im Laboratorium bei der Untersuchung der Bronchialmuskeln angewendet wurde[1]).

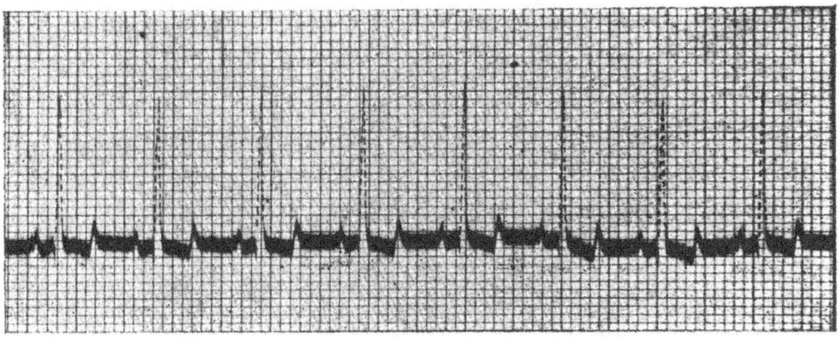

Fig. 12. Hund. Oberflächliche Chloroformnarkose.

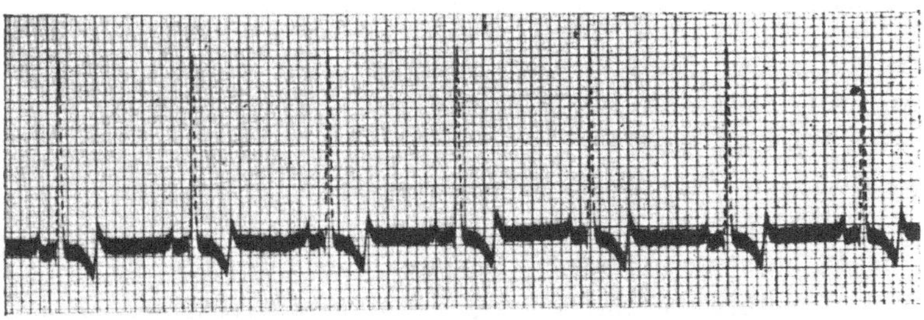

Fig. 13. Hund. Tiefe Chloroformnarkose.

Mit dieser Vorrichtung, deren Beschreibung wir hier übergehen dürfen, ist man imstande, bei einem Hunde auf solche Weise die Atmung künstlich zu erhalten, dass das Tier bei übermässiger Luftzufuhr jedes erwünschte Quantum Chloroform bekommt. Das Aufhören der eigenen Atembewegungen des Tieres bietet nun keine Schwierigkeit mehr für die weitere Verabfolgung von Chloroform, die, wenn man

1) Siehe: Über die Wirkung der Bronchialmuskeln, nach einer neuen Methode untersucht, und über Asthma nervosum. Pflüger's Arch. f. d. ges. Physiol. Bd. 51 S. 367. 1892 und Onderzoekingen physiol. Laborat. Leiden, 2. R. I p. 28.

es wünscht, leicht so weit getrieben werden kann, dass das Tier bei einem Übermaass von O und einem Minimum von CO_2 durch eine reine Chloroformvergiftung getötet wird.

Ist die Narkose tief, so wird die Leitung von den Vorkammern nach den Kammern erschwert; es treten einige Vorkammerkontraktionen ein, denen keine Kammerkontraktionen folgen, wodurch das Vorhandensein von Herzblock erwiesen wird. Schliesslich kann eine vollständige Dissoziation oder Allorhythmie der Tätigkeit von Kammern und Vorkammern entstehen, welche Erscheinung man in „Le Télécardiogramme" — Fig. 1 der Tafel — abgebildet findet. Auch die Entstehung atypischer Herzkontraktionen scheint durch eine tiefe Narkose befördert zu werden.

Alle Veränderungen im Elektrokardiogramm, die wir als die Folge tiefer Narkose haben kennen lernen, werden merkwürdigerweise durch Vagusreizung während der Narkose verstärkt. Namentlich trifft dies vom Herzblock zu, der regelmässig eintritt, wenn man unter tiefer Narkose den Vagus reizt.

Die in „Le Télécardiogramme" reproduzierten Beispiele von Herzblock und das von Fig. 2 unserer Taf. XI sind sämtlich durch Vagusreizung bei tiefer Narkose erhalten, und es liegt die Vermutung nahe, dass wir zur Erklärung dieser Erscheinung der kombinierten Wirkung des Chloroforms und der durch den Herzstillstand hervorgerufenen Blutdruckabnahme Rechnung tragen müssen.

Schliesslich gestatten wir uns die Bemerkung, dass der deutlich und leicht zu konstatierende Einfluss, den das Chloroform auf die elektromotorischen Erscheinungen des Herzens ausübt, vielleicht später, wenn die Anwendung des Saitengalvanometers allgemeiner geworden sein sollte, auch eine praktische Bedeutung für den Chirurgen wird bekommen können, der vor und vielleicht auch während der Narkose seiner Patienten sich über ihre Herztätigkeit zu erkundigen wünscht.

4. Das menschliche Elektrokardiogramm.

Während bei der Registrierung des menschlichen Elektrokardiogrammes dieselbe Art von Drahtverbindung und dieselbe Methode der Widerstandsmessung angewendet worden sind wie bei der Untersuchung des Frosch- und des Hundeherzens, haben wir für die Verbindung der Versuchspersonen mit dem Galvanometer andere

Elektroden gebraucht. Diese sind schon früher beschrieben[1]) und wiederholt im hiesigen physiologischen Laboratorium verwendet worden, aber bis jetzt fehlte eine Angabe ihres Widerstandes.

Als Elektrodenwiderstand wurde von uns der Widerstand gemessen, der zwischen zwei amalgamierten Zinkplatten vorhanden war (siehe Fig. 14). Eine der beiden Platten war in die Na Cl-Lösung der Tonzelle *P* eingetaucht, wo sie die menschliche Hand vertrat, während die andere Platte *Z* sich wie beim gewöhnlichen Registrieren in der $ZnSO_4$-Lösung befand, womit der Glaszylinder *G* gefüllt war. Bei der Widerstandsmessung haben wir uns keine Mühe gegeben, die Polarisation zwischen dem Zink und der Na Cl-Lösung vollständig aufzuheben. Dennoch wurde für unseren Zweck der Polarisationsstrom in genügendem Maasse herabgemindert, indem wir die Stromesrichtung in der Elektrode schnell und wiederholt umkehrten. Auch wurden verschiedene Stromstärken angewendet.

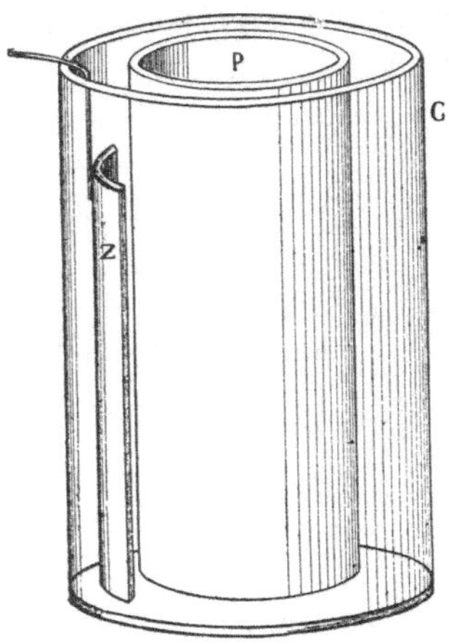

Fig. 14.

Eine Anzahl von Messungen bei zwei verschiedenen Tonzellen ergaben als Minimum 0,72 Ohm, als Maximum 1,09 Ohm, welche Beträge ohne Bedenken in Bezug auf den Widerstand des menschlichen Körpers vernachlässigt werden dürfen, da letztere unter den Verhältnissen, unter denen wir arbeiten, 1000—2000 mal grösser war.

Um die verschiedenen Formen von Elektrokardiogrammen leicht miteinander vergleichen zu können, ist in Fig. 4 von „Le Télécardiogramme" ein Schema[2]) gegeben, das einer früher mittels des Kapillar-Elektrometers angestellten Untersuchung entnommen worden ist. Dieses Schema musste mit Hilfe einer Anzahl von Messungen

1) Siehe W. Einthoven und K. de Lint, Über das normale menschliche Elektrokardiogramm. Pflüger's Arch. f. d. ges. Physiol. Bd. 80 S. 140. 1900.

2) Siehe auch: Über die Form des menschlichen Elektrokardiogrammes. Pflüger's Arch. f. d. ges. Physiol. Bd. 60 S. 101. 1895 und die galvanometrische Registrierung des menschlichen Elektrokardiogrammes, zugleich eine Beurteilung der Anwendung des Kapillarelektrometers in der Physiologie. Ibidem Bd. 99 S. 472. 1903.

und Berechnungen aus einer willkürlich gewählten kapillar-elektrometrischen Kurve konstruiert werden, und mag es auch prinzipiell durchaus mit einem saitengalvanometrischen Elektrokardiogramm übereinstimmen, selbstverständlich weicht es doch in einigen Einzelheiten von letzterem ab.

Anstatt des Schemas nehmen wir deshalb lieber eine wirklich mit dem Saitengalvanometer registrierte Kurve als Basis unserer Vergleichungen an (siehe Fig. 15).

Während diese wieder dieselben fünf Spitzen *P*, *Q*, *R*, *S* und *T* aufweist, bemerken wir ausdrücklich, dass wir ebensowenig mit der Kurve von Fig. 15 als mit dem früheren Schema eine Form anzugeben meinen, die als Durchschnittsform aller menschlichen Elektrokardiogramme gelten könnte[1]). Wir wünschen nur eine Vergleichungsbasis zu haben und wählen dazu selbstverständlich eine

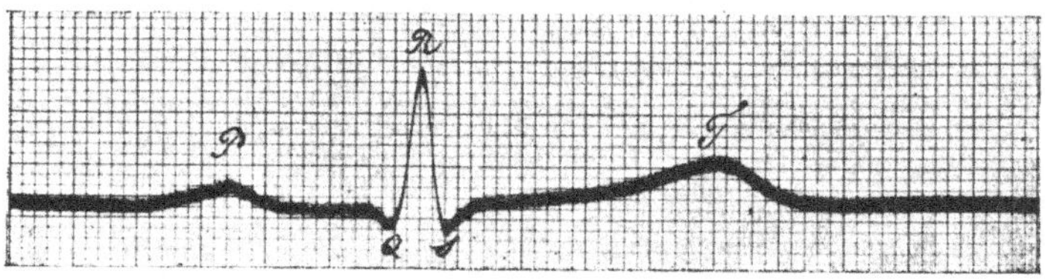

Fig. 15. *Me.* Stromableitung von rechter Hand und linkem Fuss. Absz. 1 mm = 0,01 Sek. Ordin. 1 mm = 10^{-4} Volt.

Form, die uns zweckmässig erscheint, und mit welcher zahlreiche andere normale Elektrokardiogramme Ähnlichkeit aufweisen.

Um die Form der Spitzen besser hervortreten zu lassen, ist in unserem Musterelektrokardiogramm die Geschwindigkeit der empfindlichen Platte bis zum Vierfachen des gewöhnlichen Betrages gesteigert, während die Empfindlichkeit des Galvanometers unverändert geblieben ist. In Fig. 15 haben wir also 1 mm einer Abszisse = 0,01 Sekunde und 1 mm einer Ordinate = 10^{-4} Volt.

1) In Nagel's Handbuch der Physiologie des Menschen Bd. 1 S. 253 nennt Hofmann das obenerwähnte Schema „Normalform des menschlichen Elektrokardiogramms". Der Ausdruck „Normalform" könnte zu Irrtümern veranlassen. Von vielen normalen Personen mit gesundem Herzen werden Elektrokardiogramme erhalten, deren Form nicht unbedeutend von der schematischen Form und auch von der oben abgebildeten Vergleichsbasis abweicht, während all diese Kurven doch normale Elektrokardiogramme genannt werden müssen.

Das Elektrokardiogramm des Hundes von Fig. 5 ist in einem Koordinatensystem abgebildet, das völlig mit dem obenstehenden von Fig. 15 übereinstimmt, so dass beide Kurven, die des Menschen und die des Hundes unmittelbar miteinander verglichen werden können. Welche Unterschiede sie untereinander aufweisen, ist schon im vorigen Abschnitt besprochen worden, so dass wir jetzt darauf nicht zurückzukommen brauchen.

Eine Frage, welche geraume Zeit unbeantwortet geblieben ist, bezieht sich auf die kleinen unregelmässigen Schwingungen, die, unabhängig von den fünf beschriebenen typischen Spitzen, in vielen Elektrokardiogrammen des Menschen sowohl wie des Hundes vorkommen. Bei Gelegenheit einer früheren Untersuchung war schon ausgemacht worden, dass die erwähnten Schwingungen nicht durch Bodenerschütterungen oder durch andere technische Unvollkommenheiten der Versuche entstehen, sondern dass sie tatsächlich der Ausdruck von Potentialschwankungen sind, deren Ursprung im lebendigen Körper liegt. Gleichwohl war noch unentschieden geblieben, ob letztere durch das Herz oder durch andere Organe hervorgerufen werden.

Die Entscheidung ist später leicht und gleichsam von selbst erfolgt. Aus der grossen Anzahl von Elektrokardiogrammen, die unter den verschiedensten Verhältnissen registriert worden sind, geht mit genügender Sicherheit hervor, dass die besagten unregelmässigen kleinen Potentialschwankungen durch elektromotorische Wirkungen in den Skelettmuskeln verursacht werden.

Im vorigen Abschnitt erwähnten wir schon, dass die Stellung der Saite unruhig wird, sobald man ein Elektrokardiogramm eines Hundes schreibt, der in den Tonzellen der Elektroden stehend untersucht wird. Kleine sichtbare Zitterungen des Tieres, welche vielleicht noch durch die gewöhnliche für das Stehen erforderliche Muskelanstrengung verstärkt werden, rufen Schwankungen der Saite hervor, die, sobald man das Tier ruhig niederlegt, schon bedeutend abnehmen. Um diese Saitenschwankungen ganz aufhören zu lassen, braucht man das Tier nur so weit zu narkotisieren, dass es ruhig schläft. Wird der Hund bequem niedergelegt und namentlich gut warm gehalten, so dass er keine Neigung zum Zittern zeigt, so reicht schon eine oberflächliche Narkose für den Zweck aus.

Bei der Registrierung des menschlichen Elektrokardiogrammes wurde die Versuchsperson in möglichst bequemer Haltung auf einen

Stuhl gesetzt oder zu Bett gelegt und um zu verhindern, dass sie — sich für die Untersuchung des eigenen Herzens interessierend — unwillkürlich ihre Haltung in dem Augenblick änderte, wo die photographische Aufnahme stattfinden sollte, wurde der Registrierapparat, ohne dass sie selbst es bemerkte, in Bewegung gesetzt.

Wurde ein Telekardiogramm geschrieben, wobei der Patient sich im Universitäts-Krankenhause befand, während das Galvanometer im physiologischen Laboratorium aufgestellt blieb, so konnten wir natürlich leicht der besagten Anforderung genügen. Aber auch wenn der Patient im Laboratorium untersucht wurde, bot sich keine Schwierigkeit dar, weil er in ein anderes Zimmer gebracht werden konnte, als wo das Galvanometer sich befand. Dennoch blieben in der Regel die Saitenschwankungen nicht ganz aus, während sie bei einigen Patienten, die an einem krankhaften Zittern litten, sogar stark hervortraten und dadurch die Beurteilung des Elektrokardiogrammes erschwerten. Unter diesen Verhältnissen dürfte man von einer Narkose unzweifelhaft gute Dienste erwarten[1]).

Einfluss der Stellen, von denen der Strom abgeleitet wird.

Wir müssen jetzt den Formunterschieden, die das Elektrokardiogramm bei Veränderung der Stromableitung aufweist, einige Zeilen widmen.

Waller[2]) teilte bekanntlich den Körper in zwei Teile, von denen der eine das Potential der Herzbasis, der andere das der Herzspitze annehmen sollte. Zum ersteren Teile rechnete er den Kopf und den rechten Arm, zum letzteren den linken Arm und die beiden Beine. Stromableitung zwischen zwei zu verschiedenen Teilen gehörigen Stellen sollte grosse Potentialschwankungen verursachen und folglich eine günstige Kombination genannt werden dürfen, während Stromableitung zwischen zwei zum selben Teile gehörigen Stellen eine ungünstige Kombination ergeben sollte.

1) Bei einer späteren Gelegenheit hoffen wir von den frequenten Potentialschwankungen, die durch die Kontraktion der willkürlichen Muskeln verursacht werden, Gebrauch zu machen, um die verschiedenen Arten des Zitterns voneinander zu unterscheiden. Wahrscheinlich wechselt der Rhythmus der Reize, die eine Muskelkontraktion herbeiführen, je nachdem der Ursprung dieser Reize mehr peripherisch oder mehr zentral liegt.

2) A. a. O.

Die Wahrnehmungen mit dem Saitengalvanometer stimmen mit dieser Vorstellung, die auf der früheren Untersuchung mit dem Kapillarelektrometer beruht, nicht völlig überein. Namentlich wenn der Strom von der linken Hand und einem der Füsse abgeleitet wird, treten oft bedeutende Potentialschwankungen auf. Dass Waller letztere Kombination zu den ungünstigen rechnet, muss wahrscheinlich dem Umstande zugeschrieben werden, dass dabei besonders die stumpfe Spitze *T*, die infolge ihrer längeren Dauer besser als die anderen Spitzen durch das Kapillarelektrometer wiedergegeben wird, klein ist. Die um so viel schärfere Spitze *R* kann im saitengalvanometrischen Elektrokardiogramm, das die richtige Form der Potentialschwankungen abbildet, viel höher sein, während diese Spitze, weil sie von nur kurzer Dauer ist, in einer kapillarelektrometrischen Kurve nicht zu ihrem Rechte kommt. Hier könnte sie sogar unter gewissen Verhältnissen übersehen werden.

Welche enormen Beträge die Potentialschwankungen bei Stromableitung von der linken Hand und dem linken Fusse erreichen können, zeigt sich besonders deutlich in pathologischen Fällen von Hypertrophie des rechten und von Hypertrophie des linken Herzens. Man findet die dabei erhaltenen Kurven in den Fig. 17—20 von „Le Télécardiogramme" abgebildet, während auch in den Fig. 18, 21, 24 und 25 dieser Abhandlung Beispiele von Elektrokardiogrammen gegeben werden, die bei derselben Ableitung registriert worden sind und das Vorhandensein beträchtlicher Potentialschwankungen nachweisen.

Bei unserer Untersuchung sind als Stromableitungsstellen bloss die Hände und die Füsse verwendet worden. Hierbei wurden verschiedene Kombinationen gemacht, von denen jedoch die Stromableitung von beiden Füssen bald aufgegeben wurde, weil diese, wie Fig. 6 von „Le Télécardiogramme" zeigt, nur Kurven mit sehr niedrigen Spitzen lieferte. Infolgedessen war es auch, wenn eine der Elektroden an einen Fuss angelegt werden musste, ziemlich gleichgültig, welcher Fuss gewählt wurde. Wir wählten immer den linken Fuss, und so blieben uns nur noch drei Weisen von Stromableitungen übrig:

I in querer Richtung, von den beiden Händen,

II in schräger Richtung, von der rechten Hand und dem linken Fuss,

III in der Längsrichtung, von der linken Hand und dem linken Fuss.

Wir bemerken, dass beim Wechsel der Stellen, von denen der Strom abgeleitet wird, die verschiedenen Spitzen des Elektrokardiogrammes nicht immer gleichmässig vergrössert oder verkleinert werden, wodurch also die Form der Kurve überhaupt mehr oder weniger modifiziert wird. Während die Entstehung dieser Form im Zusammenhang mit der Weise, wie die Kontraktionswelle im Herzmuskel fortschreitet, erst im folgenden Abschnitt ausführlicher behandelt werden wird, dürfen wir hier doch als fast selbstredend bemerken, dass die durch die Veränderung der Stromableitung hervorgerufenen Unterschiede unter anderem auch durch die Lage des Herzens im Körper bedingt werden. Es muss sogar in vielen Fällen die Lage des Herzens durch die elektrische Untersuchung bestimmt werden können. Dergleichen Bestimmungen sind schon früher ausgeführt worden [1]), wobei aber weniger Aufmerksamkeit der allgemeinen Form der Kurven als der Höhe der wichtigsten Spitzen gewidmet wurde. Doch genügten letztere schon, um konstatieren zu können, dass z. B. bei v. d. W. die Herzachse mehr von hinten nach vorn gerichtet ist als bei de Lt., und dass die Herzachse bei Bm. mehr von oben nach unten und weniger von rechts nach links gerichtet ist als bei v. d. W.

Jetzt, wo wir im Saitengalvanometer einen um soviel bequemeren und schneller funktionierenden Apparat besitzen, kann auch die Bedeutung der Kurvenform überhaupt zu ihrem vollen Rechte kommen, wodurch kleine Lageabweichungen des Herzens viel genauer bestimmt werden können.

Es ist uns jedoch hauptsächlich darum zu tun, die W i r k u n g des Herzens besser kennen zu lernen, und es leuchtet ein, dass, wenn schon durch eine Lageabweichung dieses Organs eine Formveränderung des Elektrokardiogrammes herbeigeführt wird, es einigermassen schwierig halten muss, aus dieser Form zugleich auch die Wirkung des Herzens zu beurteilen.

Die Aufgabe kann am besten gelöst werden, wenn man von der Person, deren Herzwirkung untersucht wird, Elektrokardiogramme bei mehr als einer Weise von Stromableitung aufnimmt und also trachtet, sich von dem Einfluss der Lageabweichungen des Herzens möglichst unabhängig zu machen. In „Le Télécardiogramme“ ist der Kürze halber von einem Patienten meistens nur eine Kurve ver-

1) Vgl. W. E i n t h o v e n und K. d e L i n t, a. a. O.

öffentlicht, aber ausnahmslos sind doch immer von jedem Kranken die Elektrokardiogramme bei den drei obenerwähnten Ableitungen I, II und III aufgenommen worden.

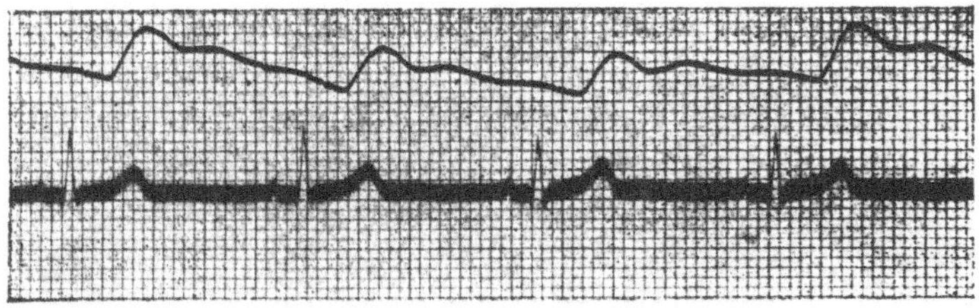

Fig. 16. *Ei.* Karotispuls und Elektrokardiogramm. Ableitung I.

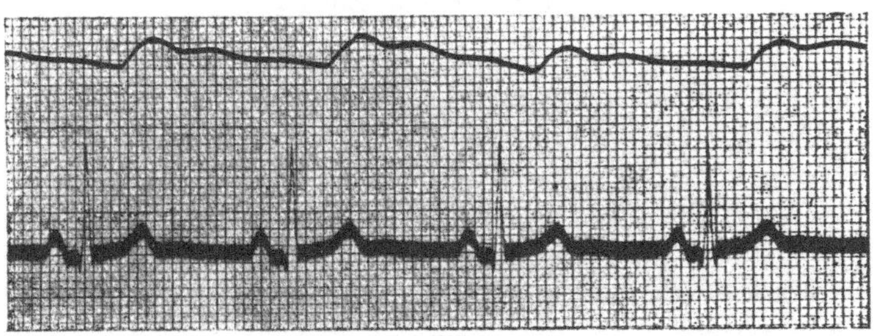

Fig. 17. *Ei.* Karotispuls und Elektrokardiogramm. Ableitung II.

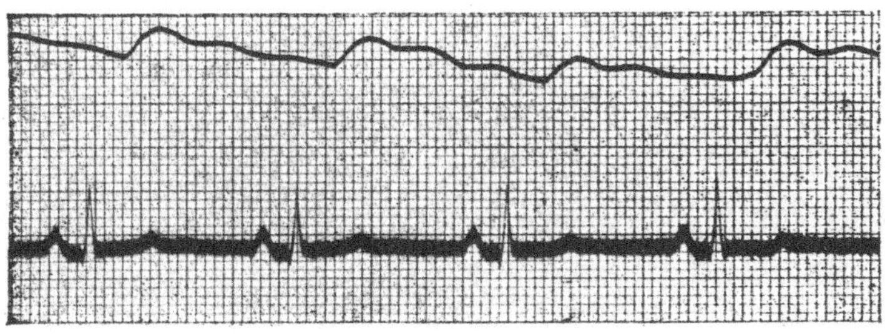

Fig. 18. *Ei.* Karotispuls und Elektrokardiogramm. Ableitung III.

Wir haben uns immer an die Regel gehalten, bei jeder zu untersuchenden Person diese drei Ableitungen anzuwenden. Sie erscheinen uns bei einer über viele Personen sich erstreckenden Untersuchung am zweckmässigsten, weshalb wir die Besonderheiten, welche sie aufweisen, hier des näheren besprechen werden.

Erstens sei erwähnt, dass beim Menschen wie beim Hunde die Spitzen meistens bei Ableitung II am grössten sind. Zuweilen ist die hierbei erhaltene Kurve den bei den Ableitungen I und III erhaltenen sehr ähnlich.

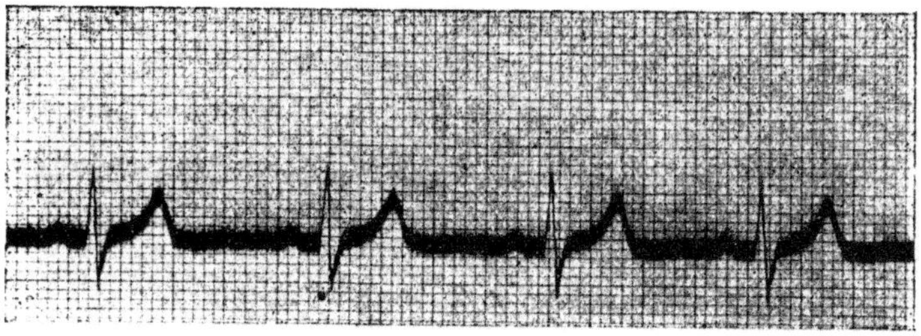

Fig. 19. *Fl.* Ableitung I.

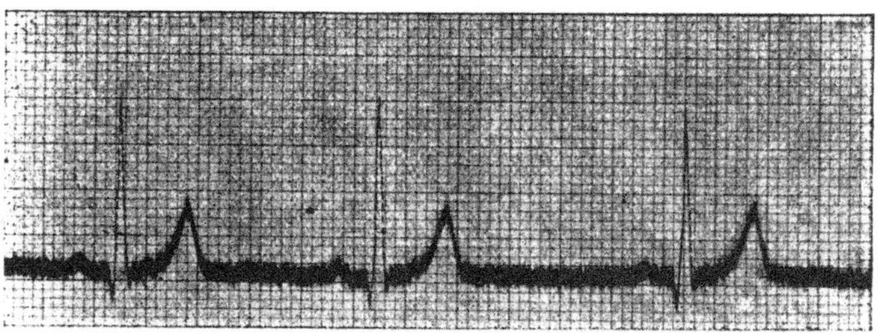

Fig. 20. *Fl.* Ableitung. II.

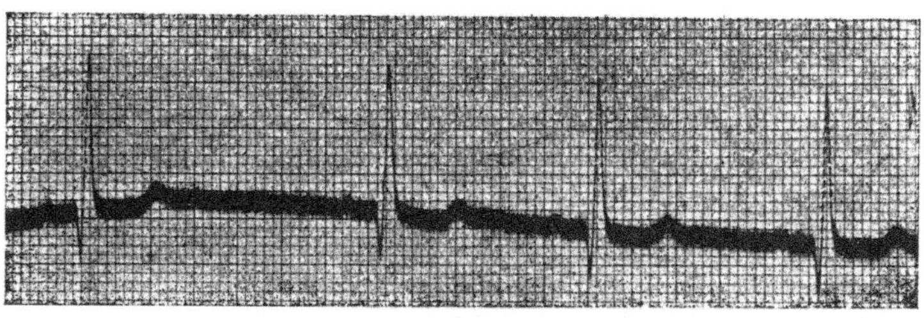

Fig. 21. *Fl.* Ableitung III.

Als Beispiel mögen die drei auf vorangehender Seite abgebildeten, bei den genannten Ableitungsweisen registrierten Kurven von Ei. dienen [1]).

1) Wenn nicht ausdrücklich eine andere Angabe gemacht wird, ist bei allen hier reproduzierten menschlichen Elektrokardiogrammen das Koordinatensystem so gewählt, dass 1 mm einer Abszisse $= 0{,}04$ Sek. und 1 mm einer Ordinate $= 10^{-4}$ Volt ist.

Man sieht, dass in jeder der drei Figuren die fünf Spitzen *P*, *Q*, *R*, *S* und *T* sichtbar sind. In Fig. 17, bei Ableitung II, sind alle Spitzen am grössten. In Fig. 16, bei Ableitung I, ist namentlich die Spitze *Q* sehr klein, während in Fig. 18, bei Ableitung III, die Spitze *T* im Verhältnis zu den anderen Spitzen die stärkste Verkleinerung erlitten hat.

Im Gegensatz zu *Ei.* weist *Fl.* bei den drei gebräuchlichen Ableitungsarten drei stark voneinander abweichende Formen von Elektrokardiogrammen auf. Dieselben sind in den obenstehenden Fig. 19, 20 und 21 abgebildet.

Man sieht, dass die wichtigsten Spitzen *R* und *T* wieder bei Ableitung II am grössten sind (siehe Fig. 20), während die Kurve bei Ableitung I (siehe Fig. 19) sich durch eine tiefe Spitze *S* von

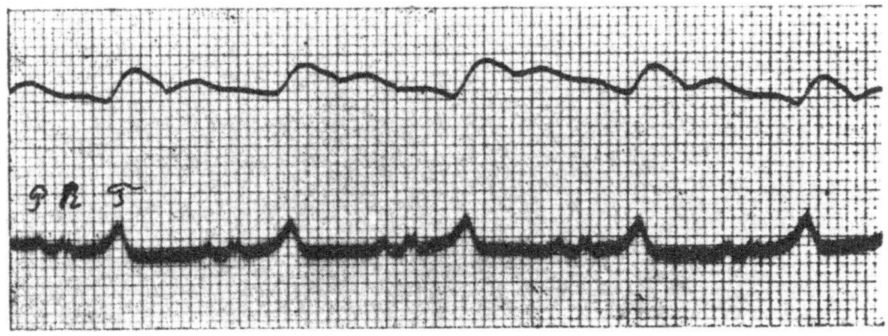

Fig. 22. *Wi.* Karotispuls und Elektrokardiogramm. Ableitung I.

Fig. 20 unterscheidet. Die Kurve bei Ableitung III ist wieder durch die geringe Grösse der Spitze *T* und namentlich durch eine sehr tiefe Spitze *Q* gekennzeichnet.

Die wichtigsten Spitzen im Elektrokardiogramm sind, ausser der Vorkammerspitze *P*, die beiden Kammerspitzen *R* und *T*. Dass ihre Bedeutung nur beurteilt werden kann, wenn man bei derselben Person mehr als eine Ableitung anwendet, ist z. B. aus dem Elektrokardiogramm von *Wi.* ersichtlich, das bei Ableitung I erhalten wurde und in Fig. 22 abgebildet ist. Die Spitze *R* ist hier sehr eigentümlich geformt und viel kleiner als *T*. Wir werden sogleich noch sehen, wie die Spitze, die wir hier *R* nennen, aus der Verschmelzung der drei im Musterelektrokardiogramm angegebenen Spitzen *Q*, *R* und *S* hervorgegangen ist. Während in der zu unserer Verfügung stehenden Sammlung von Elektrokardiogrammen eine solche Spitze *R* nur äusserst selten vorkommt, stellt *Wi.* bei anderer Ableitung ein Elektrokardiogramm dar, dessen Form mit der der meist vorkommenden Elektrokardiogramme übereinstimmt. Als Beweis hierfür wird in Fig. 23 die bei Ableitung II von ihm aufgenommene Kurve reproduziert.

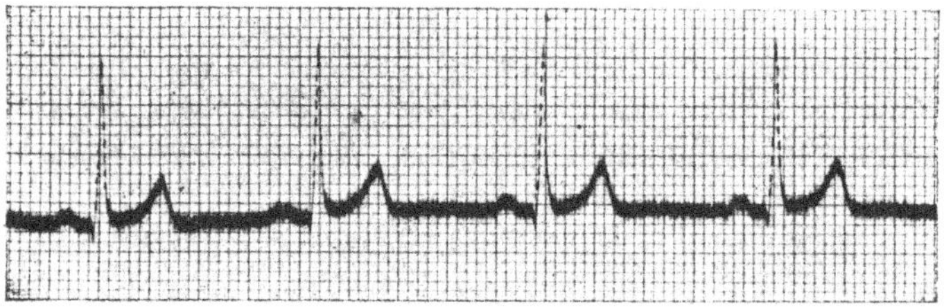

Fig. 23. *Wi.* Ableitung II.

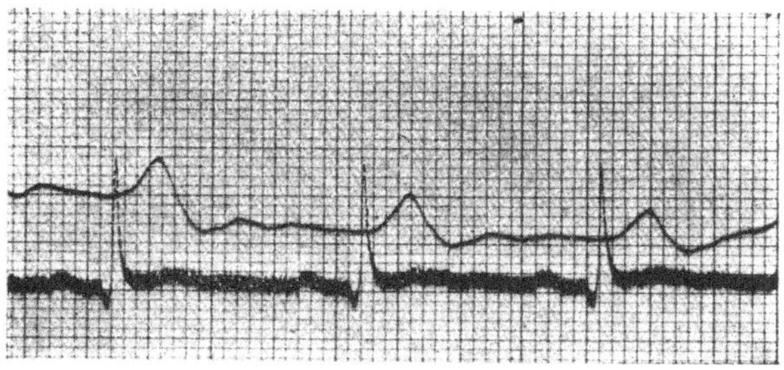

Fig. 24. *Ca.* Karotispuls und Elektrokardiogramm. Ableitung III.

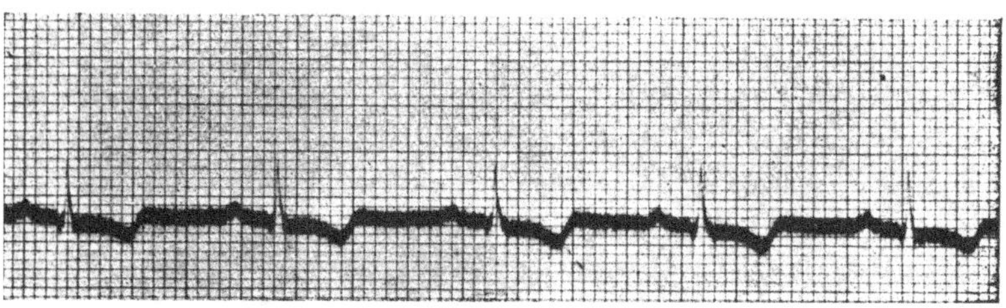

Fig. 25. *Va.* Ableitung III.

Die Spitze *T* ist in normalen Herzen bei Ableitung I und II immer ziemlich gross, während sie bei Ableitung III in der Regel klein ist, ja oft ganz verschwindet oder negativ wird. Eine kleine Spitze *T* bei Ableitung III findet man schon in den obenstehenden

Fig. 18 und 21 abgebildet. Weiter sind in den Fig. 24 und 25 die Elektrokardiogramme von *Ca.* resp. *Va.* bei derselben Ableitung III reproduziert. Ersteres gibt ein Beispiel von dem fast vollständigen Verschwinden, letzteres von dem Negativwerden der Spitze *T.* Sowohl *Ca.* wie *Va.* weisen bei Ableitung I und II keine nennenswerten Besonderheiten in ihrem Elektrokardiogramm auf, und es darf hier ausdrücklich erwähnt werden, dass alle oben besprochenen Kurven von Personen erhalten worden sind, deren Herz keine krankhaften Abweichungen zeigte.

Selbstverständlich muss zwischen den bei den drei verschiedenen Ableitungsweisen von derselben Person erhaltenen Elektrokardiogrammen ein enger Zusammenhang bestehen, und zwar derartig, dass, sobald zwei Formen bekannt sind, man immer die dritte daraus berechnen können muss. Muss doch der bei Ableitung II (von der rechten Hand und dem linken Fuss) und Ableitung I (von der rechten und der linken Hand) sich zeigende Unterschied der elektrischen Spannungen gleich sein der elektrischen Spannung bei Ableitung III (von der linken Hand und dem linken Fuss), was sich folgendermaassen kurz formulieren lässt:

Ableitung II — Ableitung I = Ableitung III.

Wie schon in „Le Télécardiogramme“ erwähnt wird, würde diese Berechnung nicht nur als Kontrolle auf die Genauigkeit der verrichteten Arbeit nützlich sein können, sondern sie wäre auch bei der Identifizierung der in verschiedenen Elektrokardiogrammen mit denselben Buchstaben bezeichneten Spitzen verwendbar. Die Aufgabe mag aber noch so einfach erscheinen, bei der Ausführung stösst man auf Schwierigkeiten, deren wichtigste Ursache gerade in dem Umstande liegt, dass die mit denselben Buchstaben bezeichneten Spitzen oft n i c h t in identische Phasen einer Herzperiode fallen.

Letzteres kann leicht nachgewiesen werden. Man beachte z. B. die obenstehenden drei Elektrokardiogramme von *Ei.*, Fig. 16, 17 und 18, und messe den Abstand zwischen den genau bestimmbaren Gipfeln der Spitzen *P*, *R* und *T*. Bei Ableitung I, Fig. 16, beträgt der Abstand zwischen den Gipfeln der Spitzen *P* und *R* durchschnittlich 2,8 mm, während der nämliche Abstand bei Ableitung III, Fig. 18, einen Durchschnittsbetrag von 3,7 mm erreicht. Wenn also der Gipfel der Spitze *P* bei beiden Kurven in dieselbe Phase einer Herzperiode fällt, und wenn dabei — was wir vorläufig wohl annehmen dürfen — die untersuchten Herzperioden gleich gross sind, so ist es unmöglich, dass auch *R* bei beiden Ableitungen dieselbe Phase der Herztätigkeit darstellt[1]).

Dieselbe Behauptung kann auf den Abstand zwischen den Spitzen *R* und *T* gegründet werden. Bei Ableitung I beträgt dieser 6,4 mm, bei Ableitung III 7,1 mm.

In den Elektrokardiogrammen vieler anderen Personen werden entsprechende Abstandsunterschiede wahrgenommen, z. B. in denen von *Fl.* (siehe die Fig. 19, 20 und 21). Bei Ableitung I beträgt der Abstand zwischen *R* und *T* 6,3 mm, bei Ableitung III 7,9 mm. Um die gemessenen Zeitwerte genauer kennen zu lernen, kann man die Bewegungsgeschwindigkeit der empfindlichen Platte vergrössern. So sind z. B. die Elektrokardiogramme von *Me.* in Koordinatensystemen geschrieben, bei denen 1 mm einer Abszisse einer Zeit von 0,01 Sekunde entspricht. Bei Ableitung I beträgt der Abstand zwischen *P* und *R* 13,3 mm, bei Ableitung III 15,5 mm. *RT* ist bei Ableitung I 21,8 mm, bei Ableitung III 23,3 mm, welche Beträge sämtlich Durchschnittswerte einer Anzahl von Messungsergebnissen darstellen, die untereinander nur sehr geringe Differenzen aufweisen.

Diese Messungen, die mit einer grossen Anzahl anderer vermehrt werden könnten, führen alle zu übereinstimmenden Resultaten, nämlich, dass die Abstände zwischen den Gipfeln der Spitzen *P*, *R* und *T* bei Ableitung III grösser sind als bei Ableitung I. Die gefundenen Unterschiede sind verhältnismässig gross und rechtfertigen die Folgerung, dass besagte Spitzen n i c h t in identische Phasen der Herzperioden fallen.

Auch noch durch eine andere Betrachtung kann unsere Folgerung bestätigt werden. Dazu vergleichen wir die in den Elektrokardiogrammen von *Fl.* vorkommenden und in den Fig. 19, 20 und 21 abgebildeten Spitzen *Q* miteinander. Wenn diese Spitzen bei den drei Ableitungen in identische Phasen von Herzperioden fielen, so müssten sie bei den Ableitungen II und III gleich sein, da bei Ableitung I die Spitze $Q = 0$ ist. Wir sehen aber, dass die Spitze *Q*, die bei Ableitung II durchschnittlich 2,3 mm hoch ist, bei Ableitung III

---

1) Auch wenn die Herzperioden nicht vollkommen gleich gross sind, trifft diese Behauptung zu, wenn nur der Unterschied zwischen den Perioden so gering ist, dass er gegen die Abstandsunterschiede der Spitzen vernachlässigt werden darf. Und letzteres trifft in der Regel tatsächlich zu.

fast die doppelte Höhe, und zwar durchschnittlich 4,5 mm erreicht, welche Ungleichheit endgültig beweist, dass die Phasen, in welche die Spitzen *Q* fallen, nicht identisch genannt werden dürfen.

Dasselbe können wir schliessen aus den Dimensionen der Spitzen *S*. Wenn diese Spitzen bei den drei Ableitungen in identische Phasen von Herzperioden fielen, würde man aus den Kurven der Ableitungen I und II für die Ableitung III eine Kurve berechnen, in der neben *R* eine aufwärts gerichtete Spitze *S* von 4 mm Höhe vorhanden wäre. Da diese in der wirklichen Kurve fehlt, muss man wieder folgern, dass die Phasen, in welche die Spitzen *S* fallen, nicht identisch sind.

Aber wenn wir auch als bewiesen annehmen müssen, dass die gleichnamigen Spitzen in den bei den drei verschiedenen Ableitungen erhaltenen Elektrokardiogrammen nicht in identische Phasen der Herzperioden fallen, so ist dennoch damit die Möglichkeit nicht ausgeschlossen, dass man aus den Dimensionen der bei den Stromableitungen I und II erhaltenen Kurven die Kurve konstruieren kann, die bei Ableitung III zum Vorschein kommt. Diese Konstruktion würde man jedoch nur dann mit Erfolg ausführen können, wenn man bei den Ableitungen I und II über Elektrokardiogramme verfügen könnte, bei denen die Herzperioden als in jeder Hinscht gleich betrachtet werden dürften.

Ausserdem muss noch wenigstens ein Punkt der ersten Kurve mit einem Punkt der zweiten identifiziert werden, und schliesslich wäre man noch gezwungen, äusserst genaue Zeitmessungen zu verrichten, weil an einigen Stellen, wo die Kurve jäh steigt oder fällt, wie bei der Spitze *R*, ein Fehler in der Zeitmessung von einigen Tausendsteln einer Sekunde einen Fehler in der berechneten Ordinate von mehreren Millimetern veranlassen würde.

Diese Betrachtungen mögen genügen, um zu zeigen, mit wieviel Schwierigkeiten die wirkliche Ausführung einer Konstruktion verbunden sein würde. Aber glücklicherweise ist die Konstruktion auch nicht nötig. Sie würde ihren Zweck verfehlen, weil sie doch nie als Kontrolle auf die Genauigkeit der Registriermethode angewendet werden könnte. Denn die Konstruktion wird gerade in bezug auf Sicherheit viel zu wünschen übrig lassen, während das Registrieren mit den Apparaten, wie dieselben nun einmal eingerichtet sind, bequem, fast ohne Anstrengung und Zeitverlust mit grösserer

Genauigkeit, als für den Zweck erforderlich ist, ausgeführt werden kann.

Verzichten wir aus den obenerwähnten Gründen auf eine auf Einzelheiten eingehende genaue Konstruktion, so kann es dennoch zur Beurteilung der Kurvenformen nützlich sein, die bei den Ableitungen I und II erhaltenen Elektrokardiogramme mit dem bei Ableitung III erhaltenen zu vergleichen. Man gewinnt dann leicht die Überzeugung, dass die Formulierung Ableitung II — Ableitung I = Ableitung III in vielen Fällen, wenn auch nicht genau, so doch ungefähr stimmt.

Vergleicht man z. B. die Fig. 16, 17 und 18 miteinander, so wird man, wenn man wenigstens keine genauen Messungen verlangt, leicht konstatieren können, dass die Höhe der Spitze *P* bei Ableitung III dem Unterschiede der Spitzen *P* bei den Ableitungen II und I gleich ist. Kurz ausgedrückt ist $P_{III} = P_{II} - P_I$.

Was für *P* zutrifft, ist in diesen Elektrokardiogrammen von *Ei.* auch wahr für die übrigen Spitzen *Q*, *R*, *S* und *T*. Für *P* und *T* gilt diese Regel bei weitaus den meisten Personen; als Beispiele davon dürfen wir auf die Elektrokardiogramme von *Fl.* in den obenstehenden Fig. 19, 20 und 21 und auf die von *M.* in den Fig. 5, 7 und 8 von „Le Télécardiogramme" weisen.

Der geringen Höhe, welche die Spitze *T* bei Ableitung III bei den meisten Personen aufweist, entspricht ausnahmslos eine fast völlig gleiche Höhe von T_I und T_{II} bei denselben Personen, während bei anderen, die eine negative Spitze T_{III} aufweisen, T_{II} auch immer kleiner ist als T_I.

Für die nahe beisammenstehenden Spitzen *Q*, *R* und *S* kann keine Regel festgestellt werden. Zuweilen entsprechen sie ungefähr der oben gegebenen Formulierung, wie z. B. die Fig. 16, 17 und 18 zeigen, zuweilen aber ist die Phasendifferenz bei ihrem Auftreten zu gross, wie schon aus den Fig. 19, 20 und 21 hervorgegangen ist.

Einfluss der Atembewegungen.

Jetzt gehen wir zur Besprechung einiger Umstände über, die bei derselben Person die Form des Elektrokardiogrammes zu modifizieren imstande sind, und dazu untersuchen wir erstens, ob auch Veränderungen in der Kurve konstatiert werden können, die denselben Rhythmus wie die Atembewegungen haben.

Während in den Elektrokardiogrammen vieler Personen nichts oder nahezu nichts von einem Einfluss der Atembewegungen wahrgenommen werden kann, weisen andere sehr deutliche rhythmische Abweichungen auf. Diese betreffen ausnahmslos das System der drei Spitzen *Q*, *R* und *S*, das in der Phase der tiefsten Einatmung gleichsam abgeplattet und in der Regel nach unten gedrückt wird. Bei vielen nimmt man kaum etwas anderes als eine Verkleinerung der Spitze *R* wahr, bei anderen sieht man, namentlich bei Ableitung III, dass das System der genannten drei Spitzen bis auf zwei aufwärts gerichtete dicht nebeneinanderliegende kleine Spitzen reduziert wird, während bei wieder anderen nur die Spitze *S* tiefer wird.

Ein Beispiel der ersten Gruppe ist *Tj.*, dessen Elektrokardiogramm in Fig. 3 der Taf. XI abgebildet ist. Hierbei ist Ableitung II angewendet worden, während mit dem Elektrokardiogramm zu gleicher Zeit der Ictus cordis registriert ist. Die Linie, die den Iktus angibt, zeigt auch deutlich den Rhythmus der Atembewegungen, und zwar so, dass eine Verschiebung nach oben einer Einatmung, eine Verschiebung nach unten einer Ausatmung entspricht.

Man sieht, dass in der Phase der tiefsten Einatmung, die viermal im Photogramm sichtbar ist, die Spitze *R* eine Höhe von 11 mm erreicht, während sie dreimal am Schluss einer Ausatmung 14 mm hoch wird. Dieser Unterschied von 3 mm wird bis etwa 5 mm oder 0,5 Millivolt vergrössert, wenn durch Körperanstrengung die Atembewegungen frequenter und tiefer werden.

Um keine übermässig grosse Anzahl von Abbildungen zu bekommen, ist das Photogramm, auf dem dieser grössere Unterschied sichtbar ist, hier nicht reproduziert worden, ebensowenig wie die Kurve, die bei Ableitung I hergestellt ist, und auf der man einen geringeren Höhenunterschied konstatiert. Dagegen ist in Fig. 4 der Taf. XI das Elektrokardiogramm derselben Person bei Ableitung III wiedergegeben, und dort sieht man nach je vier Herzschlägen, also im Rhythmus der Atembewegungen, eine verhältnismässig sehr kleine, nur 4 mm hohe Spitze *R*. Die maximale Spitze *R* am Schlusse der Ausatmung erreicht 8 mm, d. h. also die doppelte Höhe.

Ein Beispiel der Erscheinung, dass in der Phase der tiefsten Einatmung das System der drei Spitzen *Q*, *R* und *S* bis auf zwei aufwärts gerichtete, dicht nebeneinander liegende kleine Spitzen reduziert wird, findet man in dem in Fig. 5 der Taf. XI reproduzierten Elektrokardiogramm von *v. d. W.* Es kommen, wie man sieht, bei *v. d. W.* nur drei Herzschläge in einer Atemperiode vor.

Schliesslich wird in Fig. 6 der Taf. XII ein Beispiel der drittens erwähnten Erscheinungen gegeben, nämlich, dass bei der Einatmung die Spitze *S* tiefer wird. In der von *Le.* bei Ableitung I registrierten Kurve sieht man bei *i* nach je vier Herzschlägen[1]) eine deutliche Vergrösserung der Spitze *S*.

Wird von *Le.* eine Kurve bei Ableitung III registriert, so zeigt sich die rhythmische Variation im Elektrokardiogramm auf andere Weise. Wie aus Fig 7 der Taf. XII ersichtlich ist, ist hier nach je vier Herzschlägen bei *i* die Spitze *R* nicht nur etwas kleiner, sondern am Gipfel auch ein wenig breiter.

Wie muss dieser Einfluss der Atmung auf die Form des Elektrokardiogrammes erklärt werden?

Zunächst schliessen wir die Möglichkeit aus, dass durch die Atembewegungen selbst, sei es durch Muskelwirkung, sei es durch Verschiebung der Elektroden, Potentialunterschiede hervorgerufen werden. Denn wenn das geschähe, würde die Kurve, die eine Reihe von aufeinanderfolgenden Elektrokardiogrammen wiedergibt, in ihrer Gesamtheit rhythmisch auf und nieder gehen. Wir sehen aber, dass die Linie, welche die Herzpausen verbindet, einen derartigen Rhythmus nicht aufweist, sondern sogar, wie mit Hilfe des Quadratmillimeternetzes leicht konstatiert werden kann, in vielen Photogrammen vollkommen gerade verläuft.

Als zweite Möglichkeit, der wir Rechnung tragen müssen, nennen wir den Einfluss der durch die Senkung des Diaphragmas oder die Ausdehnung des Thorax verursachten Lageveränderung des Herzens. Es wäre gar nicht befremdlich, dass diese durch die Atembewegungen herbeigeführte rhythmische Ortsveränderung des Herzens die Form des Elektrokardiogrammes auch rhythmisch modifizierte; allein offenbar ist der Lagewechsel bei den meisten Menschen ungenügend, merkliche Formveränderungen des Elektrokardiogrammes hervorzurufen. Dass er auch die wirklich vorhandenen und deutlich zu konstatierenden rhythmischen Veränderungen desselben nicht verursacht, wird unseres Erachtens, wo nicht mit Sicherheit bewiesen,

---

1) In der Figur ist aus Versehen der mittlere Buchstabe *i* eine Herzperiode zu früh eingetragen.

so doch sehr wahrscheinlich gemacht durch den Umstand, dass nur die Spitze *R* oder das System der drei Spitzen *Q*, *R* und *S* modifiziert wird, während *P* und namentlich auch die Spitze *T* nicht merklich an Grösse ab- oder zunehmen.

Als dritte Möglichkeit bringen wir einen rhythmisch wirkenden Einfluss zur Sprache, der, vom zentralen Nervensystem ausgehend, das Herz durch die Vagi und die Akzeleratoren erreichen und dann eine modifizierte Kontraktionsweise desselben veranlassen könnte. Aber auch diese dritte Möglichkeit kommt uns nicht sehr wahrscheinlich vor. Erstens zeigen sich die Abweichungen im Elektrokardiogramm fast ohne Phasenunterschied gerade im Stadium der tiefsten Einatmung, was vielmehr für die Existenz eines direkten mechanischen Zusammenhanges zwischen den elektromotorischen Erscheinungen des Herzens und den Atembewegungen spricht, als für einen Zusammenhang, der auf dem Umwege des O- und CO_2-Gehaltes des Blutes und der nervösen Zentralorgane hervorgerufen werden könnte. Aber zweitens haben wir auch Gelegenheit gehabt, einen Patienten zu untersuchen, der in hohem Grade die Erscheinung von Cheyne-Stokes aufwies. Zeiten von oberflächlichen, kaum merklichen Atembewegungen wechselten regelmässig mit Zeiten, in denen der Kranke sich stark dyspnoisch zeigte und tiefe, kräftige, frequente Atembewegungen ausführte. Es wurden von dem Manne *Ko.* bei Ableitung I zwei Telekardiogramme geschrieben; ersteres in einem Augenblick heftiger Dyspnoe, letzteres in einem Augenblick von Apnoe. Von beiden Photogrammen, die merkwürdigerweise nicht oder kaum voneinander unterschieden werden können, reproduzieren wir nur ersteres, das bei Dyspnoe aufgenommen wurde (siehe Fig. 8, Taf. XII).

Man sieht an der Kurve, dass die heftigen Atembewegungen, die der Patient machte, und bei denen er natürlich seine in die Tonzellen getauchten Arme nicht stillhalten konnte, nicht den geringsten Einfluss, weder auf den ruhigen Nullstand des Galvanometers noch auf die Form des Elektrokardiogrammes ausgeübt haben. Durch dieses Beispiel wird bewiesen, dass rhythmische Funktionsstörungen des verlängerten Markes noch keine rhythmischen Veränderungen in der Herztätigkeit herbeizuführen brauchen.

Wie schon oben bemerkt wurde, macht der Umstand, dass die Abweichungen im Elektrokardiogramm sich fast ohne Phasenunterschied gerade im Stadium der tiefsten Einatmung zeigen, es sehr wahrscheinlich, dass ein direkter mechanischer Zusammenhang zwischen den elektromotorischen Erscheinungen des Herzens und den Atembewegungen besteht. Wir suchen diesen Zusammenhang im negativen interpleuralen Druck, der während der Einatmung verstärkt wird und überhaupt einen deutlichen Einfluss auf die Zirkulation ausübt. Das rechte Herz wird wegen seines schwächeren Muskelsystems diesen Einfluss stärker empfinden als das linke, und wenn die Tätigkeit der einen Herzhälfte mehr oder weniger verändert wird als die der anderen, da wird — wie die Kurven von Patienten mit Hypertrophie des rechten und Hypertrophie des linken Herzens in „Le Télécardiogramme" bewiesen haben — besonders das System der drei Spitzen *Q*, *R* und *S* im Elektrokardiogramm modifiziert. Die Tatsache, dass in Fällen, wo ein deutlicher Einfluss der Atembewegungen auf die Form des Elektrokardiogrammes besteht, letzteres auch wirklich eine Modifizierung der drei Spitzen *Q*, *R* und *S* aufweist, bestätigt unsere Meinung, dass der negative interpleurale Druck dabei eine wichtige Rolle spielt.

Einfluss gesteigerter Herzfrequenz.

Wir gehen jetzt zur Besprechung des Einflusses über, der durch eine veränderte Herzfrequenz auf die Form des Elektrokardiogrammes ausgeübt wird. Über diesen Gegenstand ist schon früher bei der kapillar-elektrometrischen Untersuchung ausführlich verhandelt worden [1]).

Die jetzt von uns erhaltenen Resultate brauchen nur kurz erwähnt zu werden, wobei ein paar Beispiele zur Erläuterung genügen. Die drei gebräuchlichen, bei einer Siebenzahl von Personen sowohl im Zustande der Ruhe als unmittelbar nach starker Körperanstrengung angewendeten Stromableitungen I, II und III geben uns die Verfügung über 42 Reihen von Elektrokardiogrammen. Während bei Ableitung I die Formunterschiede der Kurve vor und nach der Körperbewegung nicht in die Augen fallen, zeigen sie sich bei den Ableitungen II und III konstant und recht deutlich.

In den untenstehenden Fig. 26 und 27 reproduzieren wir als Beispiele von bei Ableitung II erhaltenen Kurven die Elektrokardiogramme von *Gö.*, Fig. 26, im Zustande der Ruhe, Fig. 27 unmittelbar nach kräftiger Körperanstrengung. Man sieht, dass in

1) Vgl. Einthoven und de Lint, a. a. O.

Fig. 27 die Herzfrequenz gesteigert ist, und dass die Vorkammern sich schon wieder in einer neuen Herzperiode kontrahieren, bevor die Kammersystole der vorigen Periode abgelaufen ist, so dass man eine Superposition von Vorkammer- und Kammersystole bekommt, wobei erstere sich dachziegelähnlich über letztere legt.

Die wichtigste Veränderung in der Kurvenform besteht in einer Vergrösserung der Spitzen *P* und *T*. Zwar bleiben auch *Q*, *R* und *S* nicht unverändert und tritt der Einfluss der Atembewegungen auf

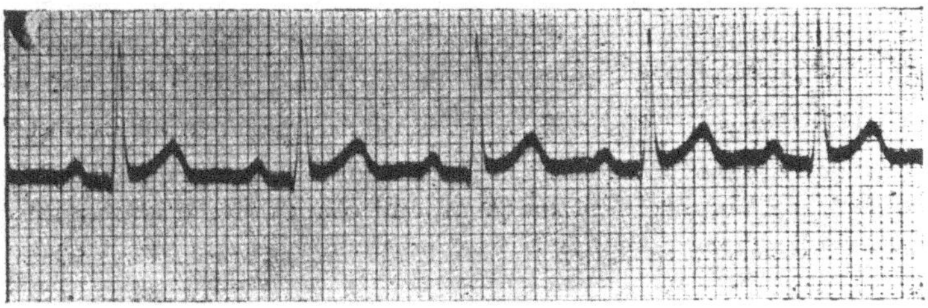

Fig. 26. *Gö.* Ableitung II. Ruhe.

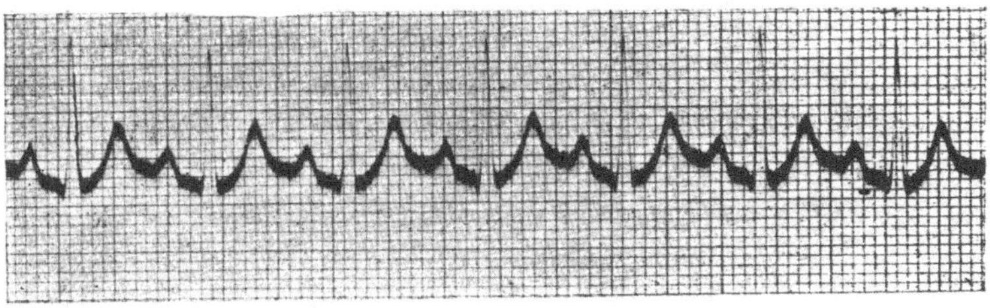

Fig. 27. *Gö.* Ableitung II. Nach kräftiger Körperanstrengung.

das System dieser drei Spitzen deutlicher hervor, aber die Veränderungen, welche sie erleiden, sind nicht so auffallend wie die der erstgenannten Spitzen.

In den Fig. 28 und 29 werden die bei Abteilung III erhaltenen Elektrokardiogramme von *Ra.* wiedergegeben, und zwar in Fig. 28 im Zustande der Ruhe, in Fig. 29 nach kräftiger Körperanstrengung. Man bemerkt ausser der Zunahme der Herzfrequenz einige wichtige Veränderungen in der Kurvenform. Erstens ist ebenso wie bei Ableitung II die Spitze *P* vergrössert; zweitens sehen wir, dass die Spitze *T*, die im Zustande der Ruhe (Fig. 28) negativ ist, nach

Körperanstrengung (Fig. 29) das Zeichen wechselt und bis gut 2 mm über die Abszissenachse reicht, welche Veränderung grundsätzlich auch mit der bei Ableitung II übereinstimmt.

Schliesslich konstatiert man eine bedeutende Vertiefung der Spitze *S*, und zwar in höherem Grade als bei Ableitung II. Diese starke Vertiefung stimmt sehr gut zu den Ergebnissen der oben

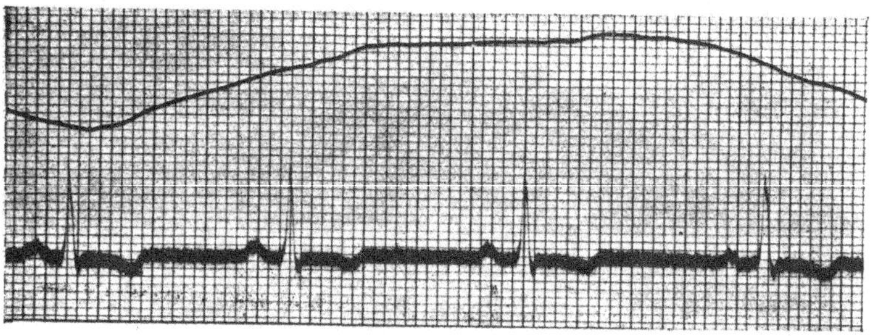

Fig. 28. *Ra.* Atembewegungen und Elektrokardiogramm. Ableitung III. Ruhe.

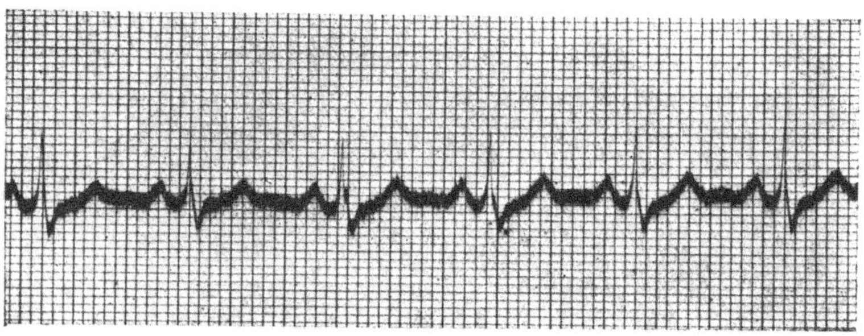

Fig. 29. *Ra.* Ableitung III. Nach kräftiger Körperanstrengung.

schon erwähnten kapillar-elektrometrischen Untersuchung, wobei wir den Strom von der Regio cordis bei der Herzspitze und der rechten Hand ableiteten.

Die sich bei gesteigerter Herzfrequenz zeigenden Formveränderungen lassen in bezug auf Deutlichkeit nichts zu wünschen übrig, und obgleich eine endgültige Erklärung des Zusammenhangs zwischen der modifizierten Herztätigkeit und der Formveränderung des Elektrokardiogrammes vorläufig noch nicht gegeben werden kann, gestatten wir uns doch, hier diesbezüglich auf einiges aufmerksam zu machen.

Erstens weisen wir auf die Vergrösserung der Spitze *P* bei den Ableitungen II und III hin. Diese Vergrösserung kann wohl nichts anderes bedeuten, als dass die Kraft der Vorkammerkontraktionen zugenommen hat.

Die Vertiefung der Spitze *S* bei Ableitung III weist darauf hin, dass die Wirkung der linken Kammer mehr zugenommen hat als die der rechten, und dieser Schluss gründet sich auf die schon oben angeführten, in „Le Télécardiogramme“ erwähnten Beobachtungen, die sich auf die Hypertrophie jeder der beiden Herzhälften gesondert beziehen.

Schliesslich muss noch die Vergrösserung der Spitze *T* sowohl bei Ableitung II wie bei Ableitung III genannt werden. Die Erklärung dieser Vergrösserung bietet ziemlich grosse Schwierigkeiten. Wir können jedoch einiges Licht auf die Erscheinung fallen lassen, indem wir auch andere Verhältnisse, unter denen die Höhe der Spitze *T* verändert wird, einer Betrachtung unterziehen.

So erinnern wir erstens daran, dass durch verschiedene Einflüsse, welche die Herztätigkeit beim Hunde beeinträchtigen, wie reichliche Blutentziehung, tiefe Chloroformnarkose und oft auch Vagusreizung, die Spitze *T* sich senkt: eine niedrige Spitze *T* wird negativ, eine negative Spitze *T* wird stärker negativ. Sodann sehen wir beim Menschen in pathologischen Verhältnissen, dass in einer Anzahl von Fällen von Insuffizienz, Dilatation, Myodegeneratio cordis, wobei die Herztätigkeit überhaupt mangelhaft ist, die Spitze *T* auch bei den Ableitungen I und II klein und zuweilen negativ wird. Eine Vergrösserung von *T*, so wie dieselbe bei gesteigerter Herzfrequenz nach Körperanstrengung erscheint, ist also der durch beeinträchtigte oder mangelhafte Herztätigkeit herbeigeführten Veränderung entgegengesetzt. Wir kommen hierauf sogleich noch zurück.

Während im folgenden Abschnitt bei den Schlussbetrachtungen einige Zeilen dem näheren Zusammenhang gewidmet werden mögen, der überhaupt zwischen der Herzmuskelkontraktion und der Form des Elektrokardiogrammes besteht, schliessen wir diesen Abschnitt mit einer kurzen Erörterung einiger

Pathologischen Fälle,

die als eine weitere Ergänzung der Abhandlung über „Le Télécardiogramme“ betrachtet werden dürfen. Wie bei allen Personen, deren Elektrokardiogramme in jener Abhandlung zur Sprache gebracht wurden, sind auch jetzt wieder bei jedem der untersuchten Patienten die drei Ableitungsweisen I, II und III angewendet worden.

Wir fangen mit einem Patienten *d. Wa.* an, der eine Stenosis des Ostium aortae mit Hypertrophie des linken Herzens hatte, welche letztere Abweichung vermuten liess, dass er bei Ableitung III eine negative Spitze *R* aufweisen würde. Untenstehende Fig. 30 beweist, dass diese Vermutung richtig ist, wodurch die schon früher

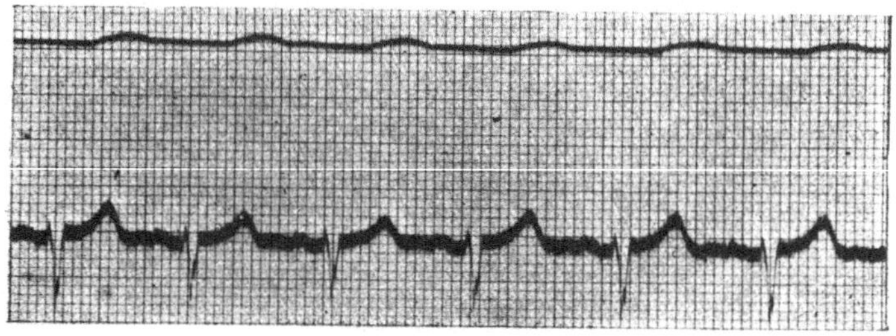

Fig. 30. *d. Wa.* Karotispuls und Elektrokardiogramm. Ableitung III. Hypertrophie des linken Herzens.

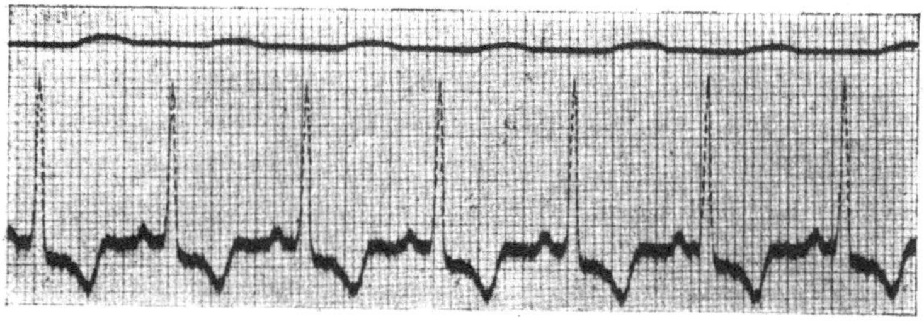

Fig. 31. *d. Wa.* Karotispuls und Elektrokardiogramm. Ableitung I. Hypertrophie des linken Herzens.

ausgesprochene Behauptung, dass R_{III} bei Hypertrophie des linken Herzens nach unten gerichtet ist, von neuem bestätigt wird.

Von wie grosser Bedeutung es ist, die Untersuchung der elektrischen Erscheinungen des Herzens immer bei allen drei Ableitungen zu verrichten, können die Kurvenformen lehren, die unser Patient bei den verschiedenen Ableitungen darstellt. So wird z. B. sowohl bei Ableitung I wie bei Ableitung II von ihm eine Kurve registriert, in der die Spitze *R* positiv und die Spitze *T* negativ ist. Man findet das bei Ableitung I erhaltene Elektrokardiogramm in der

Fig. 31 abgebildet, in der also merkwürdigerweise *R* und *T* den gleichnamigen Spitzen der Ableitung III (Fig. 30) gerade entgegengesetzt sind.

In „Le Télécardiogramme" werden drei Patienten mit einer Hypertrophie des linken Herzens erwähnt, die, wie aus den Fig. 18, 19 und 20 jener Abhandlung hervorgeht, sämtlich bei Ableitung III eine stark negative Spitze *R* aufweisen. Bei Ableitung I wird bei allen drei Patienten die Spitze *R* positiv und erreicht dabei sogar ziemlich bedeutende Höhen: bei *B. H. S.* 13×10^{-4} Volt, bei *C. de G.* 14×10^{-4} Volt, bei *J. v. V.* 14×10^{-4} Volt.

Bei einer Patientin *A. B.* mit Hypertrophie des rechten Herzens und, wie aus Fig. 17 von „Le Télécardiogramme" hervorgeht, mit einer positiven Spitze R_{III}, deren Höhe den enormen Betrag von 2,7 Millivolt erreicht, ist R_I negativ bis zu einem Betrage von 1,1 bis 1,2 Millivolt.

Diese Beispiele mögen genügen.

Widmen wir jetzt noch einige Zeilen der Spitze *T*. Dieselbe ist in normalen Elektrokardiogrammen bei Ableitung III meistens niedrig und zuweilen negativ, wie wir oben schon mit Beispielen in den Fig. 18, 21, 24, 25 und 28 erörtert haben. Dagegen sind T_I und T_{II} in normalen Herzen immer positiv. Findet man bei den Ableitungen I und II eine niedrige oder eine negative Spitze *T*, so hat man es mit einem kranken Herzen zu tun, dessen pathologische Abweichung oft nur als „Insuffizienz" oder „Myodegeneratio cordis" qualifiziert werden kann.

Der Patient *d. Wa.*, der in obenstehender Fig. 31 eine negative Spitze T_I aufweist, hat wirklich ein insuffizientes Herz, während in ein paar anderen Fällen, wo die Diagnose nur auf „Myodegeneratio cordis" lautete, bei allen drei Ableitungen die Spitze $T = 0$ oder schwach negativ war.

Wir reproduzieren in Fig. 32 das Elektrokardiogramm der einen Patientin *H. d. B.* bei Ableitung II, wobei die Spitze *T* so gut wie vollständig abgeplattet ist, während Fig. 33 das Elektrokardiogramm des anderen Patienten *v. H.* bei Ableitung I wiedergibt, wobei dann und wann eine schwach negative Spitze *T* erscheint.

Bei dem Patienten *F. d. J.* wurde eine rekurrierende, akute septische Endocarditis diagnostisiert, während wir aus der negativen Spitze T_I (siehe Fig. 34) schliessen dürfen, dass dabei zugleich die Tätigkeit des Herzmuskels beeinträchtigt war.

Eine seltene Form der Spitze T_{II} wurde bei *Ch. N.* gefunden, der einen angeborenen, schwer genauer zu bestimmenden Herzfehler hat, und dessen Elektrokardiogramm bei Ableitung II in Fig. 35 reproduziert ist.

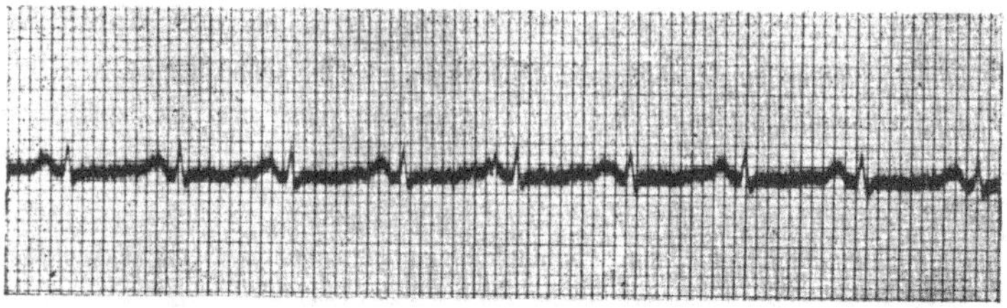

Fig. 32. *H. d. B.* Pericarditis adhaesiva. Insufficientia cordis. Ableitung II.

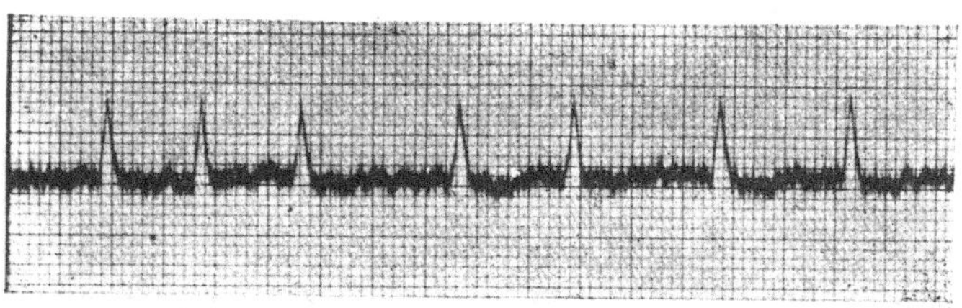

Fig. 33. *v. H.* Myodegeneratio cordis. Ableitung I.

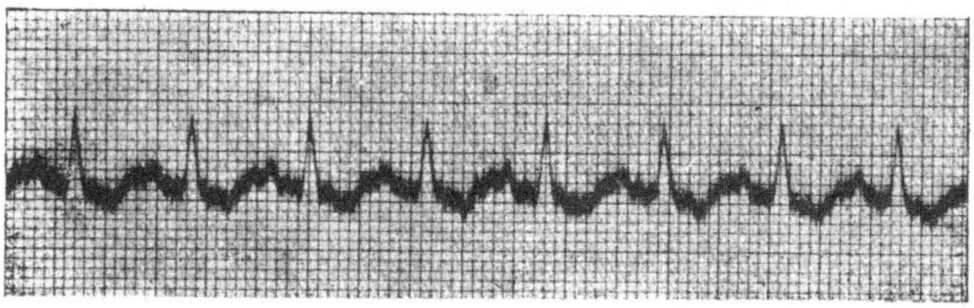

Fig. 34. *F. d. J.* Akute septische Endocarditis. Ableitung I.

In „Le Télécardiogramme" wurde in Fig. 24 die bei Ableitung III erhaltene Kurve dieses Patienten abgebildet, die zwar eine eigentümliche Form von R_{III} aufweist, von der aber T_{III} nicht zu besonderen Bemerkungen Anlass gibt. Bei demselben Patienten ist T_I negativ.

Ein Patient mit Herzblock und vollständiger Dissoziation der Vorkammer- und Kammerkontraktion ist schon in „Le Télécardiogramme" beschrieben worden, aber wegen der Seltenheit dieser Krankheit darf hier noch die Untersuchung eines zweiten ähnlichen Patienten *Ca.* erwähnt werden [1]). In Fig. 9 der Taf. XII sieht man in der oberen Kurve das Phlebogramm der V. jugularis, in der unteren das Elektrokardiogramm bei Ableitung II. Die in letzterer Kurve mit *a* bezeichneten Vorkammerspitzen werden darin leicht und gleichsam von selbst aufgefunden, während man sich in den unzähligen Spitzen des Phlebogrammes nur mühsam auskennt.

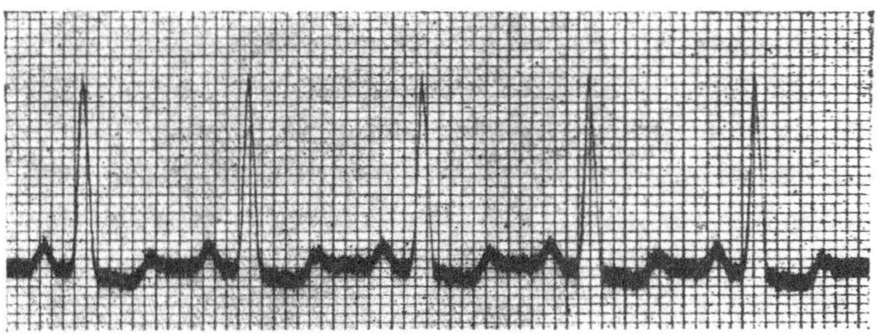

Fig. 35. *Ch. N.* Angeborener Herzfehler. Ableitung II.

Durch die Form des Elektrokardiogrammes geleitet haben wir diejenigen Spitzen des Venenpulses, die als eine Folge der Vorkammerkontraktion aufgefasst werden müssen, mit a_1 bezeichnet, was wir ohne die Hilfe der auf elektrischem Wege erhaltenen Kurve unmöglich mit derselben Bestimmtheit hätten tun können. Tatsächlich gibt uns das Elektrokardiogramm zur Unterscheidung der Vorkammer- und Kammertätigkeit ein genaueres und zuverlässlicheres Mittel an die Hand als die gewöhnliche mechanisch-graphische Methode.

In der Form des Elektrokardiogrammes bemerken wir als etwas Besonderes die nach unten gerichtete Spitze R_{II} und die eigentümlich geformte Spitze T_{II}, die deutlich aus zwei Teilen, einem negativen und einem darauffolgenden positiven Teil besteht. Dass diese Besonderheiten für die Krankheit von Stokes-Adams nicht charakteristisch sind, geht aus einer Vergleichung mit den früher veröffentlichten Elektrokardiogrammen der anderen Patientin *S. v. G.*

1) Dieser Patient wurde uns durch freundliche Vermittelung von Dr. Hijmans van den Bergh aus Rotterdam zugeschickt, dem wir dafür gern unsern besten Dank abstatten. Die übrigen Patienten befanden sich alle im hiesigen Universitäts-Krankenhause und wurden uns von Prof. Nolen für die Untersuchung zur Verfügung gestellt. Auch dem sagen wir dafür herzlich Dank.

hervor (siehe „Le Télécardiogramme"). Bei derselben Ableitung II sind bei *S. v. G.* die Spitzen *R* und *T* positiv und geben zu besonderen Bemerkungen keinen Anlass.

Schliesslich reproduzieren wir in Fig. 10 der Taf. XII noch den Carotispuls und das Elektrokardiogramm desselben Patienten *Ca.* bei Ableitung III. Aus der Negativität von R_{III} darf auf das Vorhandensein einer Hypertrophie des linken Herzens geschlossen werden.

5. Schlussbetrachtungen.

Die bequeme Handhabung des einmal aufgestellten Saitengalvanometers und die direkte Brauchbarkeit der registrierten Kurven, die keinen zeitraubenden Messungen und Berechnungen unterzogen zu werden brauchen, hat die Herstellung einer grossen Anzahl von Photogrammen veranlasst. Wir verfügen jetzt über gut 500 photographische Aufnahmen, die zusammen ungefähr 5000 einzelne Elektrokardiogramme enthalten. Zwar ist der Grund zu unserer Kenntnis des Elektrokardiogrammes mit Hilfe des Kapillarelektrometers gelegt worden und werden die mit diesem Instrument erhaltenen Resultate im allgemeinen durch die Untersuchung mit dem Saitengalvanometer bestätigt, allein es braucht uns doch auch nicht Wunder zu nehmen, dass nach der grossen Erweiterung, welche die Untersuchung durch die Anwendung des Saitengalvanometers erfahren hat, auf einige Erscheinungen ein anderes Licht gefallen ist und einige der früher ausgesprochenen Meinungen über die Bedeutung der verschiedenen Kurvenspitzen jetzt geändert werden müssen.

Dies hat besonders für die Vorkammerspitze *P* Geltung. Früher hielten wir es für wahrscheinlich[1]), dass die beiden Spitzen *P* und *Q* durch die Vorkammersystole verursacht würden, während jetzt mit genügender Sicherheit bewiesen ist, dass *Q* zum Kammerelektrogramm gehört, während die Atriumkontraktion nur durch *P* repräsentiert wird. Viele Elektrokardiogramme lassen darüber keinen Zweifel mehr zu.

So erinnern wir an die Kurven, die in einer Anzahl von besonderen Fällen registriert wurden: den Fällen von Herzblock, wobei mehr als eine Vorkammerkontraktion erforderlich war, eine Kammersystole herbeizuführen, den Fällen vollständiger Dissoziation

---

1) Diese Ansicht hat Hofmann in Nagel's Handbuch der Physiologie Bd. 1 S. 253 übernommen.

der Vorkammer- und Kammersystole und endlich den Fällen verstärkter Vorkammersystole bei Stenosis valvulae mitralis. Man findet sowohl in den vorigen Abschnitten dieser Abhandlung wie in „Le Télécardiogramme" viele Beispiele der in diesen besonderen Fällen erhaltenen Elektrokardiogramme, die teilweise vom Hunde und teilweise vom kranken Menschen herrühren, und deren Deutung in bezug auf den betreffenden Punkt vollkommen klar und einfach ist.

Was die Form des Kammerelektrogrammes anbelangt, bemerken wir, dass es wünschenswert ist, darin zwei Teile zu unterscheiden, von denen der erste durch die drei Spitzen Q, R und S, der zweite durch die Spitze T gebildet wird.

Wie müssen diese Spitzen erklärt werden?

In den vorigen Abschnitten haben wir uns im allgemeinen auf die Feststellung einiger Erscheinungen beschränkt, wobei wir zu gleicher Zeit auf das Zusammentreffen gewisser Veränderungen in der Herztätigkeit mit charakteristischen Formen des Elektrokardiogrammes aufmerksam machen konnten. Auf diese Weise konnte nicht nur die Bedeutung der Vorkammerspitze P konstatiert werden, sondern auch die Vergrösserung von R_{III} bei Hypertrophie des rechten Herzens, das Negativwerden der Gruppe Q_{III} R_{III} S_{III} bei Hypertrophie des linken Herzens, die Erhöhung von T_{II} bei verstärkter Herztätigkeit nach Körperanstrengung, das Sinken von T_{II} bei beeinträchtigter Herztätigkeit und bei Myodegeneratio cordis, die völlig veränderte Form des Elektrokardiogrammes bei einer atypischen Herzkontraktion usw..

Es kommt uns vor, dass diese Resultate eine grössere Sicherheit gewähren als die Ergebnisse, die man erzielt, wenn man bei einem Hunde die verschiedenen Abteilungen des Herzens künstlich reizt, wie Kraus und Nicolai getan haben, die den Thorax ihres Versuchstieres öffneten und während der Registrierung des Elektrokardiogrammes elektrische und mechanische Reizungen anwendeten.

Jetzt müssen wir noch die Bedeutung der verschiedenen Spitzen des Elektrokardiogrammes von einem anderen Gesichtspunkte aus betrachten und versuchen sie im Zusammenhang mit der

Fortpflanzung der Kontraktionswelle durch den Herzmuskel

zu erklären. Das Elektrokardiogramm lehrt uns unmittelbar nur den Weg der negativ-elektrischen Welle im Herzen kennen. Setzt man voraus, dass der Zusammenhang zwischen dieser Welle und der Erregung oder der Zusammenhang zwischen der Negativität und der Kontraktion aufgehoben ist, so kann man aus der Form des Elektrokardiogrammes nicht auf die Wege schliessen, welche die Erregung und die Kontraktionswelle zurücklegen.

Wir dürfen aber annehmen, dass die Kontraktionswelle auf der Stelle, wo sie anlangt, immer mit einer Negativität der dort befindlichen Muskelfasern verbunden ist. Die Kontraktion ist die Folge der Erregung, und in der Regel werden Erregung, Negativität und Kontraktion so innig zusammenhängen, dass, wenn der Weg der negativ-elektrischen Welle durch den Herzmuskel bekannt ist, zugleich der Weg angegeben ist, den die Erregung und die Kontraktionswelle nehmen.

Unter diesen Bedingungen kann aus der Form des Elektrokardiogrammes auch die Reizleitung durch den Herzmuskel bestimmt werden. Unseres Erachtens hat sogar für die Lösung dieses Problems die elektrische Untersuchungsmethode viele Vorzüge vor der mechanischen.

Wie schon Waller und Bayliss und Starling versucht haben, aus der Form des Elektrokardiogrammes auf die Reizleitung im Herzen zu schliessen, findet man in der Dissertation von Dr. de Vogel[1]) erwähnt.

Schlüter[2]), der unter der Leitung Langendorff's arbeitete, wendete eine andere Methode als seine Vorgänger an. Er legte auf dem isolierten Säugetierherzen oder auf dem blossgelegten Herzen im lebendigen Tiere die Nerven von zwei physiologischen Rheoskopen an, den einen näher der Herzbasis, den anderen näher der Herzspitze, und registrierte die auf jeden der Herzschläge folgenden Wadenmuskelkontraktionen. Die Messung der Zeitunterschiede zwischen den Kontraktionen des näher der Herzbasis angelegten Präparates *b* und denen des näher der Herzspitze angelegten *s* ergab keine konstanten Resultate. Bald zog *b* sich eher zusammen als *s*, bald erfolgte das Umgekehrte. In der Regel war der Verlauf so, dass im Anfang der Untersuchung *b* vor *s*, in späteren Stadien *s* vor *b* kam.

---

1) A. a. O.

2) Franz Schlüter, Die Reizleitung im Säugetierherzen. Pflüger's Arch. f. d. ges. Physiol. Bd. 89 S. 87. 1902.

Dies veranlasst Schlüter, die normaliter von der Basis nach der Spitze verlaufenden Wellen „rechtläufige" zu nennen, im Gegensatz zu den „rückläufigen", die von der Spitze nach der Basis gerichtet sind und abnormal sein sollen.

Wir glauben, dass der Weg, den die Kontraktionswelle durch das Herz nimmt, nicht als einfach von der Basis nach der Spitze führend oder umgekehrt aufgefasst werden darf. Das Verbindungsbündel von *His*, das den Reiz der Vorkammern auf die Kammern überbringt und in der letzten Zeit der Gegenstand ausführlicher Untersuchungen war, leitet vermutlich den Reiz zu gleicher Zeit nach einer Anzahl in den Herzkammern sehr verbreitet liegender Stellen.

Nach den Untersuchungen Tawara's[1]) besteht das atrioventrikuläre Verbindungsbündel aus einem System von Muskelfasern, die einen sich baumförmig verzweigenden Strang bilden, und die von ihrem Ursprung im Septum atriorum an bis zu den Endausbreitungen an den Wänden der Herzkammern immer durch Bindegewebe von den übrigen Herzmuskelfasern getrennt sind. Auf ihrem ganzen Verlaufe treten diese Fasern nirgendwo mit der Herzmuskulatur in Verbindung, während erst ihre Endausbreitungen, die sogenannten Fasern von Purkinje oder deren Äquivalente, die über eine grosse Oberfläche in den Kammerwänden verbreitet liegen, mit diesen letzteren verschmelzen.

Völlig in Übereinstimmung mit diesem anatomischen Bau ist die Fortpflanzung der Kontraktionswelle im Herzen, wie dieselbe aus der Form des Elektrokardiogrammes abgeleitet werden muss[2]). Der Reiz, dessen Ursprung in den grossen Venen liegen kann, veranlasst zuerst die Kontraktion der Vorkammern (Spitze *P*). Die zwischen der Vorkammer- und der Kammerkontraktion verlaufende Zeit ist dazu nötig, den Reiz durch das atrioventrikuläre Verbindungsbündel nach den Endausbreitungen dieses langen Fasersystems zu leiten.

---

1) S. Tawara, Das Reizleitungssystem des Säugetierherzens. Gustav Fischer, Jena 1906.

2) Im Hinblick auf die Fragen bezüglich der neurogenen und myogenen Theorie der Herztätigkeit darf hier daran erinnert werden, dass Tawara in dem Atrioventrikulärbündel von Kalbsherzen einen Nervenstamm beschreibt, der sich mit dem Muskelbündel aufs innigste verflechtend verläuft und sogar in der Kammerscheidewand Ganglienzellen besitzt. Bei Menschen und Hunden konnte er auf dieser Stelle keine nennenswerten Nervenfasern finden, aber er hält ihr dortiges Vorhandensein doch nicht für ausgeschlossen.

Während dieser Zeit schreibt das Saitenbild des Galvanometers eine horizontale Linie. Vorkammern und Kammern befinden sich in Ruhe, und die durch das Verbindungsbündel fortschreitende Kontraktionswelle ist an und für sich zu schwach, bei der für die Registrierung eines zweckmässigen Elektrokardiogrammes erforderlichen starken Saitenspannung einen merkbaren Ausschlag des Galvanometers zu erzielen.

Von den Endausbreitungen des Fasersystems geht der Reiz auf die Kammerwand über, wo er nicht speziell entweder an der Basis oder an der Spitze anlangt, sondern wo er direkt über eine grosse Oberfläche verbreitet wird.

Die Kontraktion fängt also in den Kammern auf vielen Stellen zugleich oder fast zugleich an, was im ersten Teil des Kammerelektrogrammes, dem System der Spitzen *Q*, *R* und *S*, zum Ausdruck kommt. Gelangt der Reiz zuerst an eine nahe der Spitze oder der linken Kammer liegende Stelle, so wird sich eine Spitze *Q* bilden, während diese Spitze fehlen muss, wenn die entgegengesetzten Stellen der Kammern zuerst getroffen werden.

Dass die Fasern des Atrioventrikularbündels den Reiz auch nach näher der rechten Kammer und der Herzbasis liegenden Stellen leiten, wird durch die Spitze *R* dargetan, die als eine der konstantesten aufwärts gerichteten Spitzen angesehen werden muss, während das Vorhandensein der Spitze *S* zeigt, dass bald darauf wieder die Kontraktion der der linken Kammer und dem Apex näher liegenden Teile des Herzens die Oberhand gewinnen kann.

Bei Hypertrophie des rechten Herzens, wobei R_{III} ungemein hoch ist, leiten die Fasern des Verbindungssystems den Reiz besonders nach Stellen, die sich der Herzbasis nähern, während bei Hypertrophie des linken Herzens und einer nach unten gerichteten Spitze R_{III} die Stelle, wo der Reiz ankommt, näher der Herzspitze liegt.

Der Ruhestand des Galvanometers zwischen dem System der Spitzen *Q*, *R* und *S* auf der einen und der Spitze *T* auf der anderen Seite weist auf einen Kontraktionszustand hin, an dem die ganze Muskelmasse der beiden Herzkammern sich gleichmässig beteiligt. Hört dieser Kontraktionszustand auch in der ganzen Muskelmasse im selben Moment auf, so bildet sich keine Spitze *T*, wie bei Degeneration und Insuffizienz des Herzens vorkommt (siehe Fig. 32 und 33).

Bleibt die rechte Herzhälfte länger im Kontraktionszustande als die linke, so entstehen die aufwärts gerichteten Spitzen T_I und T_{II}, die in normal funktionierenden Herzen stets vorkommen. Bleibt die Basis länger kontrahiert als die Spitze, so bildet sich eine aufwärts gerichtete Spitze T_{III}, während sich eine nach unten gerichtete Spitze T_{III} entwickelt, wenn die Spitze länger kontrahiert bleibt als die Basis (siehe z. B. Fig. 25).

Bei normalen Herzen findet man sowohl eine positive wie eine negative Spitze T_{III}. T_I und T_{II} sind normaliter immer positiv, während sie bei beeinträchtigter Herztätigkeit niedriger, bei verstärkter Herztätigkeit nach Körperanstrengung höher werden. Die dabei sich zeigenden Besonderheiten sind schon in den beiden vorhergehenden Abschnitten beschrieben worden.

Das atypische Elektrokardiogramm.

Schon in „Le Télécardiogramme" ist darauf hingewiesen worden, dass bei einigen Personen neben den gewöhnlichen Systolen atypische Herzkontraktionen vorkommen, die oft mit dem Aussetzen des Pulses verbunden sind und stets durch eigentümlich gebildete Elektrokardiogramme wiedergegeben werden. Letztere sind meistens besonders auffallend, weil sie durch grosse und verhältnismässig lange andauernde Potentialunterschiede erzeugt werden.

Die Formen des atypischen Elektrokardiogrammes weichen bei verschiedenen Personen voneinander ab, und es kommt sogar vor, dass bei derselben Person bald die eine, bald die andere Form registriert wird. In der Regel besteht das Elektrogramm der atypischen Herzkontraktion aus einem einfachen zweiphasigen Aktionsstrom, der durch ein allmähliches Fortschreiten der Kontraktionswelle von einem Ende der Herzkammern nach dem anderen erzeugt wird. Der Reiz geht nicht von den Vorkammern auf die Kammern über, sondern fängt unmittelbar in den Kammern selbst an, und zwar entweder dicht bei der Basis oder dicht bei der Herzspitze, während er vermutlich von den Kammern nach den Vorkammern fortgepflanzt wird.

Als Beispiel reproduzieren wir in den drei untenstehenden Figuren 36, 37 und 38 die bei den üblichen drei Ableitungsweisen registrierten Elektrokardiogramme von *A. v. Y.*

A. v. Y. ist eine Patientin mit Myodegeneratio cordis; auch in Fig. 23 von „Le Télécardiogramme" ist eine Kurve von ihr abgebildet. Die eigentümliche Verdoppelung der Spitze T_{II}, worauf in besagter Abhandlung aufmerksam gemacht wurde, ist auch in Fig. 37 deutlich zu sehen.

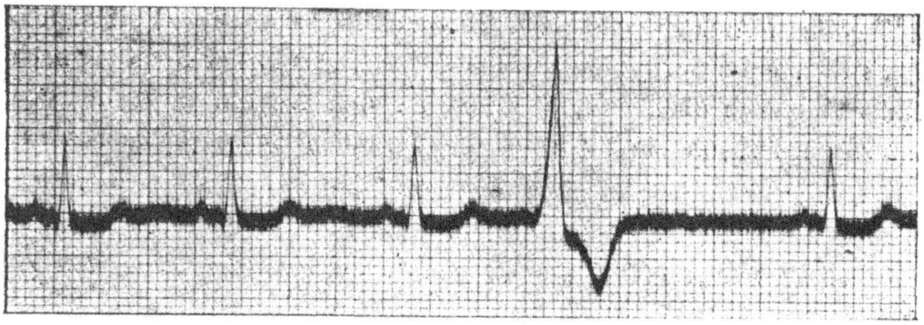

Fig. 36. *A. v. Y.* Atypische Herzkontraktion. Ableitung I.

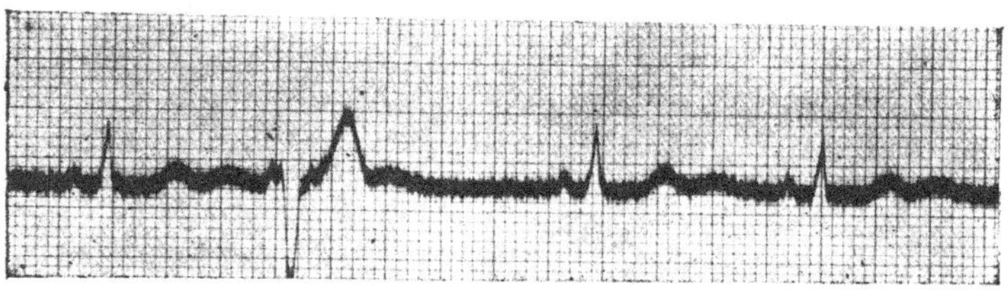

Fig. 37. *A. v. Y.* Atypische Herzkontraktion. Ableitung II.

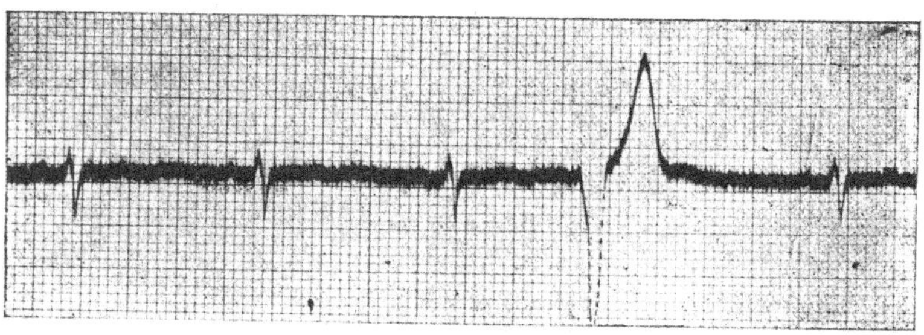

Fig. 38. *A. v. Y.* Atypische Herzkontraktion. Ableitung III.

Der mit der atypischen Herzkontraktion verbundene zweiphasische Aktionsstrom erzeugt eine einfach gebildete Kurve mit zwei grossen Spitzen, von denen eine nach oben, die andere nach unten gerichtet ist. Fig. 36, die bei Ableitung I registriert worden ist, zeigt, dass der Ursprung der Kontraktionswelle dichter bei der rechten als bei der linken Herzhälfte liegt, während man mit Hilfe der bei Ableitung III registrierten Fig. 38 dartun kann, dass der Ursprung sich mehr der Spitze als der Basis nähert.

Die geringe Höhe der Spitzen in Fig. 37 (Ableitung II) stimmt zu der Annahme, dass die Kontraktionswelle rechts bei der Herzspitze ihren Anfang genommen hat. Von hier schreitet sie allmählich nach dem entgegengesetzten Ende des Herzens in der Richtung nach links und nach oben fort, während an den Kurven nicht deutlich zu sehen ist, ob sie auch auf die Vorkammern fortgepflanzt wird.

Als zweites Beispiel einer atypischen, mit der oben beschriebenen übereinstimmenden Herzkontraktion erinnern wir an die Fig. 26, 27, 28 und 29 von „Le Télécardiogramme“, welche die Kurven von *R.*

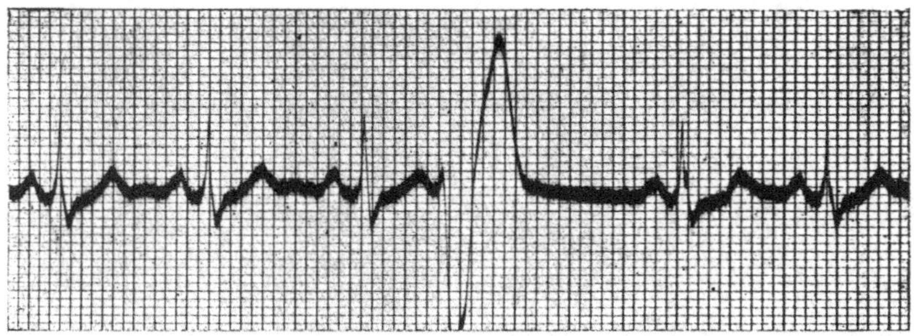

Fig. 39. *R.* Atypische Herzkontraktion. Ableitung III.

bei Ableitung I und II wiedergeben. Wir ergänzen diese Abbildungen durch eine bei Ableitung III von derselben Person registrierte Kurve (Fig. 39).

Die atypischen Elektrokardiogramme von *R.* stimmen in fast jeder Hinsicht mit denen von *A. v. Y.* überein und beweisen, dass auch hier wieder eine Kontraktionswelle rechts bei der Spitze ihren Anfang genommen hat und nach einer Endstelle links bei der Basis allmähich fortgeschritten ist. Nur ist in den Kurven von *R.* bei Ableitung I und II ein Haken zu bemerken, der die Vermutung rechtfertigt dass die Kontraktionswelle an jener Stelle von den Kammern auf die Vorkammern übergegangen ist.

Der Patient *S. K.* mit Herzbigeminie hat regelmässig wiederkehrende atypische Herzkontraktionen, deren Kontraktionswelle im Gegensatz zu denen der beiden obenerwähnten Personen von der Herzbasis, wo sie beginnt, nach der Spitze fortschreitet.

In Fig. 30 von „Le Télécardiogramme" ist eine Kurve von *S. K.* bei Ableitung II reproduziert, während zur Vervollständigung in den untenstehenden Fig. 40 und 41 die Kurven bei den Ableitungen I und III abgebildet werden.

In Fig. 40 ist wie gewöhnlich 1 mm einer Ordinate $=10^{-4}$ Volt, aber wegen der grossen Ausschläge, die das Galvanometer bei Ab-

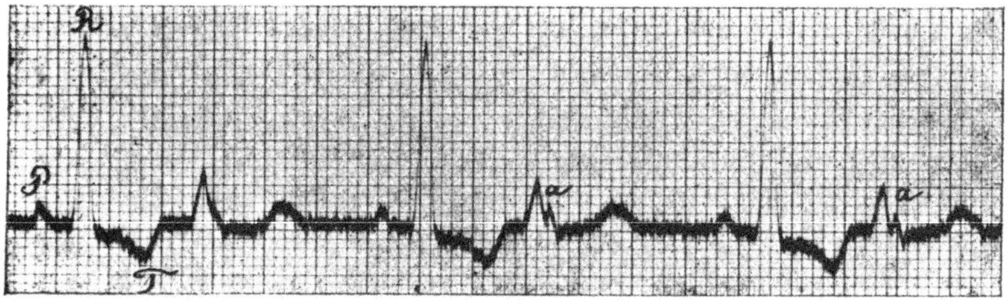

Fig. 40. *S. K.* Atypische Herzkontraktionen. Ableitung I.

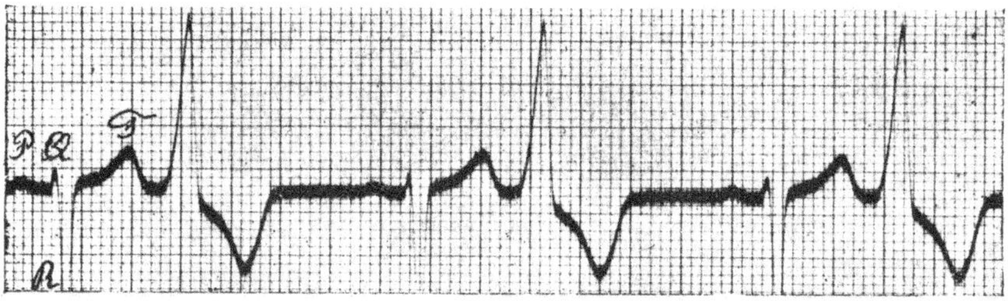

Fig. 41. *S. K.* Atypische Herzkontraktionen. Ableitung III.
Absz. 1 mm = 0,04 Sek. Ordin. 1 mm 2×10^{-4} Volt.

leitung III machte, wurde bei der Registrierung von Fig. 41 die Saitenspannung verdoppelt. In dieser Figur entspricht deshalb, wie in Fig. 30 von „Le Télécardiogramme", 1 mm einer Ordinate einem Potentialunterschied von 2×10^{-4} Volt. In jeder der drei besagten Figuren ist eine der gewöhnlichen Systolen durch die Buchstaben *P*, (*Q*), *R*, (*S*), *T* angedeutet.

Die geringe Höhe der Spitzen des atypischen Elektrokardiogrammes in Fig. 40 bei Ableitung I weist darauf hin, dass die Welle nahezu rein von der Basis nach der Spitze geleitet wird, während der Haken bei *a* zeigt, dass an dieser Stelle wahrscheinlich der Reiz von den Kammern auf die Vorkammern übergeht.

Die atypischen Herzkontraktionen der drei obenerwähnten Personen, die uns bei den üblichen Stromableitungen neun verschiedene Elektrogramme gegeben haben, stimmen mit allen anderen von uns beobachteten Extrasystolen darin überein, dass die Reizleitung einen ungewöhnlichen Weg durch den Herzmuskel nimmt (siehe z. B. auch die Fig. 25 und 31 von „Le Télécardiogramme"). Der Reiz geht dabei nicht von den Vorkammern auf die Kammern über.

Eine Extrasystole, die durch eine atypische Kammerkontraktion charakterisiert ist, muss ihren Ursprung entweder in dem Kammermuskel selbst oder in einem nahe dem Kammermuskel befindlichen Teil des Atioventrikularbündels nehmen. Es kommt uns vor, dass die von einigen Forschern gemachte Unterscheidung von Extrasystolen, die in den grossen Venen und den Vorkammern entstehen, nicht aufrecht erhalten werden kann, weil es an jeder Veranlassung zu einer abnormalen Reizleitung im Kammermuskel fehlt, sobald der Reiz auf dem gewöhnlichen Wege von den Vorkammern zu den Kammern übergeht.

Sogar wenn der Reiz an einer nahe den Vorkammern befindlichen Stelle des Atrioventrikularbündels entsteht, kann die weitere Leitung durch das Bündel auf normale Weise stattfinden, so dass die Ankunft des Reizes in die Kammern und die Reizleitung durch den Kammermuskel nicht von der Norm abzuweichen brauchen.

Letzteres wird durch die Elektrokardiogramme der Patienten mit der Krankheit von Stokes-Adams dargetan (siehe Fig. 2 und 3 der Tafel von „Le Télécardiogramme" und Fig. 9 und 10 der dieser Abhandlung beigefügten Taf. II).

Wir müssen bei diesen Krankheitsfällen, bei denen eine totale Dissoziation der Vorkammer- und Kammertätigkeit eingetreten ist, annehmen, dass der Zusammenhang zwischen den Vorkammern und dem Atrioventrikularbündel aufgehoben ist, und dass der Reiz ausser in den grossen Venen oder in den Vorkammern auch noch in dem Atrioventrikularbündel selbst entsteht. Dennoch haben wir es hier mit gewöhnlichen Kammersystolen zu tun, wie die Form des Kammerelektrogrammes zur Genüge beweist.

Dagegen entsteht, wie schon oben erörtert wurde, bei der durch atypische Herzkontraktion gekennzeichneten Extrasystole der Reiz in oder nahe dem Kammermuskel selbst, und zwar entweder nahe der Herzbasis (siehe Fig. 41) oder nahe der Spitze (siehe Fig. 38 und 39).

Die Formen der Elektrokardiogramme, die man bei atypischer Herzkontraktion bekommt, machen den Eindruck, als ob dabei die Reizleitung im Herzmuskel verlangsamt ist. Wäre diese Verlangsamung wirklich vorhanden, so würde schon allein dadurch ein Charakteristikum für die atypischen Herzkontraktionen gegeben sein. Es kommt uns aber vor, dass eine Verlangsamung der Leitung nicht mit Sicherheit bewiesen werden kann, und dass die eigentümlich gedehnte Kurvenform aus dem langen Wege, den die Kontraktionswelle von der Spitze nach der Basis oder umgekehrt zurücklegen muss, zu erklären ist.

Die Kraft der atypischen Herzkontraktionen.

Wie schon im Abschnitt 3 bemerkt worden ist, hat man allen Grund, anzunehmen, dass bei der Vergleichung einiger nahezu dieselbe Form besitzenden Elektrokardiogramme die Höhe der Spitzen einigermaassen einen Maassstab für die Kraft der Herzkontraktionen angibt.

Dieser Maassstab geht verloren, sobald wir zwei verschieden gebildete Elektrokardiogramme miteinander vergleichen müssen, und in diesem Falle sind wir, wenn wir mit Hilfe unserer galvanometrischen Kurven die Kraft einer atypischen Herzkontraktion unmittelbar aus der einer normalen Systole ableiten wollen.

Dennoch kann unser Zweck, die Kraft einer atypischen Herzkontraktion kennen zu lernen, leicht erreicht werden. Dazu braucht man nur einen kleinen Umweg einzuschlagen. Erst vergleiche man einige in derselben Kurvenreihe geschriebenen atypischen Elektrokardiogramme miteinander. Man sieht dann, dass diese oft in nahezu jeder Hinsicht miteinander übereinstimmen, woraus man schliessen darf, dass die Kontraktionen, denen sie entsprechen, auch eine gleiche Kraft entwickelt haben.

Nun kann der Effekt einer atypischen Herzkontraktion mit der einer normalen mittels des Pulses verglichen werden, wenn nur die atypische Kontraktion sich in einem Augenblick entwickelt, wo unter gewöhnlichen Verhältnissen eine normale Systole erfolgen würde.

Allerdings sind die atypischen Kontraktionen in der Regel verfrüht und dürfen alsdann wegen ihres unzeitigen Eintrittes Extrasystolen genannt werden; allein bisweilen ist die Verfrühung so gering, dass sie kaum noch in Betracht gezogen zu werden braucht.

VIII
On vagus currents examined with the string galvanometer

This paper was chosen as an example of Einthoven's studies on neural action currents recorded by means of the string galvanometer. From a cardiological point of view it is important to note, that Einthoven shows in this paper that electrical variations occur in the divided vagus nerve which are synchronous with the heart beat, in conjunction with the respiratory rhythm which was already known.

The two papers on action currents in the sympathetic nerve (126, 135) have been mentioned in chapter 1; in this connection the study with Jolly on retinal action currents (93) must also be mentioned.

ON VAGUS CURRENTS EXAMINED WITH THE STRING GALVANOMETER. By W. EINTHOVEN (in collaboration with A. FLOHIL and P. J. T. A. BATTAERD). (From the Physiological Laboratory of Leyden.)

(*Received for publication 6th July 1908.*)

THE demarcation current which may be derived from the peripheral end of a divided vagus nerve shows a negative variation whenever the lungs are expanded. This phenomenon was first demonstrated by Lewandowsky[1] with the aid of a Deprez-d'Arsonval galvanometer; later Alcock and Seemann[2] studied it more in detail with the capillary electrometer. In a research made by means of the string galvanometer we have been able completely to confirm the results of the above-mentioned authors, and also to obtain evidence of the presence of another source of stimuli

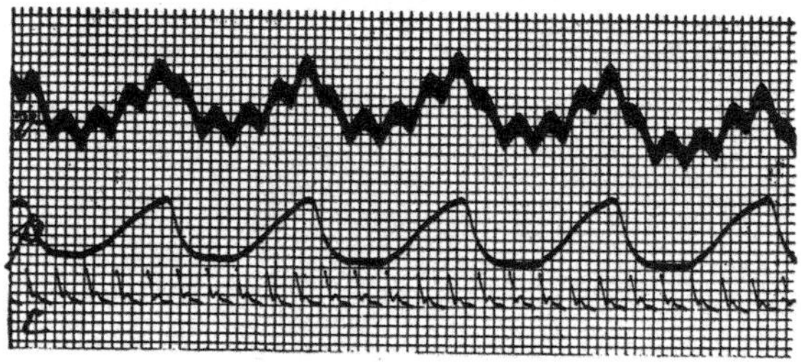

Figure showing the electrical changes in the vagus nerve which accompany the respiratory and heart movements.
v, electrovagogram; *p*, respiration record (ascent of curve, inspiration; descent, expiration); *c*, pulse record.

situated in the heart—the vagus shows rhythmic action currents which synchronise with the heart-beats.

A vagus nerve in the neck of an anæsthetised dog is isolated for a considerable distance and divided at a spot high up in the neck. The current is led off from the peripheral cut end of the nerve by means of a pair of non-polarisable electrodes, one of which is brought in contact with the cross-section, the other with the surface, the space between the electrodes being

[1] Max Lewandowsky, "Ueber Schwankungen des Vagusstromes bei Volumänderungen der Lunge," Pflüger's Arch. f. d. ges. Physiol., Bd. lxxiii., S. 288, 1898.
[2] N. H. Alcock and John Seemann, "Ueber die negative Schwankung in den Lungenfasern des Vagus," Pflüger's Arch. f. d. ges. Physiol., Bd. cviii., S. 426, 1905.

about 1·5 cm. The demarcation current of the nerve is compensated in the usual way, and the electrodes are connected with the galvanometer in such a manner that a decrease of the demarcation current, or an action current, causes the image of the string to move in an upward direction. In the accompanying figure, 1 mm. of the abscissa corresponds to 0·2 sec.; 1 mm. of the ordinates, to 2·7 microvolts. The upper curve (v) represents the action currents of the vagus nerve, and may be called the "electro-vagogram"; the middle one (p) reproduces the respiratory movements of the animal in such a way that every inspiration corresponds to an ascent and every expiration to a descent of the curve. This pneumogram is obtained by causing the dog to breathe into a large bottle and transmitting the oscillations of the pressure of the air in the bottle to a suitably placed recording Marey's tambour. The lower curve (c) indicates the sphygmogram of the crural artery.

It can be seen that the electrovagogram exhibits undulations having a double rhythm, viz.: (1) synchronous with the respiratory movements, (2) synchronous with the heart-beats of the animal. That these undulations are caused by the real action currents of the nerve and not by current escape from other organs, can be proved in different ways.

In the first place we may rely on the method employed, which does not appear subject to this source of error. We have further repeatedly submitted it to the usual proofs of control. Thus, if the nerve is ligatured peripherally to the electrodes or is killed by means of a drop of ammonia, the rhythmic oscillating image of the string is brought completely to rest.

In the dog, the respiratory oscillations of the right vagus are larger than those of the left one; while, on the other hand, the heart-beat oscillations of the left vagus surpass those of the same nerve on the right side. In the rabbit the vagus nerve shows exclusively respiratory oscillations, the depressor nerve solely heart-beat oscillations.

The excitatory state of the vagus endings in the lungs is determined by the volume of these organs and not by the intrapulmonary pressure. If during the cessation of the natural respiratory movements of the animal the lungs are insufflated artificially, the electrovagogram shows an undulation in the same direction as if the animal is making a natural inspiration. Nevertheless the insufflation is accompanied by an increase, the natural inspiration by a decrease of the intrapulmonary pressure.

The experiments which we have performed on the effects of insufflating and deflating the lungs have given evidence of the presence of two kinds of pulmonary vagus fibres: those having expiratory and those having inspiratory effects. The latter act more weakly, are sooner tired, and are killed more easily by injuries than the former, so that the two kinds of fibres can be separated from each other as to their action. Especially is it easy to isolate the effect of the expiratory fibres. The theory of Hering[1]

[1] E. Hering, "Die Selbststeuerung der Athmung durch den Nervus Vagus," Wiener Sitzungsberichte, 2 Abt., Bd. lvii., S. 672, 1868.

and Breuer[1] on the self-regulation of the respiratory movements obtains in this way fresh support.

The connection of the respiratory and the heart-beat undulations in the electrovagogram also throws light on the association which virtually exists between the heart's action and the respiratory movements. This association finds inter alia its expression in the constant ratio between the number of respiratory movements and the number of heart-beats per minute. It is well known that this ratio usually remains unaltered with variations in pulse frequency. Since we now learn that the beating heart sends rhythmic stimulations along the vagus to its centre, we may reasonably ask whether these stimulations may not reach the respiratory centre and there cause with each variation of the pulse frequency a proportional variation of the frequency of the respiratory movements. In this way an automatic regulation of the respiratory movements would be promoted by the heart's action.

Yet another automatic regulation may be pointed out, viz. that of the heart's action by itself. We must in all probability look to this regulation as furnishing the cause of the vagal tonus, this tonus being thus maintained automatically by the action of the heart itself.[2]

[1] J. Breuer, ibid., Bd. lviii., S. 909, 1868.
[2] A more detailed description of our experiments will appear in Pflüger's Archiv f. d. ges. Physiol.

IX
The different forms of the human electrocardiogram and their signification

It was already explained in chapter 1 why this publication was selected instead of the subsequent, much better known, paper by Einthoven, Fahr and de Waart (102). The latter deals, however in more detail, only with the equilateral triangle and the resultant vector ("manifest potential"), and perhaps is also somewhat more explicit regarding the schematic character (and therefore limited validity) of the equilateral triangle. On the other hand, the present paper, which embodies a lecture given to the Chelsea Clinical Society in London, gives an almost comprehensive review of Einthoven's work on electrocardiography up to 1911. Thus the equilateral triangle, which is introduced here for the first time, is shown in its true perspective.

Even the paper by Einthoven, Fahr and de Waart left some doubts and unanswered questions. It is fortunate, that in the next reprint (X) parts of correspondence with Lewis and Wilson can be presented, which bear on these problems and elucidate Einthoven's thoughts.

THE DIFFERENT FORMS OF THE HUMAN ELECTROCARDIOGRAM AND THEIR SIGNIFICATION.[1]

BY PROFESSOR WILHELM EINTHOVEN, M.D.,
OF LEYDEN.

THE application of electrocardiography to clinical examination gives valuable data in two different ways. In the first place, it shows the time relations between the action of the ventricles and the auricles. The difference in time between the contraction of these two parts of the heart can be measured easily and accurately. Diseases such as Stokes-Adams's, in which the auricles have a rhythm different from that of the ventricles, and which sometimes give difficulties when examined by the older methods, are always immediately recognised, electrocardiographically. And further may be mentioned that a new insight has been obtained into several other diseases, among which auricular fibrillation takes a prominent place.

But this evening we shall pass over this first group of symptoms, and we shall limit our attention to the second one, which is concerned with the form of the EKG. If this form is perfect, it must be the exact expression of the changes in potential difference which take place between two parts of the human body. It is self evident that a perfect form can only be obtained by means of a perfect instrument, and it need not be mentioned that such an instrument does not exist. The capillary electrometer is not rapid enough when made sufficiently sensitive, and therefore not suitable for clinical purposes. The oscillograph suffers from the same fault, although in a less degree, and has, moreover, the great disadvantage that the movements of the recording mirror are oscillatory. On the contrary, the string galvanometer is in general sufficient for clinical purposes, and by means of this instrument we are able to approximate the exact form of the EKG. so closely that the remaining divergences from it become practically imperceptible.

Not every model of the string galvanometer is equally suitable. Even if we have at our disposal a good instrument in all other respects, the correctness of the work done with it depends in a high degree upon the qualities of a small part of the apparatus, the string, and we have further to take into consideration the magnification and the sensitiveness used.

How is the clinician to know if the curves which he has obtained with the instrument are reliable reproductions of the electrical variations under investigation? He can, it is true, correct the curves obtained by means of data determined from the properties of the instrument, and which are to be found by means of control curves. But such a correction requires a fairly detailed calculation and a reconstruction of the curve, for which reason he will be loth to apply it. And happily this is unnecessary in most cases. It is only necessary to record a control curve in such a way that an equal resistance from a rheostat is introduced into the galvanometer circuit in place of the body resistance, which usually has a value of from 1000 to 2000 ohms.

The tension of the string must be so regulated that an excursion of the image of the string of 1 mm. is equal to 10^{-4} volts. At a given moment a constant potential difference is thrown into the circuit. If the string reaches its new position of equilibrium within about 0·01 second or less, the instrument is rapid and at the same time sensitive enough for recording EKG.'s with sufficient accuracy. The deviations from an ideal EKG. which a curve recorded under these conditions exhibits are so small that in the great majority of cases they may be neglected.

To prove this we reproduce in Figs. 1 and 2 two EKG.'s which were taken from the same person by lead I. The sensitiveness of the galvanometer was accurately adjusted in both records, so that 1 scale division corresponded to 10^{-4} volts. All other conditions were also kept the same as nearly as possible, with the one exception that in recording Fig. 2 a magnification was used twice as large as in Fig. 1. Therefore the string was stretched twice as much in Fig. 2, and in accordance with this the duration of a deflection was reduced to half.

It is possible to determine the duration of a deflection to a certain degree by means of Fig. 3, which was recorded immediately after Fig. 2 upon the same photographic plate. A resistance of 2300 ohms was introduced into the galvanometer circuit from a resistance box, this resistance being equal to that found for the body of the person investigated under the conditions of the experiment. The introduction of a potential difference of 3×10^{-3} volts causes a deflection of 3×10 scale divisions, and each deflection is completed in about 0·5 scale divisions—i.e., 0·01 second. The control curve for Fig. 1, which is not reproduced here, shows deflections requiring twice as much time for their completion—i.e., 0·02 second.

Notwithstanding this important difference in deflection time, Figs. 1 and 2 show EKG.'s whose forms agree in all details, and whose various peaks have the same absolute heights within the errors of adjustment—i.e., within a few tenths of a scale division.

We are now justified in making the following conclusion. If the movements of the string could be made 10 or 100 times faster, the sensitiveness remaining the same, or even if, theoretically spoken, an instrument were available with an infinitely small deflection time, the form and dimensions of the recorded EKG.'s would not be thereby perceptibly changed.

On the other hand, if the movements of the string are sufficiently retarded, the form of the EKG. will also be altered. This is illustrated by Fig. 4. This reproduces the EKG. of the same person taken under the same conditions. The sensitiveness of the galvanometer is, just as in Figs. 1 and 2, accurately regulated so that a deflection of the image of the string of 1 mm. corresponds to 10^{-4} volts. But the

[1] A paper read before the Chelsea Clinical Society on March 19th, 1912.

string moves much more slowly, and we now see that all the peaks of the EKG. are reduced in size, whilst the ratio of the peaks to one another is markedly changed.

Allow me to make a comparison here of the requirements to be demanded of the galvanometer and the accommodation of the eye. A definite adjustment of the eye corresponds to a definite distance from an object that must be focussed sharply. Therefore two objects at different distances from the eye can not form absolutely sharp images at the same time, but the physician knows that if the image of an object at 6 metres distance is sharp, the diffusion circles caused by points farther removed are so small that they may be neglected. The accommodation for infinite distance does not differ practically from the accommodation for 6 metres. In the same way we may say that an EKG. recorded with a galvanometer, of which the deflection time is about 0·01 second, does not differ practically from the same EKG. recorded with a galvanometer whose deflection time is infinitely small.

Within these limits the form of the EKG. is independent of the instrument used, and every EKG., when and where it may have been recorded, is immediately comparable with every other EKG.

A parallel can be drawn between image formation in the eye and the recording of the EKG. in still another direction. Suppose that the accommodation of the eye is faultless in a certain case. Even then the retinal image will not be absolutely sharp and exact. The errors of spherical and chromatic aberration, and of defective centration inherent in all optical systems are also found in the eye; and, moreover, the diffraction of the light rays suffices to exclude the formation of an exact image. In the same way there are sources of inaccuracy in the recording of the EKG.; their influence may be decreased, it is true, but can never be completely avoided. I have here in mind not so much the dexterity of the observer, who must regulate the tension of the string exactly, so that the curves may be recorded in absolute measure, as the unavoidable changes in resistance, which the human body offers to the electrical current.

We must make a distinction between the real and the apparent resistance in measuring the resistance of the body. The real resistance is measured by means of an alternating current, in the same way as the resistance of an electrolyte is determined, whereas the apparent resistance is found by making use of a constant current. Under certain conditions the apparent resistance can have a value of more than twice as much as the real resistance, and the question arises, which resistance are we to take into account when regulating the tension of the string. For example, we wish that a deflection of the image of the string of 1 cm. shall exactly represent 1 millivolt, when the human body is in the galvanometer circuit. If the body resistance is large, the string must be relaxed a little; if on the other hand the body resistance is small, the string must be stretched somewhat more tightly, all other conditions remaining equal.

In case the difference between the apparent and the real resistance of the body reaches an important value, the sharp peak *R* of short duration will be too high in relation to the slow wave *T*, this being an error which is just the opposite of the error produced by a slow instrument.

How can we best reduce these errors and how large is the error remaining finally? In the first place we must make the resistance of the body as small as possible by putting those parts from which the current is lead off, the hands and the foot, deeply into a strong salt solution. Under these conditions the difference between real and apparent resistance is also reduced to a minimum. Further we must use an instrument with a thin string, thus with a comparatively large internal resistance, so that the variations of the body resistance will only have a small influence upon the current strength.

In regulating the tension of the string we can make use of a rheostat resistance, the value of which is the mean of the real and the apparent body resistance. The difference between these two values need not be larger than 400 ohms under the above-mentioned favourable conditions, so that the deviation from the mean will not be more than 200 ohms. If we take the resistance of the string to be 10,000 ohms the maximum error in the dimensions of the curves is 2 per cent.

These errors are much less in reality, because peak *R* is not recorded in an infinitely short time and peak *T* not in an infinitely long time. Moreover, an error of 2 per cent. in the absolute values of the potential difference is so small that it may as a rule be neglected in physiological as well as in clinical investigations. The error would be 0·4 mm. for a large peak *R* of 20 mm. height, and only 0·1 mm. for a large peak *T* of 5 mm.

Although we cannot attain an absolute accuracy at present, yet we may consider an EKG., when properly recorded, the exact expression of the changes in potential difference, just as we may consider the retinal image an exact reproduction of the object observed.

The Form of the Curve in Connexion with the Different Leads.

It is desirable to apply three leads in electrocardiographic investigations: (1) from the two hands, across the body; (2) from the right hand and left foot, obliquely; (3) from the left hand and left foot, lengthwise. The galvanometer must be connected to the human body in such a way that the image of the string is deflected upwards when the base or the right half of the heart is negative in respect to the apex or the left half.

Each of the three leads produces an EKG. of special form so that each has its own peculiar value. Lead I has the advantage of being applied easily in the clinic. The curve obtained is of especial value in judging peak *T* and certain atypical EKG.'s. With lead II the peaks are usually larger. Especially the auricular peak *P* is clearly shown and may therefore be best studied with this lead. In judging the wave *T* in cases of cardiac insufficiency lead II has the same importance as lead I. On the other hand, many atypical forms of the EKG. can be studied better with lead I than with lead II.

Lead III is most suited for diagnosing hypertrophy of the right or left ventricle. Atypical EKG.'s are also well shown by lead III. On the other hand, the wave *T* obtained by this lead is of no value in drawing conclusions as to the functioning of the heart. T_{III} has different heights in normal EKG.'s, is often negative, and often practically absent.

The Connexion between the Forms Obtained with the Three Leads.

From the nature of the case there must be a connexion between the curves obtained by the three different leads from the same person. If two forms are known, the third may be calculated from them. The difference between the electrical tensions of leads I and II must be equal to the electrical tension of lead III. This may be formulated: lead II − lead I = lead III. The formula holds good only in case the current which is flowing through the galvanometer exercises no influence upon the tensions present at the extremities. As a matter of fact, this influence is so small that we may neglect it without making a perceptible error. For the total resistance of the circuit containing the galvanometer and the human body is very large when compared to the resistance of the heart muscle. We may therefore assume *a priori* that the formula is exact.

We might attempt to make use of this formula when examining patients, for the sake of simplicity contenting ourselves with the recording of two leads. The curve of the third lead would then be constructed from the other two. Although the construction seems to be easy, yet its execution gives difficulties, the main cause of which lies in the fact that the peaks, which we generally indicate by means of the same letters, do not occur in identical phases of a heart's revolution. It is possible to show this in various ways—e.g., by comparing the distances between the peaks *P*, *R*, and *T* in the curves obtained by lead I with the corresponding distances in the curves obtained by lead II and lead III. It then appears that the peaks mentioned stand closer to one another in lead I.

A superficial examination of certain curves—for example, those of Fl. (Figs. 5, 6, 7), in which the three leads exhibit fairly large differences—might appear to favour a doubt as to the practical validity of the formula. But it is not difficult to show that the rule is also in accordance with the facts.

The simplest way to do so would be to record two or three curves by the various leads immediately under one another. Two or three large string galvanometers should be used and the images of the three strings should be projected by means of mirrors upon the same photographic plate. It seems to me that the use of a small model of the galvanometer, in which two or more strings are placed in the same magnetic

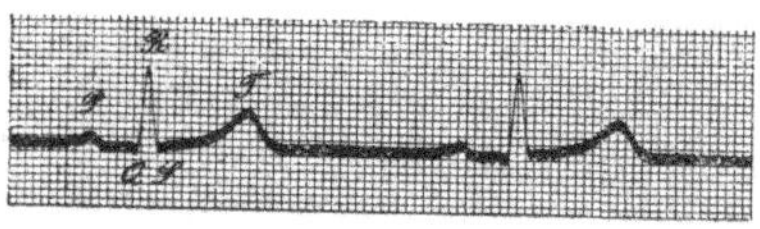

FIG. 1.—Br. Lead I. Magnification of the movements of the string 660. Absc. 1 sc. div. = 0·02 sec. Ordin. 1 sc. div. = 10^{-4} volts.

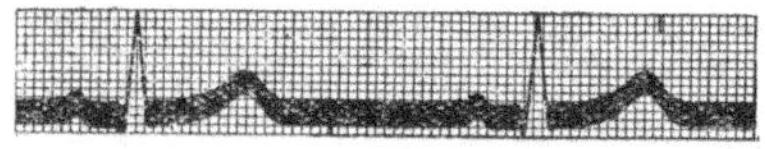

FIG. 2.—Same person and same lead as in Fig. 1. Magnification of the movements of the string about 1200. Value of abscissæ and ordinates as in Fig. 1.

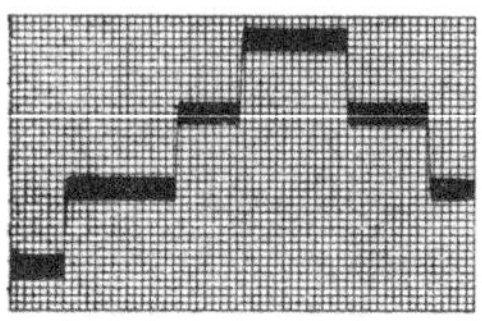

FIG. 3.—Control curve corresponding to Fig. 2. Absc. 1 sc. div. = 0·02 sec. Ordin. 1 sc. div. = 10^{-4} volts.

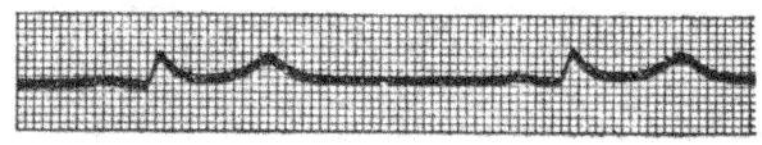

FIG. 4.—Same condition as in Fig. 1, with the exception that an extra resistance of 100,000 ohms has been introduced into the galvanometer circuit.

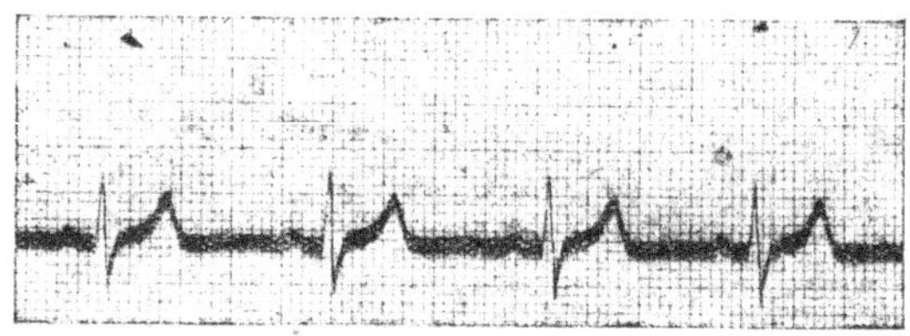

FIG. 5.—Fl., Lead I. Absc. 1 sc. div. = 0·04 sec. Ordin. 1 sc. div. = 10^{-4} volts.*

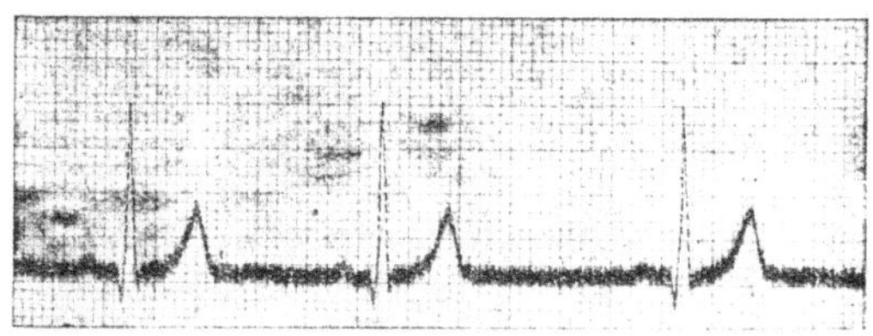

FIG. 6.—Id. Lead II.

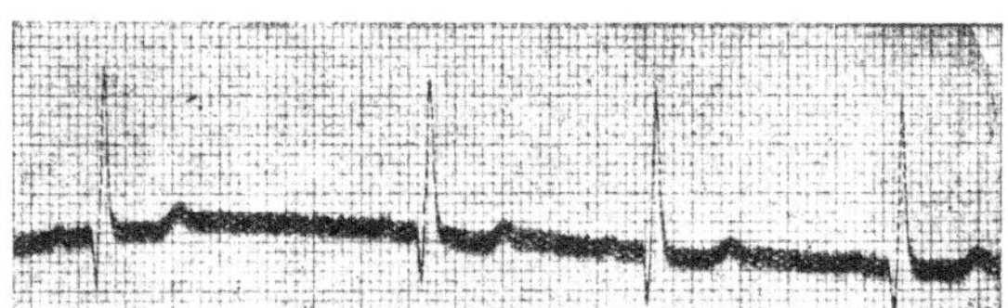

FIG. 7.—Id. Lead III.

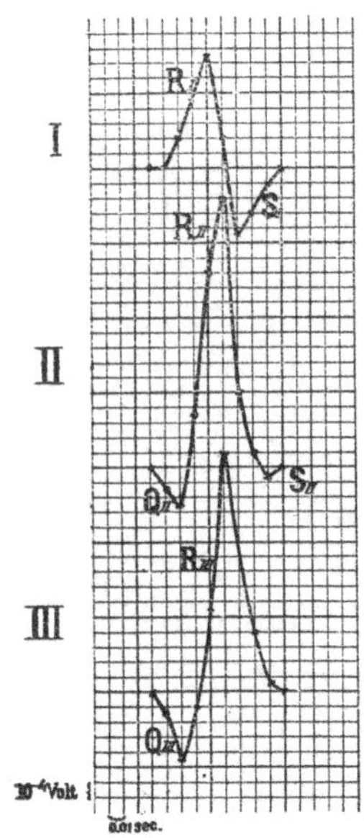

FIG. 8.—Construction of the *QRS*-group in the three leads. Each ordinate represents identical phases of a cardiac cycle. Absc. 1 sc. div. = 0·01 sec. Ordin. 1 sc. div. = 10^{-4} volts.

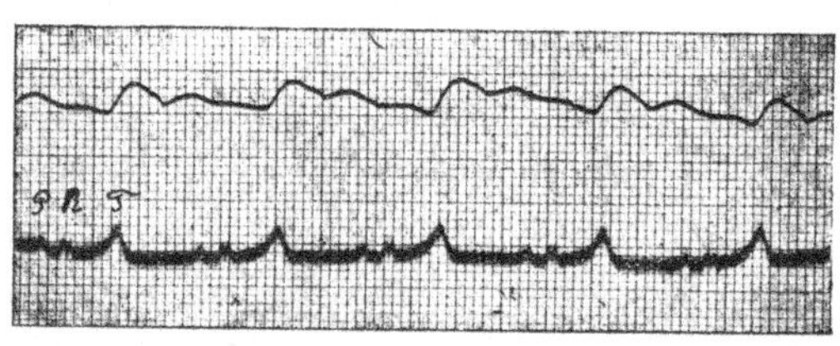

FIG. 9.—Wi. Lead I. A remarkable *QRS*-group.

* If not otherwise mentioned the abscissæ and the ordinates in all figures have the same value as in Fig. 5.

field, or the use of an oscillograph containing a number of mirrors, is not suited to this purpose, because these instruments do not reproduce the form of the EKG. accurately, whereas it is especially desirable in this case to have the form as exact as possible.

Another method has been applied by Fahr and de Waart. They have recorded the EKG., together with the heart sounds, according to the method of Kahn. The EKG.'s obtained by the three leads were taken from the same person under exactly the same conditions, the curve of the heart sounds being combined with each EKG. By this means a fixed point falling always in the same phase of a cardiac cycle could be marked, and corresponding phases in the curves of the various leads could be accurately identified.

The investigation of Fahr and de Waart shows that the ventricle EG. when obtained by leads II and III begins, as a rule, a little earlier than when obtained by lead I, whereas the summit of R_I is reached a little earlier than the summits of R_{II} and R_{III}. If we make use of these data it is not difficult to show the validity of the formula, even in complicated forms of the EKG. To illustrate this we have reproduced in Fig. 8 *QRS*-group of the EKG.'s of Fl. shown in Figs. 5, 6, and 7. The three curves are constructed in the same system of coördinates. The abscissæ have been increased 4 times more than the ordinates, so that the whole figure has been stretched in the direction of the abscissæ; one scale division of the abscissæ represents 0·01 sec., one scale division of the ordinates 10^{-4} volts. Each vertical line corresponds to one phase of a cardiac cycle and the formula lead II – lead I = lead III holds good for every phase. We see that the peaks Q_{II} and Q_{III} begin 0·01 sec. before R_I and fall in the anacrotic branch of this peak. The whole peak S_I falls in the catacrotic branch of R_{II} and R_{III}, whilst the whole of peak S_{II} only corresponds with the anacrotic branch of S_I.

Similar constructions can be made, as a rule, without great difficulty and can be applied to peaks *P* and *T* as well, but it is often difficult to attain a great degree of accuracy. This is especially true when the height of a small peak must be determined from the difference in the heights of two peaks of nearly the same size. If T_I and T_{II} are of approximately the same height, as is often the case, then the value of T_{III}, calculated by means of the formula, is very inexact.

It is thus evident that we should not content ourselves with taking only two leads, for the dimensions of a curve constructed by calculation can be determined not only more simply but also more accurately by directly recording it by the third lead. The great advantage of a construction as in Fig. 8 is the better insight obtained into the *QRS*-group.

QRS-group.

This group deserves a closer examination because it forms the beginning of the ventricular EG. and shows the path by which the excitation wave is conducted from the auricles to all parts of the ventricular wall. This group takes very different forms in normal hearts, so that it is sometimes impossible to point out the peaks *Q*, *R*, and *S*. The examination of even a small number of curves will show that the inconstant peak *Q* fails in some EKG.'s, the inconstant peak *S* fails in others. In some EKG.'s *S* is as large as *R*, and in some others both *Q* and *S* fail so that only *R* remains.

We reproduce here an EKG. of *Wi.* (Fig. 9), who possesses a normal heart. The curves obtained by leads I and II show large peaks *R*, as is often the case with normal hearts. The curve reproduced above and taken by lead I exhibits an entirely different form of the *QRS*-group. This group is here represented by a slight elevation, about as high as *P* and about one-third as high as *T*. On closer examination it is seen to consist of two small upwardly directed peaks, placed close beside one another. It is impossible to say whether they are *Q*, *R*, or *S*. The same is true of many normal as well as of many pathological curves taken with lead III. A single example of such a $(QRS)_{III}$-group may suffice (Fig. 10).

We have here again two upwardly and two downwardly directed peaks, no one of which may possibly be distinguished as *Q*, *R*, or *S*. T_{III} is negative in the EKG. of this person.

The explanation of the ventricular EG. is based upon this great variability in the *QRS*-group. As soon as the excitation wave has reached the ventricular walls through the atrio-ventricular bundle and the Purkinje fibres, the ventricular musculature begins to contract in many places at the same or nearly the same time. The atrio-ventricular bundle, according to the investigations of Aschoff-Tawara, consists of a system of muscle fibres, well likened to a tree with its branches. From their origin in the auricular septum to their arborisation in the walls of the lower chambers of the heart, these fibres are separated from the rest of the heart muscles by connective tissue. The bundle does not enter into connexion with the heart musculature excepting with its end ramifications, which are spread over a large surface in the walls of the ventricles, fusing with them at many points. The great variety of forms of the *QRS*-group is caused by small variations in the architecture and the conductivity of the bundle and the Purkinje fibres, so that the excitation wave in some hearts reaches the right side 0·01 second sooner than the left, or the base sooner than the apex, whereas the opposite sequence occurs in other hearts.

The contraction wave spreads over the whole ventricular musculature within a few hundredths of a second, and all changes in potential disappear temporarily. This happens in the time between group *QRS* and the beginning of the *T* wave.

The potential difference indicated by the galvanometer in any given moment is the resultant of the joint potential differences existing at that moment between the various parts of the heart. If we consider the phenomena from this point of view we may agree with Selenin, who regards the EKG. as the algebraic sum of the changes in potential, caused by the contraction of the right and left chambers. We also may agree with Eppinger and Rothberger, who assume that the EKG. is the resultant of the forces in the constrictor fibres and in the longitudinal fibres of the heart musculature. Neither is there any objection to the idea of the EKG. being the expression of the antagonism between base and apex. For we may divide the heart into two arbitrary parts, and the EKG will always be the resultant of the changes in potential differences in these parts. The curve must represent, under all circumstances and in every moment, the algebraic sum of all the potential differences which at that moment are developed in the heart.

Peak U.

We must now point out two peculiarities of the EKG. which up to the present have been considered worthy of only slight consideration. In the first place, the existence of a wave, which comes after the *T* wave and may have a considerable height in pathological cases. This wave *U* is also present in the curves from normal hearts, but in these cases it is very low as a rule. Lewis estimates that wave *U* is present in three-quarters of all EKG.'s taken by lead II. After an examination of my collection of EKG.'s I also conclude that the presence of peak *U* is very common, at least in half of all persons.

Figs. 11 and 12 are illustrations of EKG.'s with fairly high peaks *U*, obtained from persons with normal hearts. Fig. 11 is from a sportsman, aged 37 years, with a strong musculature; Fig. 12 is from a well-built young man, 19 years of age, of somewhat more than the average height. Wave *U* reaches a value of about $0{\cdot}5 \times 10^{-4}$ volts in both curves, but is not of equal height in all heart beats. This wave must be regarded as an inconstant one.

The significance of it and the reason for its inconstancy are for the present not known with surety. The method of recording the heart sounds, together with the EKG., has shown that the second sound is produced almost immediately after peak *T* is finished. The end of *U* lies after the second sound, so that there is no doubt that wave *U* fails wholly or partly in that phase of the cardiac cycle which follows the closing of the semilunar valves. The heart is in diastole after the closing of these valves. But the heart muscle, which does not begin to contract at all points at the same time, does not relax at all points at the same time either. A large part of the heart can have already relaxed, so that the pressure in the heart's cavities may be practically diminished to zero, and at the same time a few fibres may still be in the condition of contraction. Peak *U* will not have reached its end until these latter fibres are fully relaxed.

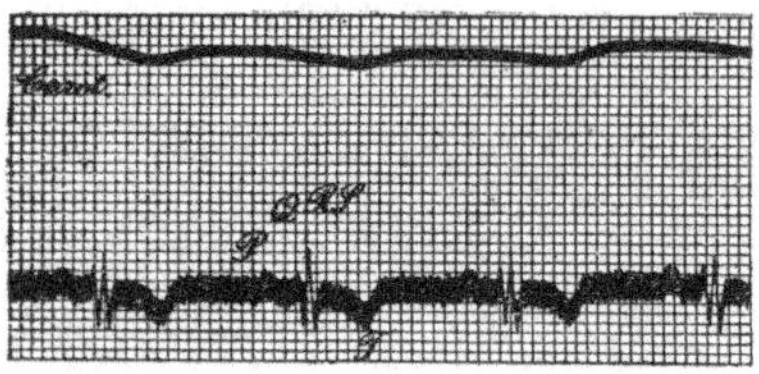

FIG. 10.—Jo. Lead III. A remarkable *QRS*-group.

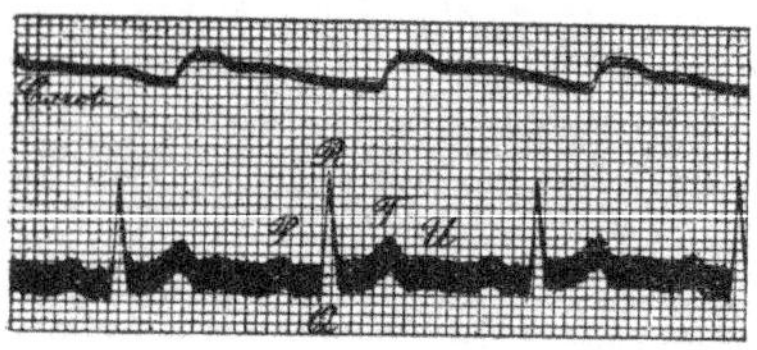

FIG. 11.—Br. Lead II. Wave *U* visible.

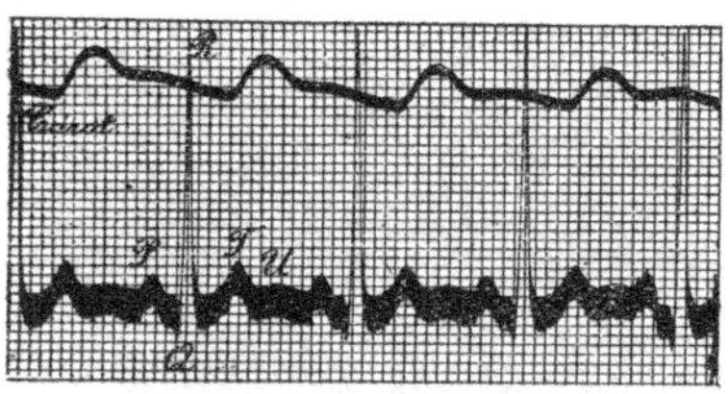

FIG. 12.—Sch. Lead II. Wave *U* visible.

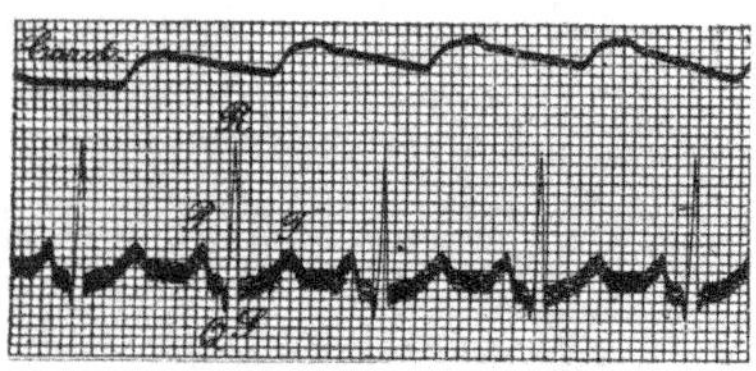

FIG. 13.—Hm. Lead II. The level of the curve between *P* and *Q* is different from the level during diastole.

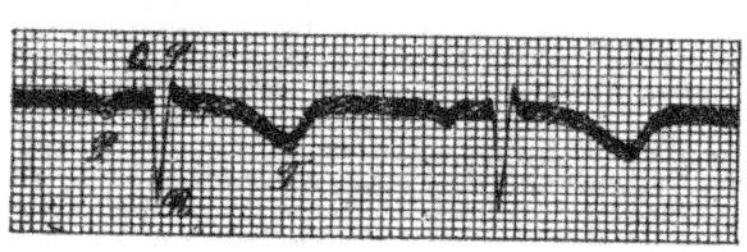

FIG. 14.—Situs inversus viscer. Lead I. Absc. 1 sc. div. = 0·02 sec. Ordin. 1 sc. div. = 10^{-4} volts.

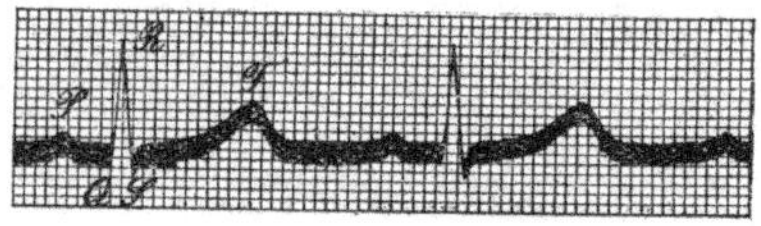

FIG. 15.—Id. The connexions of the electrodes reversed.

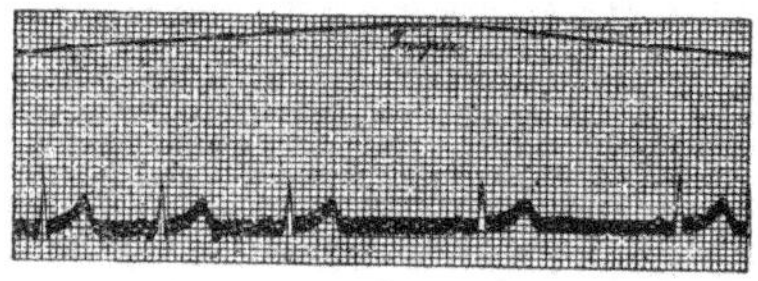

FIG. 16.—Bl. Lead I during inspiration.

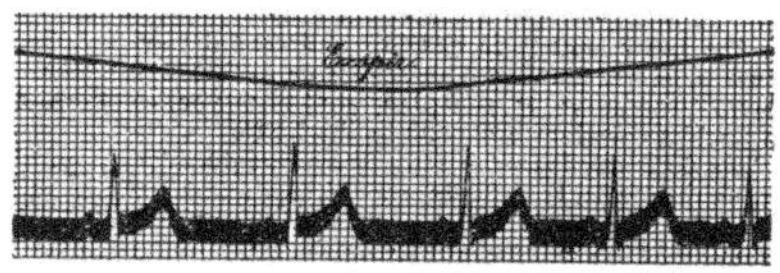

FIG. 17.—Id. Lead I during expiration.

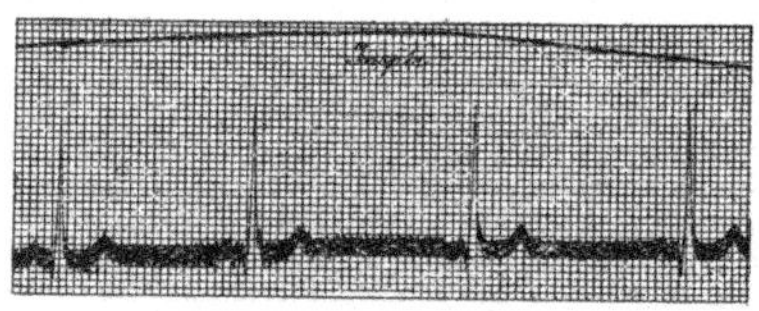

FIG. 18.—Id. Lead III during inspiration.

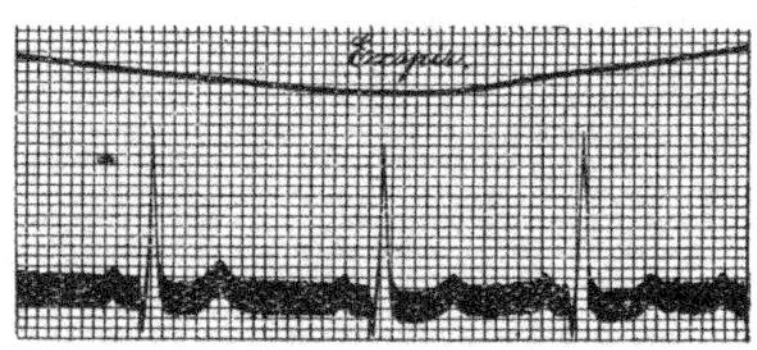

FIG. 19.—Id. Lead III during expiration.

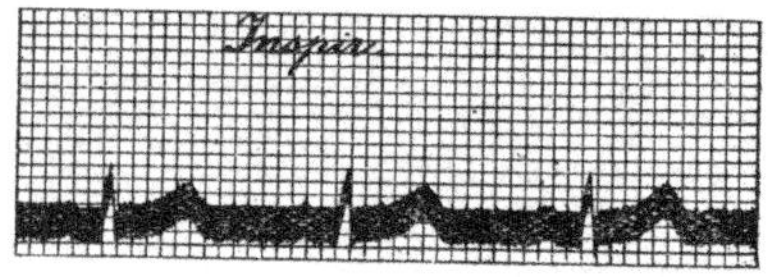

FIG. 20.—Bak. Lead I during inspiration.

The Interval between Auricular and Ventricular Contraction.

In the second place, we wish to direct attention to the position of the galvanometer in the interval between P and the QRS-group. In many cases the string takes the same position here as that held during diastole, so that a horizontal line is recorded at the level of the line of diastole. But in many other cases there is a perceptible difference in the positions of the lines. We wish to illustrate this with only one example (Fig. 13). We see in this figure that the curve between P and the QRS-group lies about 1 mm.—i.e., 10^{-4} volts lower than during diastole. To what must this be ascribed?

Is the conduction through the atrio-ventricular bundle accompanied in this case by the development of a perceptible electrical current, or is a potential difference developed even during the diastole? Have we perhaps to consider a generation of electricity effected by the same causes that produce peak U? For the present we shall not choose between the possibilities mentioned, but shall content ourselves with the information that curves like Fig. 13 are often obtained from persons with normal hearts.

The Influence of the Position of the Heart.

The position of the heart influences the form of the EKG. In electrocardiographic investigations we are chiefly interested, however, in getting a better insight into the *functioning* of the heart, and it is easy to understand that a difficulty must arise in drawing conclusions as to this point from the form of the curve, if a displacement of the organ is sufficient in itself to produce a change in the EKG.

The difficulty is best solved by making ourselves accurately acquainted with the effects of a shifting and a rotating of the heart. The easiest and at the same time the most striking example of the influence of the position of the heart upon the form of the EKG. is offered by a case of situs inversus viscerum. Waller was the first to investigate such a case, and since then a number of other cases have been published. I permit myself here, moreover, to publish a curve taken by Dr. Fahr from a boy aged 7 years by lead I. We see immediately that the peaks of Fig. 14 are exactly the reverse of a normal EKG. If we interchange the conducting wires to right and left hands we obtain a curve which cannot be distinguished from a normal EKG., as is shown in Fig. 15.

Whereas the EKG. in situs inversus may be very easily explained and gives no cause for a more extended discussion, other cases of change in position of the heart are accompanied by more complex phenomena, and these require a more detailed analysis for their understanding. We shall here discuss in particular the deviations in the position of the heart which accompany the movements of respiration.

Movements of the diaphragm participate to a greater or less extent in the respiratory movements of women as well as of men, and the heart must be displaced in the thorax whenever the diaphragm takes a higher or a lower position.

Even before the construction of the string galvanometer Samojloff demonstrated to his classes that increased respiratory movements had a perceptible influence upon the oscillations of the mercury meniscus of the capillary electrometer connected with the human body. By lead I the oscillations became larger in the phase of expiration and smaller in the phase of inspiration. Many other investigators have examined the same phenomena. In our description we shall make use of curves which were taken with the help of Vaandrager and later with the help of Fahr and de Waart. In Figs. 16 and 17 we see pieces of a curve which was taken from Bl. by lead I. The upper curve is the pneumogram.

The pneumogram was obtained by recording the movements of a Hutchinson spirometer into which the person under investigation breathed. A movement of the recording lever upwards corresponds to an inspiration, a movement downwards to an expiration. Each scale division of the ordinates represents 250 c.c. inspired or expired air; the amplitude of the oscillations of the pneumogram vary between 11·3 and 11·5 scale divisions—i.e., 2·8 to 2·9 litres. The vital capacity of the person amounted to 4·4 litres; thus the respiratory movements during the recording of the curves were about two-thirds of the vital capacity. These movements were sufficient for our purpose, and at the same time the subject could execute them with ease.

The pneumogram reproduces the changes in the volume of the thorax without practically any delay. This may be shown by means of the trembling of the subject at the height of inspiration. The effect of this trembling caused by the strong muscle contractions necessary for the excessive movements of inspiration is to be seen clearly in the EKG. As soon as the inspiration is ended the oscillations in the EKG. disappear, for the muscles relax and passive expiration begins. We may say that the end of the trembling coincides with the top of the wave of the pneumogram, if we neglect small differences in time—as, for example, differences of five scale divisions, or 0·2 second.

Apart from the form of the EKG. and the height of its peaks there is a striking variation in the heart's frequency during the movements of respiration. I should like to point out that the maxima and minima of the heart's frequency do not correspond with the crests and troughs of the pneumogram. For instance, the longest pause in the heart's action is found at the end of Fig. 16, the shortest pause at the beginning of the same figure, whereas the volume of the lungs is about the same in both places. The volume of the lungs is also the same at the beginning and at the end of Fig. 17, whereas the heart's frequency differs markedly in these places.

The explanation of this phenomenon is generally known; during very slow and deep respiratory movements the gases of the blood change sufficiently to influence the tonus of the vagi, especially at their origin in the medulla. As the maximum and minimum of vagus tonus do not correspond to the extreme positions of inspiration and expiration, the time of the greatest and the time of the least frequency of the heart will also be displaced in respect to these positions. This displacement varies largely from person to person. We have mentioned this circumstance here because it must be taken into account whenever the influence of the respiratory movements upon the form of the EKG. is discussed. For we know that the form and magnitude of peak P as well as of wave T can be materially changed by the action of the vagi.

In Figs. 18 and 19 we reproduce two pieces of a curve, which was taken from the same person by lead III. The influence of the vagi upon the form of peak P is shown very clearly in these figures. After long heart pauses P is small, sometimes diphasic, other times totally negative, whereas P has its normal form and magnitude after small pauses—i.e., with increased frequency and decreased vagus tonus.

The above mentioned facts make it evident that we meet with a difficulty when estimating the influence upon the form of the EKG. of a displacement of the heart caused by the respiratory movements. Peak P is influenced by two factors, and it is not easy to separate them from one another nor to estimate the magnitude of each alone. We shall therefore concentrate our attention upon some other peaks of the curve.

We see from Figs. 16–19 that the peaks of lead I are larger during expiration, whereas by lead III they become smaller during the same phase of respiration. If we consider these facts in connexion with the formula, lead III = lead II —lead I, we must conclude that the changes in the peaks of lead II will be very slight. And this is, in fact, the case with Bl. and with the majority of the persons investigated. The practical result of this is that we must apply this lead when examining a patient if we wish to investigate the form of the EKG. as free from the influence of the respiratory movements as possible.

Further, we wish to remark in the above figures that peaks R and T are both decreased or both increased in the same degree as well in lead I as lead III during the various phases of breathing. Thus the relative heights of the peaks remain the same, so that the curve retains its form.

But similar changes are not observed in all persons. In some persons we find differences which upon superficial examination seem to be wholly irregular and thereby puzzling. We shall first describe some of these differences separately, and shall then try to unite them all under one point of view.

In the first place we shall direct attention to the fact that the changes which peak R undergoes are, in many cases, materially larger than the corresponding changes in T. Figs. 20, 21, 22, and 23 are examples of this. Figs. 20 and 21 reproduce the EKG. of Bak. by lead I. Two pieces have been cut out of the original curve in such a way that Fig. 20 renders that portion of the record taken in inspiratory position, and Fig. 21 renders that portion taken in expiratory position. In this latter figure we see that the enlargement of peak R is materially greater than that of the T wave, whereby the curve receives quite another shape.

An even greater disparity is brought to light in Figs. 22

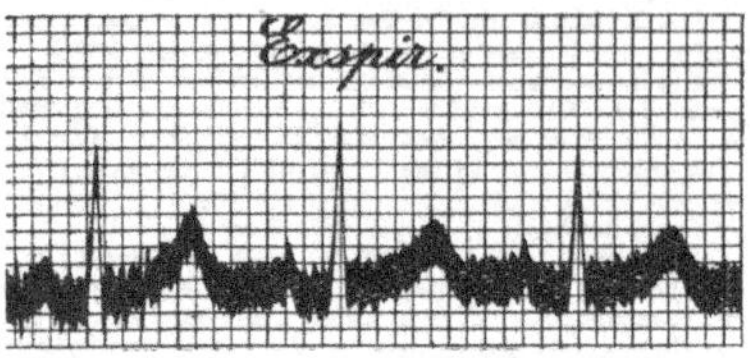

FIG. 21.—Id. Lead I during expiration.

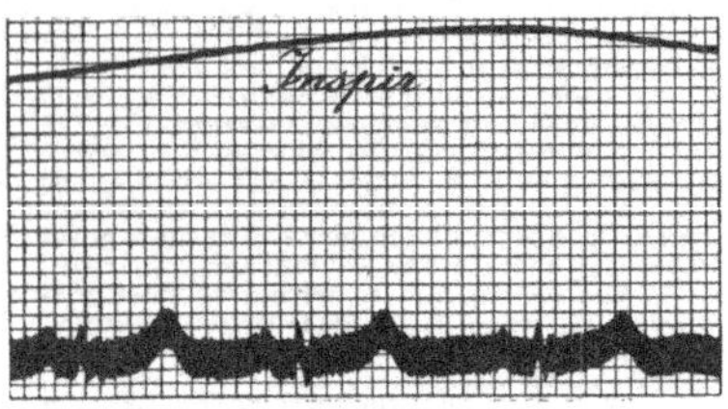

FIG. 22.—Wi. Lead I during inspiration.

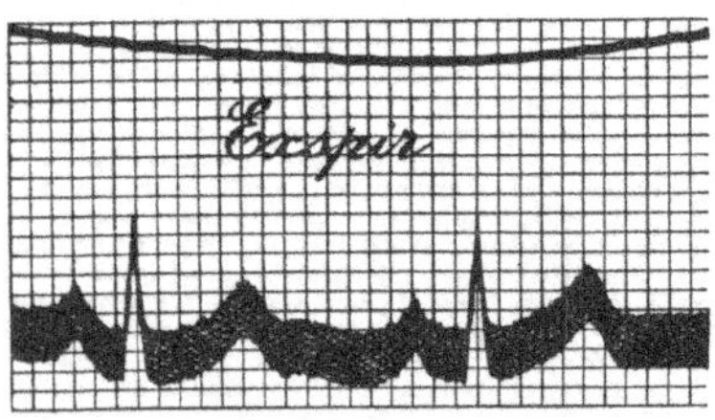

FIG. 23.—Id. Lead I during expiration.

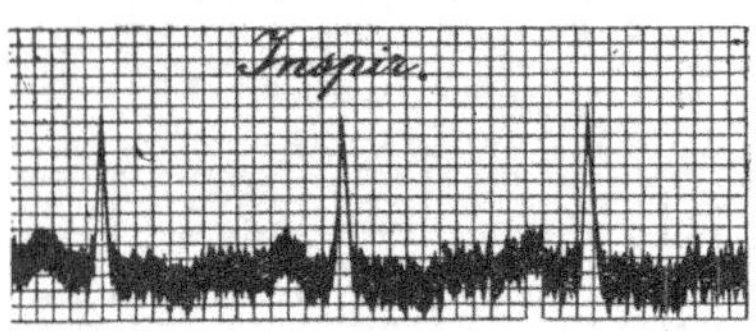

FIG. 24.—Bak. Lead III during inspiration.

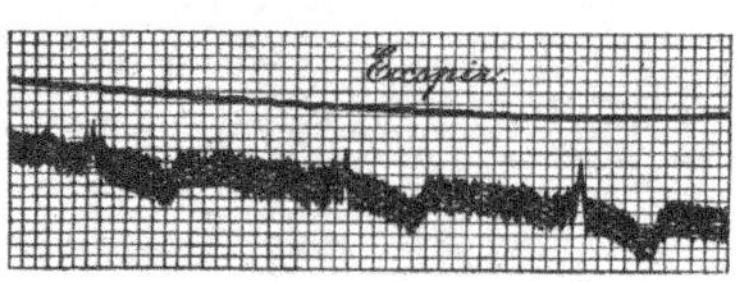

FIG. 25.—Id. Lead III during expiration.

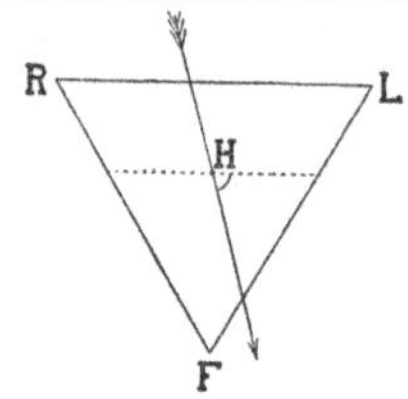

FIG. 26.—Schema of the equilateral triangle. *R* corresponds to the right hand, *L* to the left hand, and *F* to both feet. The heart, *H*, is in the centre. The arrow indicates the direction of the potential differences in the heart. $\alpha = 76°$.

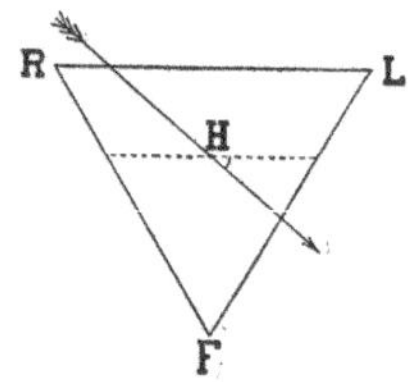

FIG. 27.—Id. $\alpha = 40°$.

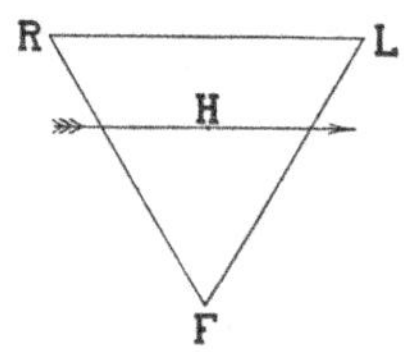

FIG. 28.—Id. $\alpha = 0°$.

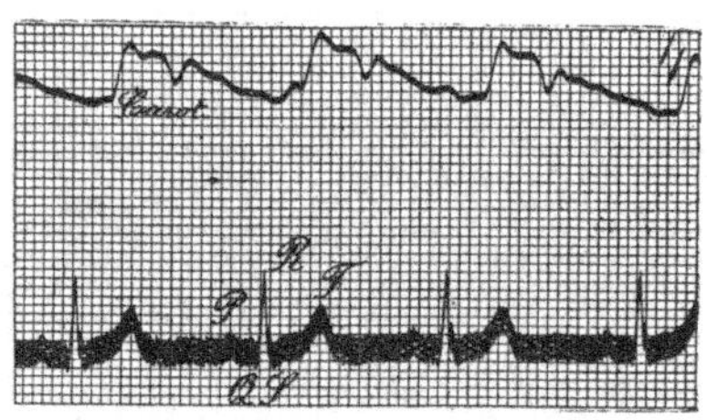

FIG. 29.—Fl Lead I, lying on his left side.

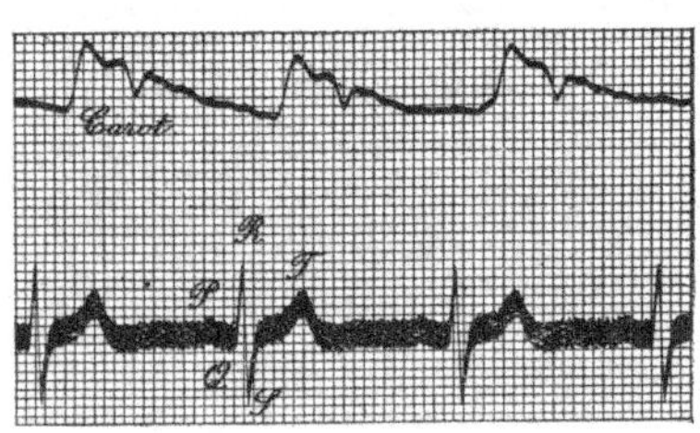

FIG. 30.—Id. with same lead, lying on his right side.

and 23, which were obtained from Wi. Here we have again two pieces of a curve taken by lead I; Fig. 22 corresponds with the inspiratory, Fig. 23 with the expiratory position of the person under investigation. In the first position *R* is larger than *T*, in the second the relation is reversed.

Another difference found is that a peak which becomes larger in lead I also increases in lead III. This phenomenon occurs whenever the peaks have opposite directions in the above-mentioned leads. Figs. 24 and 25 furnish an example of this. They reproduce the EKG. in lead III of the same person whose EKG.'s in lead I were shown in Figs. 20 and 21. Wave *T* is negative in lead III and we see that T_{III} has increased as well as T_I. Phenomena similar to those described above are to be observed in the *QRS*-group.

But we shall now try to explain the apparently so irregular effects of the respiratory movements upon the form of the EKG. In the first place we exclude the possibility that such potential differences as are shown by our curves might be due to accidental causes—as, for instance, the muscle contractions necessary for the respiratory movements, or to a displacement of the electrodes. For if such secondary causes should exercise an influence synchronous with the movements of respiration, then the curved line which reproduces a series of EKG.'s would have to rise and fall in the same rhythm as the movements of breathing. But we see that the line drawn through the heart pauses does not show such a rhythm. On the contrary, it has in many curves an absolutely straight course, as may easily be seen with the aid of the system of square millimetres.

As a second possibility to be taken into account we may mention the influence of a changing body resistance, a hypothesis pointed out by Samojloff. The electrical resistance of the organs surrounding the heart must show during breathing rhythmic changes due to changes in the blood and air content of the chest, and these changes in resistance must necessarily influence the heights of the peaks of the electrocardiogram. But this influence is obviously small, for the curve of lead II shows only slight changes as a rule, whereas the changes produced in lead III are as a rule the opposite of those in lead I. Moreover, the fact that the relation between the heights of the peak is often changed cannot be explained by a change in the resistance of the body.

As a third cause we may mention that the manner in which the heart contracts depends upon the pressure in the thorax. The negative interpleural pressure, which increases during inspiration and decreases during expiration, mechanically influences the circulation perceptibly. But this influence is also insufficient to explain the phenomena described.

The difficulties are solved at once, however, if we apply a schema in which the human body is represented by a plane, homogeneous plate in the form of an equilateral triangle, *RLF*. (Fig. 26.) From its corners the current is lead off to the galvanometer. *R* corresponds to the right and *L* to the left arm, while *F* indicates the potential of both feet. Thus, a lead from *R* and *L* corresponds to lead I, from *R* and *F* to lead II, and from *L* and *F* to lead III. A small spot *H* in the middle of the triangle represents the heart. We assume that in a given moment the potential differences in the heart are so distributed that their resultant takes the direction of the arrow drawn in the figure. This direction indicates the direction of the current in the heart. The angle which the arrow forms with the side *RL* is called α. We shall call the angle positive if, when looking towards the front wall of the chest of the patient, the arrow rotates with the hands of the clock; negative if it rotates in the opposite direction.

We now suppose that the EKG. of a patient has a simple form in each of the three leads, so that the peaks R_I, R_{II}, and R_{III} fall in corresponding phases of a cardiac cycle, and $R_{II} - R_I = R_{III}$. If we transfer the values found with the patient to the schema we are able to determine the direction of the potential difference which has been present in the heart during the recording of *R*.

The EKG. of Bak. in the position of inspiration may be taken as an illustration. In his curves the following values are found for R: $R_I = 3\cdot 2$, $R_{II} = 12\cdot 5$, $R_{III} = 9\cdot 3$ millivolts. In the homogeneous triangular plate with the heart in the centre these values can only be produced by a potential difference, having the direction of the arrow drawn —i.e., that $\alpha = 76°$.

In the position of expiration we find for the same person: $R_I = 9\cdot 2$, $R_{II} = 11\cdot 2$, $R_{III} = 2\cdot 0$; wherefrom we can calculate that under the circumstances $\alpha = 40$. (*Vide* Fig. 27.)

Thus we are able to demonstrate by means of the schema that the heart has rotated in the chest around a sagittal axis during the movement of expiration. The amount of rotation according to the schema is $\alpha_1 - \alpha = -36°$. As we have reason to believe that the real amount of rotation in the body corresponds sufficiently well for practical purposes with the amount of rotation in the schema we shall hereafter simply consider the direction of the potential difference in the body as parallel to the direction of the arrow in the schema. The way in which α can be calculated from the potential differences recorded need not be explained in details. It may suffice to state that the calculation is simple and can be executed very quickly.

The schema can show more than the direction of the potential difference only. It also makes it possible for us to compare the values of the potential differences present in the heart itself. To make this clearer we shall introduce a new term, "the manifest potential difference in the heart," and when speaking of certain peaks, *P*, *R*, or *T*, we shall indicate them with the figures *Pm*, *Rm*, or *Tm*. By these figures is meant the manifest values of the peaks.

We define the manifest potential difference in the heart as the amount shown in one of the three leads, when the direction of the current between the points of leading off is parallel to the direction of the potential difference in the heart. We here consider only potential differences in a frontal plane. Suppose that a given potential difference in the heart forms the peaks T_I, T_{II}, and T_{III}, and that the direction of the current in the schema is represented by an arrow parallel to the side RL (see Fig. 28), then T_I is the largest of the three peaks, T_{II} and T_{III} being opposite to one another, and each equal to one half of T_I. In this case $Tm = T_I$.

The manifest value of a peak can always be calculated from the height of the recorded peaks and thus can always be expressed in absolute measure—e.g., in tenths of a millivolt. This calculation is also easily and quickly made. If we apply it to peak *R* of Bak., the dimensions of which have already been given, we find $Rm = 13 \times 10^{-4}$ volts in the position of inspiration, $Rm = 12 \times 10^{-4}$ in the position of expiration.

In another person a rotation of the heart of $-12°$ was brought about by expiration, *Rm* amounting to 27×10^{-4} volts in a position of inspiration and to 26×10^{-4} volts in a position of expiration. In a third person a rotation of $-20°$ was found, whilst *Rm* kept the constant value of 20×10^{-4} volts. In all persons examined till now the rotation takes place in the same direction in expiration, whilst the manifest height of *R* keeps constant within the limits of the errors of the method.

We can investigate the direction and the manifest value for *T* in the same way as for *R*. As is to be expected, *T* is always rotated by the movements of respiration in the same direction as *R*, but the amount of rotation is not exactly the same. Moreover, the manifest value of *T* changes—a fact which points out that other factors besides the rotation of the heart are active in the formation of *T* during respiration. The vagus tonus is one of these factors.

There are good reasons for assuming that the most prominent peaks of the ventricle electrogram, *T* and *R*, are brought about by potential differences localised in approximately frontal planes. This is proved by the behaviour of peak *S* in lead I. When a person lying horizontally upon the left side turns over upon the right side whilst his EKG. is taken, we obtain the striking phenomenon that peak S_I, which is often very small or not present at all in the first position, becomes visible and sometimes reaches a prominent height in the second position. Figs. 29 and 30, both of which were taken by lead I, furnish an illustration of the production of a large peak S_I by the turning of the body on to the right side. Fig. 29, which was recorded while the patient was lying upon the left side, shows a small peak *S*, which may almost be neglected, whereas Fig. 30, which was obtained while the patient was lying upon the right side, shows a peak *S* so large that we are inclined to be astonished that both curves have been obtained from the same person, with the same lead, and with the exception of the body position, under quite the same circumstances.

The most satisfactory explanation of this, upon superficial examination, so puzzling phenomenon is to be found in the assumption that the heart rotates in the chest about the longitudinal axis of the body, when the body itself turns from the right upon the left side. If there is a potential difference in the heart having a sagittal direction, then a slight rotation of the organ about the longitudinal axis of the body can produce a material change in the height of the corresponding peak, and this will be especially well shown by lead I. If the potential difference has exactly the sagittal direction the peak entirely disappears. It is probable that the large differences in *S* in different persons, as well as its inconstancy, must, as a rule, be explained by this circumstance.

We direct attention to the fact that in Figs. 29 and 30 the peaks *P*, *R*, and *T* undergo hardly any change. If we conclude from the enormous change in *S* that a rotation of the heart has taken place round the long axis of the body, then we must also assume that the peaks *P*, *R*, and *T* are developed in approximately frontal planes, or in other words, in planes making relatively large angles with the sagittal plane, for thereby it can be most easily explained that under these circumstances the changes in these peaks are so small.

The application of the schema of the equilateral triangle accounts for a number of phenomena here treated of. First it is immediately obvious from the schema that a comparatively large displacement of the heart parallel to itself will only slightly affect the heights of the peaks recorded. This explains the fact that the EKG. of many persons is hardly perceptibly changed or is not changed at all during the ordinary movements of breathing. It also explains the fact that with the exception of peak *S*, there are only slight changes produced in the EKG., when the body is turned from one side to the other, although we must expect from the anatomical conditions that the heart has hereby taken a lower position in the chest.

The schema explains easily and satisfactorily how the various peaks of the EKG. are often unequally increased or decreased by a change in the position of the diaphragm, and why the curve of lead II shows slighter changes than the curves of leads I and III. A potential difference which is present in the heart and has a direction which in the one position of the heart makes an angle of 80°, and in the other position an angle of 40°, according to the schema, causes the formation of a peak which remains unchanged in lead II, but which is very much altered in lead I as well as in lead III. If this peak in lead II has the value $9 \cdot 4 \times 10^{-4}$ volts in the first position of the heart, it keeps this value in the second position. It increases in lead I from $1 \cdot 7 \times 10^{-4}$ volts in the first position to $7 \cdot 7 \times 10^{-4}$ volts in the second. It decreases in lead III from $7 \cdot 7 \times 10^{-4}$ volts in the first position to $1 \cdot 7 \times 10^{-4}$ volts in the second.

It is equally clear why a peak which has the same direction in leads I and III undergoes opposite changes by a displacement of the diaphragm, whereas it is either increased or decreased in both leads if it has a positive value in lead I and a negative in lead III. This is the case when α has a value between $-90°$ and $+30°$.

With the aid of the schema we are in a better position to judge the form of the EKG. under all circumstances. For instance, it is possible therewith to show that an increased frequency of the heart brought about by bodily exercise is always accompanied by a positive rotation of *T* and by an increase in the manifest value of this peak. In myodegeneratio cordis and in many cases of auricular fibrillation *T* is small in all three leads. It need not be said that *Tm* must also be small under these circumstances.

In cases of hypertrophy of the left ventricle we sometimes find the most prominent peak of the *QRS*-group in a direction represented by $\alpha = 40°$, whereas in normal hearts the value of α for this peak lies between $+40°$ and $+90°$. We see from these figures that the deformation of the EKG. in this heart affection is not, or not chiefly, caused by a change in the position of the heart. The manifest value of the most prominent peak of the *QRS*-group in hypertrophy of the left ventricle can reach the enormous value of 26×10^{-4} volts. In hypertrophy of the right heart we obtain, as is well known, EKG.'s of an entirely different form, to which, however, similar considerations may be applied. By means of the schema we can in general differentiate the real changes in the heart's action from the apparent ones which are only caused by variations in the position of the heart.

Atypical contractions may also be examined with the aid of the schema. They are of great importance in the clinic, and are worthy of a special, detailed discussion, but I must conclude now.

It gives me an especial pleasure to bring to remembrance here that the human EKG. was first recorded by a London physiologist, Augustus D. Waller, who also introduced the term "electrocardiogram" into science; and that Dr Thomas Lewis, whose extensive researches have been crowned with such exceptional success, was the first man in England who applied electrocardiography to clinical investigations.

The method of electrocardiography is still a young plant. We may reasonably expect that it will continue to bear good fruit.

XA
Correspondence with Thomas Lewis (1915)

There was some uncertainty in connection with the equilateral triangle which is brought to light by the following correspondence with Lewis. Many years of vectorcardiographical experience have now shown in retrospect that the simplification contained in the equilateral triangle can be accepted for most purposes. The question, put by Lewis, whether the theoretical electrical scheme should match anatomical conditions returns repeatedly in the history of vectorcardiography. Much later Burger opposed the equilateral triangle again on physical grounds (unequal electrical resistances inside the body, which make the assumption of a homogeneous sheet illusive). However, in practice the original model has held its place, even after, – in the context of vectorcardiography – it had been widened to a tridimensional structure including thoracic leads (contrary to Einthoven's supposition of an "infinite" distance of the electrodes from the heart, see XB).

It is obvious from Einthoven's answer to Lewis that simplicity and practical usefulness were the guidelines for his choice. This was perhaps characteristic; according to Samojloff (ref. in chapter 1) " All methods proposed by him are based on theory and at the same time are highly practical..." It can be added, that subsequently many investigators tried to equate the anatomical and the electrical axis (the latter being the direction of the manifest potential). This led to studies, in which the anatomical and the electrical axis were compared in successive phases of respiration. Lewis* investigated this in an patient with a roentgenologically recognizable bullet in the heart. Einthoven and his assistant Flohil** took roentgenograms of the heart at successive, (electrocardiographically) monitored moments during systole and in predetermined phases of respiration. The conclusion in both instances was that the directions of the anatomical and electrical axis were not identical, but that changes in the former entailed similar changes in the latter, at least in the erect position. However, this did not appear to apply to the sitting position (Lewis); moreover, rotation does not take place around a purely sagittal axis (Flohil).

* Heart 10: 257-265, 1923.
** See A. FLOHIL, Thesis Leiden 1928.

Telephone
2307 Mayfair.

27, Queen Anne Street,
Cavendish Square, W.

1st Feb. 1915

Dear Professor Einthoven,

In calculating the electrical axis of the heart beat, you use an equilateral triangle ; but in the dog it is much more nearly a right-angled triangle, the right-angle lying at the left of the shoulder.

I have been puzzled to know whether the adoption of the equilateral triangle introduces any material error in the calculation of the angle, and also to know whether it would be any advantage to reconstruct the actual triangle for a given case. What I am anxious to do is to find the axis for a given body as accurately as possible.

With kind regards,

I am,

Yours sincerely,

Thomas Lewis

Professor W. Einthoven.
Leyden.

L e y d e n , February 15th, 1915.

deze brief is onaangeteekend verzonden, maar de dissertatie en de beide manuscripten en de figuren zijn aangeteekend
WE

Dear Lewis,

When I prepared my paper „Über die Rich„ tung und die manifeste Grösse etc" I tried several triangles in be„ „half of my calculations. The most practical one is the equilateral triangle. As soon as we take an other form we shall meet with some difficulties. If we take an isosceles triangle we must begin to

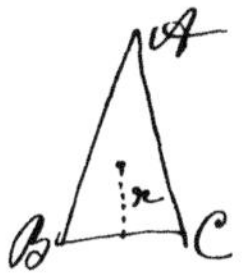

solve two questions : 1st How great is to be taken the angle A ? 2nd At which height x is the heart to be placed ?

If we take a right-angled triangle, we must begin to solve

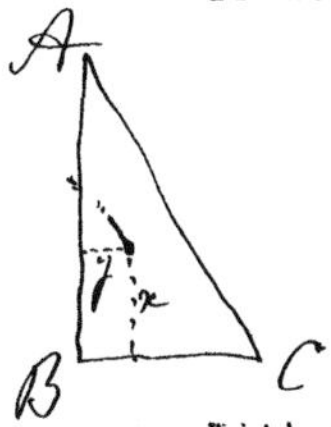

three questions : 1st How great are to be taken the acute angles ? 2nd At which height x is the heart to be placed ? 3rd How great is the dis„ tance y ?

With the equilateral triangle none of the questions arise.

Now suppose we have found out the true magnitude of the angles and the exact place of the heart in the isosceles and the right-angled triangle. Then there will rise new difficulties as soon as we try to calculate the axis of the heart beat. On the other hand the calculation of the axis in the equilateral triangle is easy.

Moreover I think that you will not make an error of any practi„

„cal value if you take the equilateral triangle for the dog as well as for man. I am sorry to say that my own work an the subject has had to be delayed and I am anxious to see the results that you may obtain.

Under separate cover I am sending to you the manuscripts of two communications, which I hope you are willing to publish in your journal „ Heart ". The first one is nearly a complete translation of a dissertation of one of my pupils Battaerd on „Further graphic researches etc." I enclose a sample of the dissertation and can af„ „ford you all the blocks required. If you perhaps might prefer the original diagrams and photo's I could send them to you too.
The second communication is one of my pupil Korteweg and myself „On the variability of the size of the pulse etc." I am joining to the type-written copy 3 diagrams, 8 tables and 6 curves. The blocks of the five last curves are to your disposal.

I have done my best to obtain a good English translation but nevertheless should like to have a proof before the communications are published.

With kind regards,

I am Yours truly

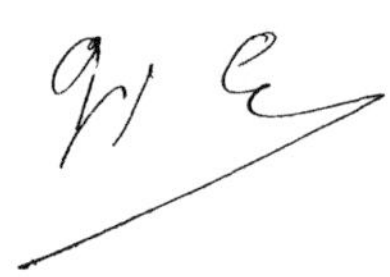

Note. This letter from Einthoven to Lewis (and equally that to Wilson) has been reproduced from the copy in Einthoven's files (Museum Boerheave). Einthoven write on it how it was sent, and added the same about the manuscripts, referred to at the end of the letter. H.A.S.

XB
Correspondence with Frank Wilson (1921)

Here again the equilateral triangle and in particular the direction of the manifest potential comes into discussion. The limits of the schematic simplification which Einthoven's triangle embodies, are more clearly defined. The difference between intrinsic and extrinsic electric effects, which Wilson quotes from Lewis, Meakins and White is not discussed in Einthoven's answer. This concept, however, was essential for much of later experimental work of Wilson and others as well as for the introduction by Wilson of the precordial leads in clinical electrocardiography. In addition to his discussion of the global, summated potential difference Einthoven makes a suggestion about the local electrical events inside the heart, which was embodied in his segmental theory, (see ch. 1 on page V). The latter was published briefly (122, 129) and incorporated in his last reviews (134, 137) but never fully studied experimentally or discussed in details and with regard to consequences. Lewis described Einthoven's suggestion in his monograph, cited above (p. 57). Soon after sending his reply to Wilson in 1921, Einthoven noted some additional remarks, presumably meant for a later publication, which was never completed.

The first half of these remarks is as follows: "1) At the locations n_1, n_2, and n_3, I have to assume the presence of an electrical source in the shape of a galvanic element or a double galvanic element, i.e. − + or + − +". 2) I have yet to make clear, that negativity is present, as long as contraction increases or decreases. In a constant state of contraction negativity is absent, e.g. in muscular tone or also, when a contraction wave has reached its peak and can be represented graphically by a horizontal stretch. (Translated from the Dutch by H.A.S.).

The letters n_1, n_2, n_3, refer to the drawing shown in XB. The analogy with Wilson* 's dipoles (sources and sinks) and Craib** 's doublets is

* F. N. Wilson: The distribution of the potential differences produced by the heart beat within the body and at its surface. Essentials of Einthoven's triangle. This paper provides an excellent illustration of Wilson's interpreting and supplementing role with respect to Einthoven. Am. Heart J. 5:599-616, 1930.
For a more extensive discussion of Wilson's own work in this field see J. Gen. Physiol. 16: 423-456, 1933.

** W. H. Craib: A study of the electrical field surrounding active heart muscle. Heart 40: 71-109. 1927-1929.
id. The electrocardiogram. Medical Research Council Special Report Series no. 147, 1930.

evident. However, the influence of the surrounding conducting medium (i.e. the body) which was the primary concern of these two authors, is not discussed in this note.

Wilson

Prof. W. Einthoven,
Physiological Institute
University of Leyden
Leyden, Holland.

Dear Prof. Einthoven;-

I have been a student of electrocardiography for some years and naturally consider myself a disciple of the master who invented the string galvanometer and introduced it to the medical world. I trust, therefore, that you will pardon my writing you in regard to some problems which have been troubling me and which relate to your published work.

First, in regard to the equilateral triangle;- This has been of very great value in picturing the events that produce the deflections of the three leads. Nevertheless, it seems to me that its applicability has been misunderstood. Let us imagine that this paper is a sheet of conducting material of infinite extent. Let us draw on its surface an equilateral triangle (ABC) and let us generate at its exact center (O) an EMF represented by the vector XY.

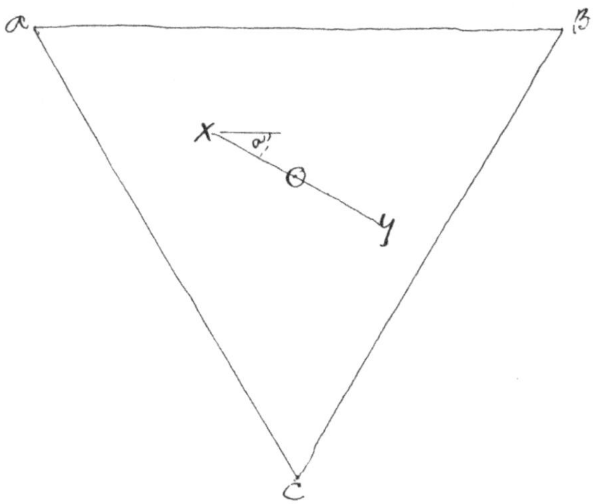

Is it not true that under these conditions the difference in potential between A and B depends upon the relations of the ratio AX/AY to the ratio BX/BY (other factors being constant are neglected) ? Now, it may undoubtedly be proven that the difference in potential between these two apices of the triangle is proportional to the cosine of the angle (a). This proof, however, is not contained in your original paper on the subject. I assume that you admitted it for the sake of simplicity, but it seems to me that this omission has led to misunderstanding as to the conditions under which the scheme of the triangle may be applied. Does the applicability of the triangle to the ordinary leads not depend upon the fact that the electrodes are applied at a considerable distance from the heart, thereby reducing

?
to a minimum the errors arising from the fact that the three points of application do not form a true equilateral triangle and from the fact that the heart does not lie at the exact center of the triangle? Is it justifiable to apply the triangle to small animals such as the frog or to other leads than those in common use even if these leads are similarly arranged? Is it justifiable to draw on the surface of the chest near the heart an equilateral triangle, to then take three electrocardiograms from the apices of the triangle, and finally apply the equations for determining the direction and magnitude of the potential difference arising in the heart? It seems to me that when the electrodes are placed near the heart the possibility of error must be great.

Second, in regard to the direction of E and the muscle activity that it represents;- Do you hold that a downward delection in all three leads indicates preponderant activity at the apex of the heart and that an upward deflection in all three leads indicates preponderant muscle activity at the base of the heart, or do you agree with Lewis that apical activity may produce an upward deflection when(as he believes to be the case) the excitation process travels from above downward from the endocardial to the epicardial surface of the heart?

In this connection I should like to call to your attention some observations made by Lewis, Meakins and White (Phil. Trans. Roy. Soc. London, Series B, vol. 205, p375). He found that, when the right-hand electrode was placed directly upon the sino-auricular node and the left-hand electrode a short distance away on the auricular muscle, the first deflection was upward indicating primary negativity of the node(See Fig. 2 of Lewis' paper) When on the other hand the right hand electrode was placed a short distance from the node ~~the first deflect~~ and the left-hand electrode still farther away, the first deflection ~~was~~ which Lewis terms the extrinsic deflection was downward. This was followed immediately by a much larger upward deflection which Lewis terms the intrinsic deflection. These conditions are diagramed below.

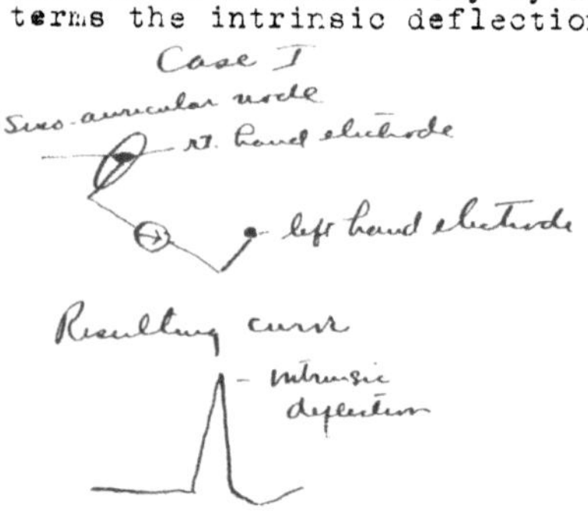

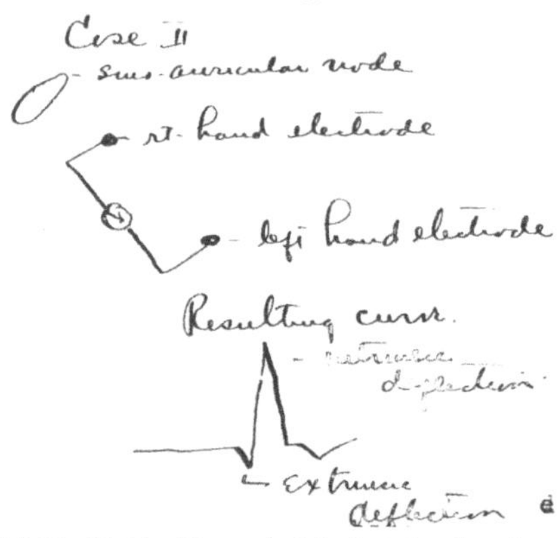

The extrinsic deflection(case II) indicates that the right hand electrode is relatively positive in spite of the fact that it lies nearest the active region. Does not the presence of this downward deflection indicate that all of the inactive muscle is not equally positive

3
with reference to the ~~inacti~~ active muscle? Does it not indicate that the muscle adjacent to the active region rather than the inactive muscle as a whole represents the positive pole of the battery of which the active muscle represents the negative pole? Are not these observations important in deciding between the two views outlined above? Are they not in favor of the view held by Lewis?

I am sending you a reprint of a paper recently published in Heart and I should value your criticism. I should also value any of your reprints which are still available, more especially those which deal with the equilateral triangle and with the construction and operation of the string galvanometer.

Please state whether I may quote from your letter should I wish to do so. I shall respect you wishes in the matter.

With most sincere regards,

Frank N. Wilson
Assoc. Prof. of Medicine
University of Michigan.

804 Lawrence St.,
Ann Arbor Mich
U.S.A.

Leiden, November 3rd, 1921.

Afschrift.

gezonden : C.3025 en M.136.

Een aantal overdrukken en deelen der „Onderzoekingen" via de [illegible].

IV 6

Dear Professor Wilson,

I apologise for having delayed so long my answer to your kind letter of a few weeks ago. I hope you will excuse me. I had to move and am not yet quite settled in my new house, where I hope to have the pleasure of meeting you at some time or other.

In regard to the equilateral triangle I fully agree with you. I assumed in my original paper „Ueber die Richtung und die manifeste Grösse d. Potentialschwankungen etc." Archiv f.d.ges.Physiol. Bd.150 p.308 and 309, in the centre of the triangle a „dipole" that is to say two points lying very close by one another and showing a potential difference.

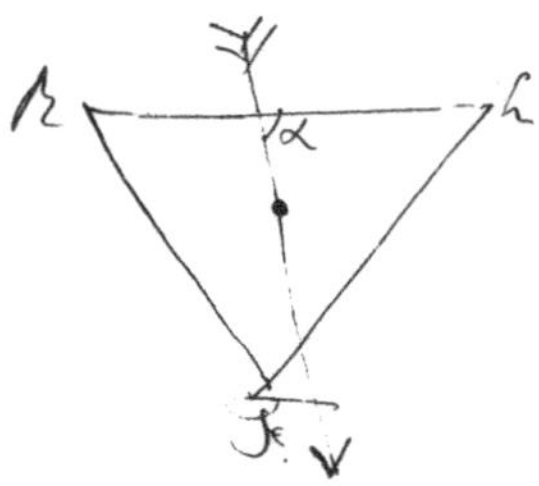

The triangle was supposed to be a homogeneous sheet of conducting material and in regard to the small distance between the two points of the dipole, of a large, let us say infinite exent.

The applicability of this scheme to the ordinary leads of the human body depends indeed on the fact that the electrodes are at a relati-

2

vely great distance from the heart. If they are placed near the heart, the errors are greater and the more so the closer they get to the heart. Even in the case of the ordinary leads from the limbs the results can not be absolutely exact.

In regard to the direction of Ē and the muscle activity that it represents : I do <u>not</u> hold, that a downward deflection in all three leads indicates preponderant activity at the apex of the heart and that an upward deflection in all three leads indicates preponderant muscle activity at the base of the heart, and I agree with Lewis that preponderant apical activity may produce an upward deflection in leads II and III.

But according to my opinion it is not quite correct to state as a strict law, that the direction in which the excitation wave travels determines the direction of the movement of the string. The potential difference that <u>at a given moment</u> exists between two leads and is indicated by the galvanometer, is not caused by the travelling of a wave but is the expression of the presence of an electromotive force <u>at the same moment</u>. I admit, that the beautiful experiments of Lewis have proved, that in the cardiac muscle the direction of the electromotive force usually corresponds to the direction in which the excitation wave travels. But it need not be so always.

The heart muscle-fibres show segmentation. There are transverse septa across the fibres, each interseptal space having its own nucleus and forming a kind of unit.

3

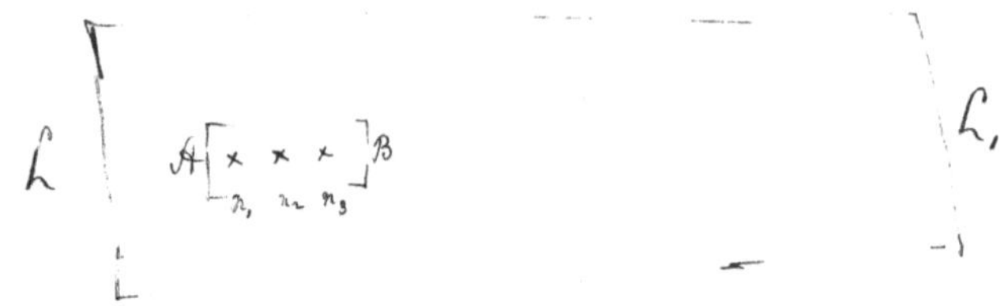

Let AB represent an interseptal space of a heart muscle-fibre and let LL_1 represent the heart or, as you like, the whole human body. Suppose there is an excitation wave travelling through the segment from A to B. At a certain moment the top of the wave showing the greatest negativity is in n_2 that is to say in the middle of the segment. At that moment A and B have the same potential and although the segment is lying asymmetrically in the heart and in the body. L and L_1 must at that same moment also be equipotential.

If the top of the wave is in n_3 , B will be negative in regard to A. Therefore L_1 will be negative in regard to L, although n_3 and even B may be nearer to L than to L_1.

If the top of the wave is in n_1 of course L will be negative in respect to L_1.

I hope to be able to study this question experimentally in the cardiac muscle, but in the mean while I may mention the phenomena which are to be seen in an ordinary frog muscle, for instance the sartorius or gastrocnemius. The fibres of those muscles may be regarded as complete syncytia and are about as long as the muscles themselves. Each fibre consists of a unit by itself, and we may consider it in the same way as we did the interseptal space of a cardiac muscle fibre.

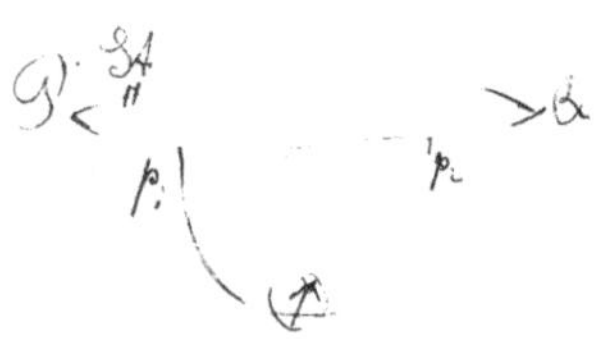

Let PQ be the sartorius, stimulate it at St and lead from p_1 and p_2 to the galvanometer. You will obtain a diphasic electro

myogram of about this form

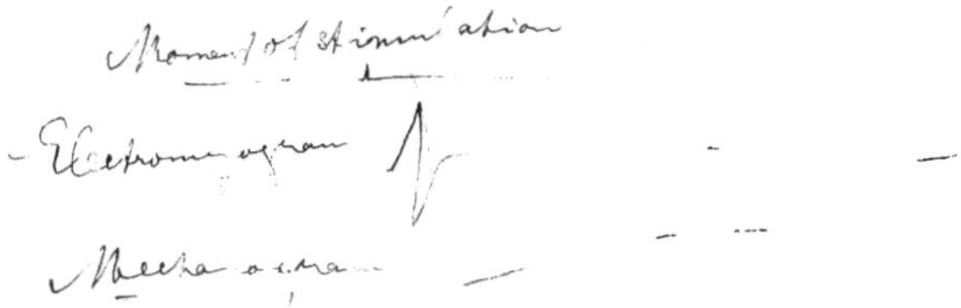

Here you have an instance of an excitation wave travelling in one direction, whilst the deflections of the galvanometer change [redacted] turning from an upward to a downward direction. This change in the direction of the deflection is not to be attributed to the decline of the excitation process in the muscle. During the recording of the whole diphasic electromyogram the muscle remains in full activity. This may be proved by considering the time relations. Within 0,04 sec. after the moment of stimulation, when the diphasic electric response has nearly come to an end, the contraction of the muscle is ~~already~~ not yet at a maximum, the relaxation only being finished a considerable time later.

We have been able to show in the laboratory that the electrical and mechanical responses of a muscle correspond more closely than is generally accepted. I enclose a curve, showing the electrical response of the gastrocnemius of a frog. You may perceive after the diphasic wave an inconspicuous, slow, long continued negative deflection, which may be compared with the T-summit of the ekg and which stops at about the moment that the contraction ceases.

I showed this curve and many other ones at a lecture that I gave in London last May, when I had the pleasure of staying with our mutual friend Lewis. I have still to publish some parts of that lecture but I doubt whether I shall have the opportunity to publish it as a

5

whole. Of course you may quote from my letter if you should wish to do so.

I have read your valuable paper on „incomplete bundle branch block" with great pleasure and am sending you a curve of a patient that may interest you in this connection. You will receive also some reprints and some volumes of the Researches of the Leyden laboratory. Vol. 3, 4 and 5 are out of print.

With kind regards I remain

yours truly

Note. Wilson made no use of this permission to quote the letter. However, he wrote around 1951 a paper, entitled "The origin and nature of the progress made in our understanding of the electrocardiogram during the last three decades", in which he reproduced the whole of Einthoven's letter. This manuscript was published posthumously in "The selected Papers by Dr. Frank N. Wilson," Heart Station, Ann Arbor, 1954. I quote from Wilson's comments: "It is now evident that Einthoven's belief that there was a very close relation between the electrical and mechanical responses of muscle, which was well supported by data he had collected, led to misinterpretation of the tracings obtained in experiments of the kind described and illustrated in his letter. The second, downwardly directed component of the diphasic curve actually corresponds to the T wave of the electrocardiogram. ---- If Einthoven had injured the muscle at the point P2 he would have obtained a monophasic response (and it is certain that the duration of this response would have been the same as that of the diphasic response), and he would have discovered his error.
---- In his discussion of the experiment on the skeletal muscle Einthoven clearly distinguishes between deflections due to the spread and those due to the decline of the excitation process ----

This brief recital of the status of knowledge of the form of the electrocardiogram thirty years ago indicates that the work of Einthoven and of Lewis, and to a lesser extent of the men who preceded them, made what has happened since in their field inevitable. The electrocardiographer of today is standing squarely on the shoulders of these two men. ----."

H.A.S.

XI
The relation of mechanical and electrical phenomena of muscular contraction, with special reference to the cardiac muscle

Einthoven regarded the close and indissoluble link between electrical and mechanical activity as a fundamental quality of cardiac and skeletal muscle. Many of his contemporaries saw or assumed to see, that contraction occurred later and ceased sooner than the action current or indeed could be absent when the latter was weak. Together with his staff he was several times engaged in studies which proved that the discrepancy, if existing at all, was slight and only apparent because of difference in sensitivity of the methods used for detection of the respective phenomena. The present paper gives a summary of his research in this field, in which related subjects like the Gaskell effect (see under VII) and muscle poisoning are included.

It should be noted that in earlier papers (see VII) and even in his last (137) Einthoven extended the relation of electrical and mechanical activity to a (limited) use of the electrocardiogram for assessing the force of the heart in different, but comparable circumstances. This idea was always cautiously handled but never abandoned. In XI it is not mentioned specifically, however.

In this connection the remark may be made, that Einthoven's interest in the estimation of the contractile force from the dextrocardiogram stemmed in first instance from the study of ventricular premature beats, which previously were said to have lost their force when there was an intermission of the pulse. On the other hand he also wished to substantiate the connection of laboratory experiments with clinical medicine, as the last paragraph of this reprint intimates.

THE RELATION OF MECHANICAL AND ELECTRICAL PHENOMENA OF MUSCULAR CONTRACTION, WITH SPECIAL REFERENCE TO THE CARDIAC MUSCLE [1]

DR. WILLEM EINTHOVEN

Professor of Physiology, University of Leyden, Holland

THE subject which I have chosen for this lecture concerns itself with the relationship between the mechanical and electrical phenomena which occur when a muscle contracts. Every

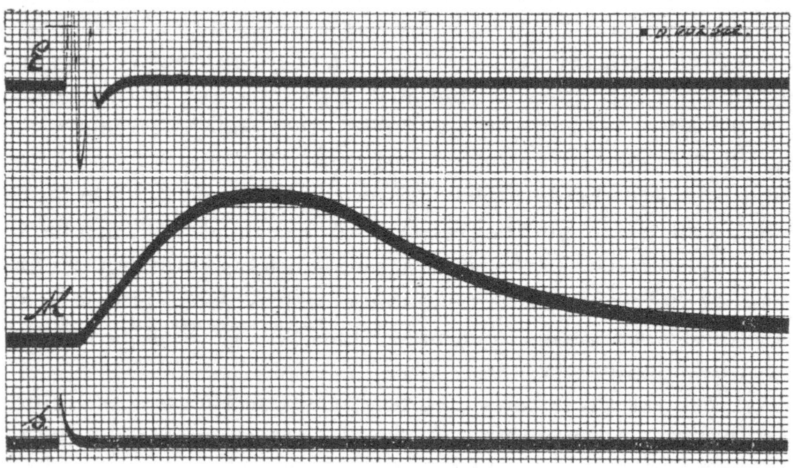

FIG. 1.—Gastrocnemius muscle of a frog stimulated by a single induction shock through the sciatic nerve. *E*, electromyogram; *M*, mechanomyogram; *S*, signal. *Hoogerwerf.*

muscle when contracting develops an electrical current which, indeed, is very weak, if you compare it with the current of an ordinary incandescent lamp, but which, nevertheless, may be measured and recorded very well by means of sensitive instruments.

The curves obtained are called *electromyograms* and are valuable means of studying the true nature of a muscular contraction.

---

[1] Lecture delivered December 6, 1924.

We shall deal with muscles in general and the cardiac muscle in particular.

When a muscle is stimulated by a single induction shock and is made to register both the mechano- and electromyogram, the curves obtained have the appearance shown in figure 1. The upper curve shows the electrogram recorded by the galvanometer; next below is the mechanogram, then follows the signal indicating the moment of stimulation.

The mechanogram is obtained by using a lever which is connected to the muscle by means of a spring. Every increase in tension of the muscle produces a movement of the lever. The muscle shortens a little, too, but this shortening is so trifling that we practically may say that the muscle increases its tension exclusively. The mode of contraction is called isometric.

A distinctly measurable time is seen to pass between the moment at which the electrogram makes its appearance and that at which the mechanogram begins to develop.

The generally accepted interpretation of the curves shown to you is as follows: the stimulus causes the development of an excitation wave which, starting from the stimulation-point, is propagated through the muscle and is the real cause of the electric current. A short time after the excitation-wave and after the development of the electric current, the mechanical action in the muscle starts; it either increases its tension or it shortens.

If you consider the curve as representing the true time relations, the interpretation given is quite conceivable,—it may, in fact, be the only possible one. There is a well-known comparison between the muscle and a steam engine. The mechanical power developed by the engine is consequent to the passage of the steam through the steam pipe. First the valve in the steam pipe has to be opened. The electric current in the muscle should be comparable to the movement of the valve, the mechanical power developed in the muscle comparable to the mechanical power of the engine.

The cardiac muscle differs in many respects from an ordinary skeletal muscle, but the principles which rule its contraction are

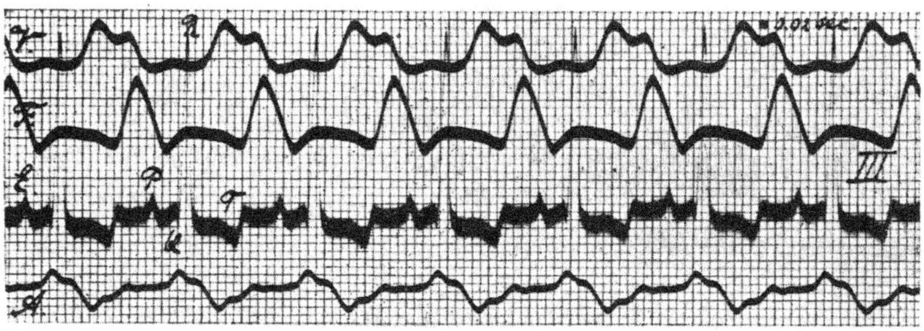

FIG. 2.—Dog. *V*, variations of pressure in the left ventricle; *A*, variations of pressure in the right auricle; *F*, pulse of the femoral artery; *E*, electrocardiogram, lead III. *Dasbach.*

the same. With every systole there is, besides the mechanical effect, the development of an electric current, and on ordinary records we can see that the electrical phenomenon precedes the development of the mechanical power.

The upper curve of figure 2 represents the variations of pressure in the left ventricle. A tube is introduced by way of the carotid artery into the left ventricle of a dog. The variations in pressure are recorded by a lever.

In a similar way the variations in pressure of the right auricle *A*, and of the arterial pulse *F* are recorded, whereas the third curve *E* represents the galvanometric record of the electric currents, developed by the cardiac muscle. The P-wave corresponds to the electric current of the auricles. You see that it precedes their increase in pressure to an amount of 2 or 3 millimetres, each millimetre corresponding to the time of 0.02 sec.

The peak *Q* and the large peak *R* correspond to the contraction of the ventricles. They precede the systole also about two millimetres.

Of course, the pulse-wave is very much later, because of the time required to propagate the wave from the heart to the artery, the pulse of which is recorded.

The comparison with the steam engine and its valve seems to be as well applicable to the heart as to the ordinary skeletal muscle. According to this view, there would only be an indirect connection between the contraction and the electric current. If there is no steam in the boiler, you may open the valve of the steam pipe, and there will be no movement of the engine. In very much the same way it might be possible, for instance in pathological cases, or by means of a poison or drug or in some other way, to inhibit or even to block the transition between the excitation wave and the contraction, and thus completely separate the two phenomena.

I shall now try to demonstrate that this view is based on insufficient evidence and that a different explanation is possible. According to the latter, the process which causes the increase of tension in the muscle is itself the cause of the electric current, and thus the electrical and mechanical phenomena are closely and inseparably connected.

At first sight this supposition seems to have very little to recommend it. The curves shown to you make it difficult to believe that two processes differing so much in time and in form should in reality be so closely coupled.

Now let us first inquire, whether in forming our opinion we may assume that the recorded curves are reliable representations of the true facts, and whether very much weight may be attached to the apparent time-interval between the electrical and mechanical phenomena. We must take into account that the registration of a movement is bound to involve some loss of time. When a body at rest of mass m is set in motion by a force f, the distance described by the body will be given by the formula

$$s = \frac{1}{2} \frac{f}{m} t^2$$

t representing the time.

The distance s represents the displacement of the marking lever and that is the quantity which can be made visible and registered. We see from the formula that when the force is small and the mass large, or rather when the ratio of the force to the mass is small, the distance s is also small, and we know moreover that some time is required for the force in a muscle to rise to a certain value. This development of force, which follows the stimulus, is a vital process and, like all vital processes, proceeds slowly and gradually. If we assume that during the first few thousandths of a second after the stimulus the force increases proportionately to t, we must conclude that the distance s, described by the lever, is proportional to t^3. And thus we see that for very small times the displacement of the lever may be imperceptible, at least by means of the instruments at our disposal.

The electrogram is less retarded than the mechanogram, since in that case the mass of the body which has to be set in motion, say the string of a string-galvanometer or the small column of mercury of the capillary electrometer, is very small in relation to the acting force.

If we don't take the utmost care in obtaining the mechanical response of a muscle as soon as possible after the stimulation, the shortening observed may be retarded enormously. This is, for instance, the case when we record an isotonic contraction.

If we try to obtain the visible contraction of the muscle as soon as possible, we meet with many technical difficulties. As the technique has improved in the course of years, the results of

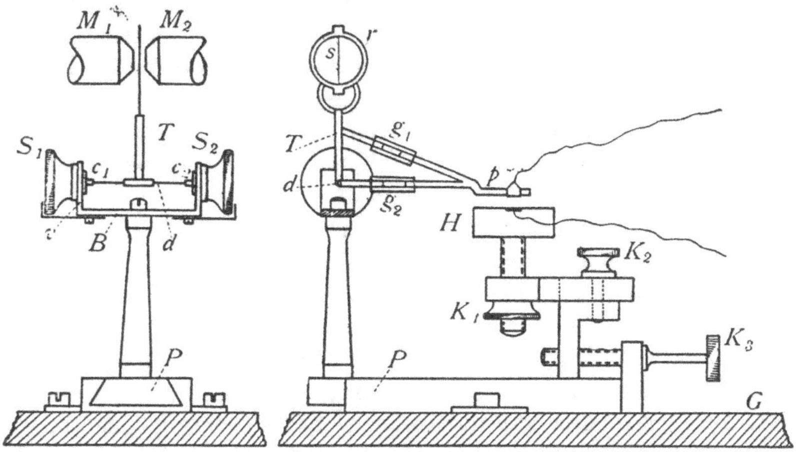

FIG. 3.—String myograph. *d*, stretched metal wire to which a right-angled triangle $T\ g_1\ g_2$ is attached. The muscle rests on the stage *H*. A quartz fibre *s* is mounted in a ring *r* and placed between the microscopes M_1 and M_2.

the measuring experiments have had to be revised. Subsequent investigators have found shorter and shorter latent periods.

Helmholtz found that the latent period of muscular contraction, *i.e.*, the time elapsing between the excitation and the visible contractile process, amounted to about one-hundredth of a second. Later it was shown by Burdon Sanderson that under favorable conditions this interval need not be more than 0.003 of a second (3σ). Koranyi and Vas tested isolated muscular fibres microscopically, and using a stroboscopic method, showed that the latent period could not exceed 1 σ.

For measuring the latent period we have used the following device (see diagram, Fig. 3). *d* is a stretched metal wire to which a right-angled triangle is attached. The muscle rests on a stage *H*. On contraction it becomes thicker and thus makes the triangle turn. At the top of its vertical side a ring *r* is attached in which a fine quartz-fibre *s* which has been made opaque is mounted. This fibre is placed between two microscopes, M_1 and M_2. The action of the triangle is by torsion and completely free of friction.

A magnification of 1000 to 2000 diameters was used, and in order to make *f* as large as possible we always worked with a fresh muscle, which was brought to its maximum contraction by a strong induction-shock. In this manner we found for the latent period about the same value as Koranyi and Vas, *viz.*, 1 σ.

Before drawing conclusions from this result, there are some points to be considered. First of all, we must remember that our apparatus is not ideal. If the mass of the triangle, in itself very small, could be reduced still further, and particularly if we could use still higher magnifications, we should undoubtedly find even smaller values for the latent period.

A second point to which we have to draw attention is the duration of the stimulus. An electric current, as used for the stimulation, can only produce an effect after having passed for some time and thus having accumulated a certain amount of energy. The stronger the current, the shorter the time required. By means of a rapidly registering measuring instrument we have been able to establish that the induction current used by us, which was derived from a simple small coil, lasts more than two-thousandths of a second. A not altogether negligible portion of this time is required for the stimulus to become effective, and thus we must conclude that the actual latent period is shorter than what is given by our registration. The interval between the electrical and the mechanical reactions in the muscle is bound to be even less, for on general physiological grounds we cannot but suppose that the electrical reaction, as also being a vital process of the muscle, requires some time to establish itself.

Taking all this into account, it does not seem at all impossible, or perhaps we may even say it becomes probable, that the two reactions develop simultaneously. In any case the apparent interval found, when the measurements are made with less perfect instruments, cannot be used as an argument in favor of the view that the two reactions which follow one and the same stimulus are two separate and separable processes.

The above experiments were made with the gastrocnemius muscle of the frog. If it is replaced by a nonstriated muscle, like that of the stomach of a frog, the latent period is found to be longer. This must be explained by the circumstance, that the processes in a nonstriated muscle are much slower, and that therefore the development of force, after the stimulus has been applied, takes place relatively slowly; f in our formula is small, hence s the displacement in the first few thousandths of a second is also small. That the latent period of a frog's stomach should reach 14 seconds, as given by some investigators is an estimate wide of the mark. In our measurements we found intervals of less than a tenth of a second, and a duration of that magnitude we think can be reconciled with the view entertained by us, since it can be entirely explained by the imperfections of our instruments.

We shall now discuss measurements made on the spontaneously beating heart, where the electrical and mechanical phenomena may be registered simultaneously, without fear of a possible current escape from the stimulus itself. By means of a device, similar to that used in the investigation of the gastrocnemius muscle of the frog, we have made measurements on the heart of the frog and of the rat. If the lead from the heart is not the most appropriate, it may happen that the electric wave at the beginning of its development is situated exactly half way between the two electrodes, in consequence of which no current is registered by the galvanometer. In that case the instrument does not indicate a current until later, when the wave has traveled a certain distance.

It is not difficult to realize the above-mentioned conditions and to register curves from a frog's heart, which show the mechanogram a considerable time before the electrogram.

For the purpose of avoiding the Eg being late, we injured in the rat's heart the apex of the ventricle over some distance and led off from the point of lesion and from a place near the base.

The demarcation-current arising was compensated in the usual way.

If we might assume that the stimulus, on its way to the ventricle along the bundle of His first reaches some of the fibres whose ends have been injured, then the negative wave, which is formed, would undoubtedly become visible in the galvanometer-curve in its first phase. The demarcation-current would immediately show its negative fluctuation. But the muscular fibres of which the heart consists have different directions and but a limited length, so that we cannot exclude the possibility of the fibres which have remained intact being first affected by the stimulus. It might be that the negative wave was found for a short space at a spot symmetrically situated with respect to the electrodes, and thus the Eg might STILL come late. That this actually happens is shown by the curves of figure 4. For if the mechanogram is registered under favorable circumstances, we may see it appear before the Eg.

By "favorable" circumstances we mean a strong magnification, say of 1000 diameters, and the force developed, the *f* of the formula as high as possible. The latter is accomplished by using a fresh, strongly beating heart.

Time-measurements can also be made with the human heart, the best method being to replace the mechanocardiogram by a registration of the heart's sounds, the phonocardiogram.

In figure 5 you see the Ecg and the apex sounds of a man recorded simultaneously. In the first sound we distinguish three parts, *viz.*, *a*, the initial vibrations being a muscular sound caused by the contraction of the muscular wall of the heart, *b* the main vibrations, *c* the end vibrations. In figure 6 you see another instance taken under the same conditions. The initial vibrations appear practically at the same time or only some few thousandths of a second after the beginning of the Ecg. The most probable conclusion is that the heart sounds actually set in at exactly the same moment as the Ecg, because the time which is needed to transfer the sound from the heart through the

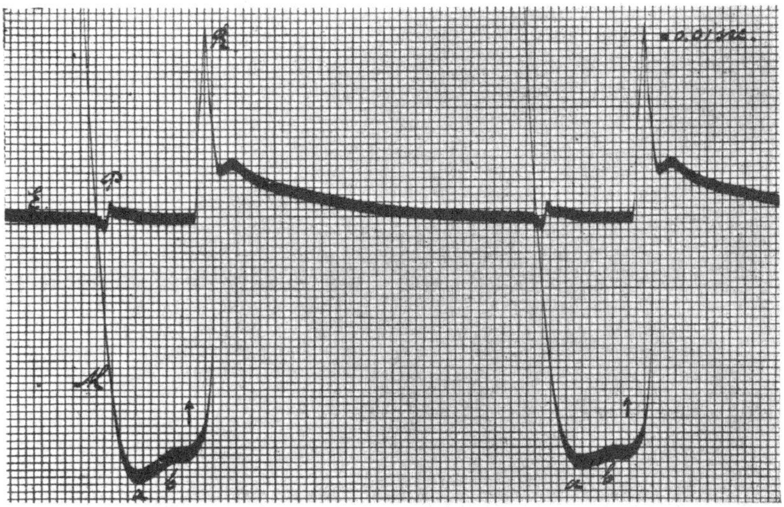

FIG. 4.—Isolated heart of a rat. *E*, electrogram; *M*, mechanogram. The arrow indicates the moment when the upstroke of the mechanogram begins. *de Jongh.*

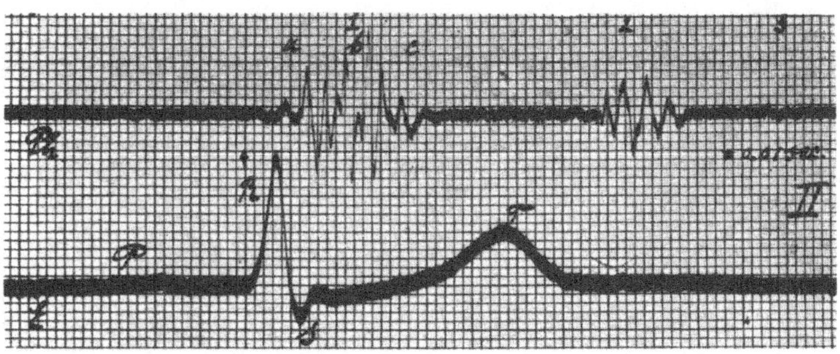

FIG. 5.—*Ph*, apex sounds and *E*, electrocardiogram of a man; 1, 2, 3, first, second, and third sound; *a*, *b*, *c*, the three parts of the first sound. The arrow indicates the beginning of the sounds as well as of the ventricular complex of the Ecg. *Battaerd.*

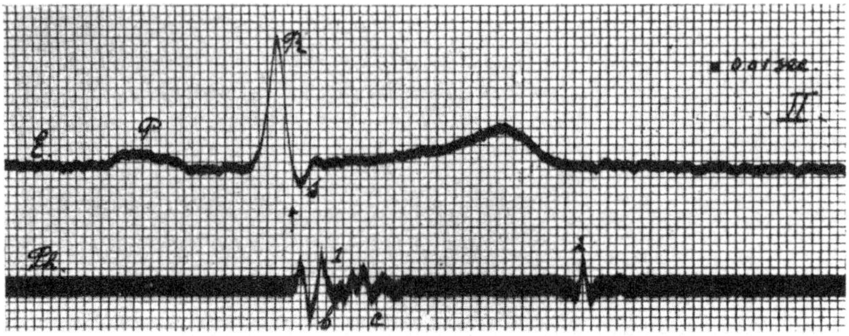

FIG. 6.—Another instance taken under the same conditions as Fig. 5. *Battaerd.*

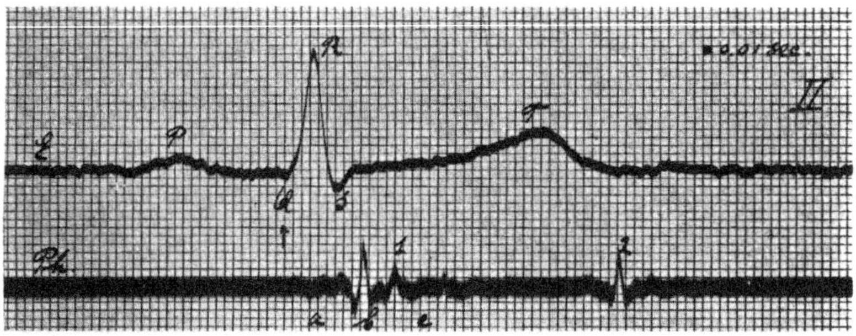

FIG. 7.—Another cycle of the same person as that of Fig. 6, taken on the same photographic plate. Here the initial vibrations of the apex sound are very weak, so that they are practically imperceptible. Therefore the sound is late with respect to the Ecg. *Battaerd.*

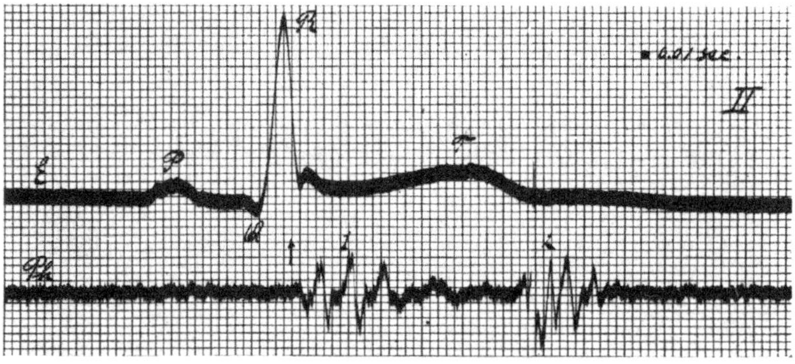

FIG. 8.—The heart sounds are taken over the valve of the pulmonary artery. They are late. *Battaerd.*

stethoscope to the microphone must be taken into account. With our apparatus, in which the sound traveled a distance of about 75 cms, the time in question amounted to 2.2 σ.

If the recording apparatus is not sufficiently sensitive, so that the initial vibrations are not visible, or if the stethoscope is not placed over the apex, the vibrations are late. This is shown in the figures 7 and 8.

Some physiologists hold the view that we, a priori have to assume, that the electric phenomena precede the mechanic ones. In nerve we have an electric response without a mechanic one. And nerve and muscle belong together. Therefore, if we don't find a difference of a 0.001 sec, there may be a difference of a 0.0001 sec. But, at any rate, there must exist a difference.

I cannot agree with this standpoint.

Physiology is an inductive science. Every physiological theory has to be based on facts, and if the facts are not well proved, we have no sufficient evidence for the theory.

There are still three groups of phenomena to be discussed: in the first place the incongruity between the electro- and mechanogram, a lack of parallelism between the two curves; in the second place, *Gaskell's* experiment, and, finally, the attempts which have been made to separate the mechanical and the electrical phenomena in the systole by means of various drugs.

First, the incongruity referred to. It is, indeed, striking, but its explanation is not difficult. We must remember that the conditions under which a contraction can be made visible, for instance, by the movement of a lever or a marker, are totally different from those for the registration of a current. The latter requires the presence of a potential-difference between two parts of the muscle, which, in its turn, must be caused by a difference in composition, in action or in metabolism. The one part may, for instance, be in condition of contraction, the other in that of relaxation. But if the whole muscle is in the same condition, either of contraction or of relaxation, and all local differences are removed, there can be no potential-difference, and the galvanometer will be free of current. We shall illustrate this with a few instances.

The above diagram represents a muscle which is stimulated at one end. The stimulus causes a contraction-wave to run along the muscle, beginning at the place of stimulation and proceeding to the other extremity of the muscle. The current is led to the galvanometer from *a* and *b*. At first, *a* becomes negative with respect to *b*, and afterwards with respect to *a*, and the galvanometer will register a diphasic current (see Fig. 10).

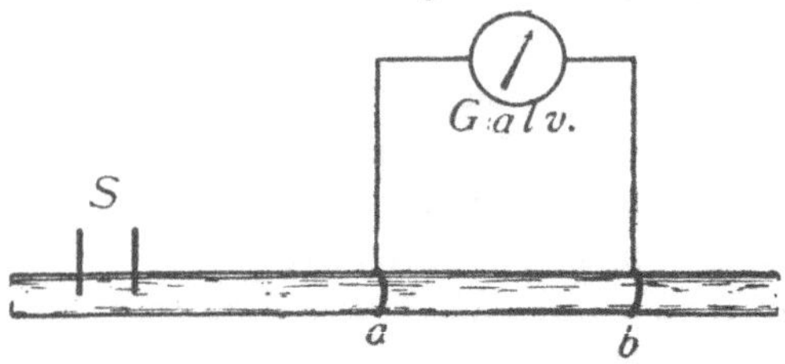

FIG. 9.—Diagram showing a muscle stimulated at *S*. The action current is led to the galvanometer from *a* and *b*.

At the moment when the current changes from the one to the other direction, that is to say, about the middle of the curve, the muscle is in full contraction, although no current can be registered at this moment. Here we have an instance showing how in a definite phase of the muscular action a contraction may exist, without being accompanied by an electric current. In this case the dissimilarity is easily understood and nobody would infer from this that there is no connection between the electric and the mechanical phenomenon.

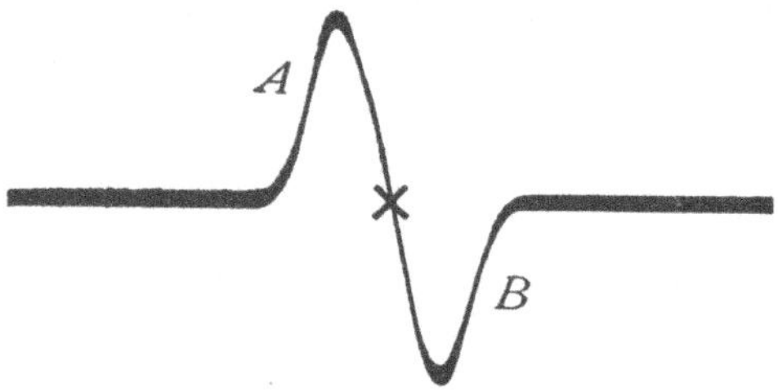

FIG. 10.—Diagram of a diphasic action current. Between the positive phase *A* and the negative one *B* there must be a moment of equipotentiality, although the muscle is in full contraction.

In the case of tetanus, we have the contraction waves blended, the curves of the Ecg and the heart sounds taken simultaneously.

With regard to the duration of the processes there is in general a parallelism that is rather satisfactory. This is shown by the curves of the Ecg and the heart sounds taken simultaneously. The duration of the systole corresponds to the time which elapses

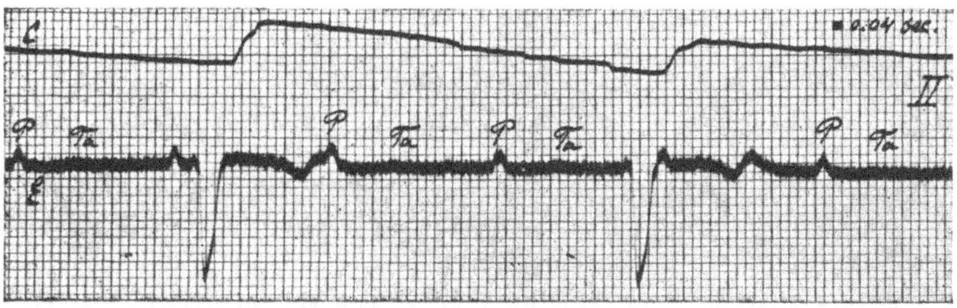

FIG. 11.—*Stokes Adams* disease with preponderance of the left ventricle. *C*, pulse of the carotid artery; *E*, electrocardiogram. *P* T_a, auricular complex. The T_a-wave is positive.

from the beginning of the first sound to the beginning of the second one, and this corresponds exactly to the duration of the ventricular complex of the Ecg, that is to say, from the beginning of the QRS-group to the end of the T-wave.

Sometimes there seems to be no parallelism. Let us consider the auricle which in the ordinary electrocardiograms seems to produce a much too short electric response. But if we have the opportunity to study the true form of the auricular complex more closely, for instance, in cases of heart block, we find the duration of the action currents considerably longer. There often

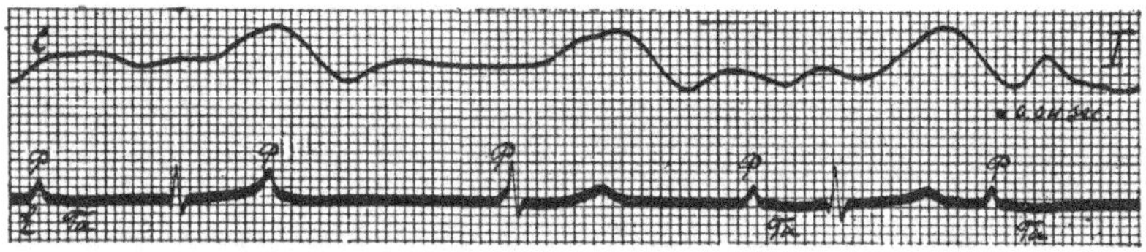

FIG. 12.—*Stokes Adams* disease. *P* T_a, auricular complex. The T_a-wave is negative.

develops after the P-summit an inconspicuous low second wave, which Hering has called T_a-wave. In figure 11 the T_a-wave is positive, in figure 12 it is negative.

Another instance of an apparent lack of parallelism between the duration of the mechanical and the electrical processes is to be found in the ventricular complex itself. In figure 13 we reproduce two electrocardiograms of the same person. The upper curve is taken from lead I. The duration of the ventricular systole is measured from the beginning of the QRS-group to the end of the T-wave and in this person amounted to 0.4 second. The bottom curve is taken from the same person but from lead III. In many persons by this lead the T-wave is positive, *i.e.*, directed upwards, in others it is negative, in yet others T_I and T_{II} are about equal, whence T_{III} practically disappears, as is the case with the present subject.

We therefore perceive here an Eg of short duration, about 2.5 scale divisions, or 0.1 second, whereas we know that the systole lasts 10 scale divisions or 0.4 of a second. The appearance of the bottom curve of the figure agrees completely in principle with the Eg of the gastrocnemius muscle of a frog: a short fluctuation of current, and during the rest of the contraction a nearly straight line.

The similarity is even closer than might be supposed on a superficial inspection of the curves, since also the Eg of the gastrocnemius muscle after the first oscillation shows a line which is not perfectly straight. In many cases an inconspicuous, slow, long-continued negative deflection could be perceived, which may be compared with the T-summit of the Ecg and which stops at about the moment that the contraction ceases (see Fig. 14).

We must return to our Ecg.

During the QRS-group there are phases in which the curve passes through the zero-line, which means that at these moments with a strongly developing systole there is no electric current. The same happens between the QRS-group and the T-summit. The line joining the two, often for a considerable length, coincides with the zero-line. This is especially the case with hearts, whose systole has been lengthened by the action of some drug.

The figure 15 here shown contains at its upper curve the mechanogram, in the second curve the electrogram of a frog's heart poisoned by veratrine. We see the duration of the systole considerably lengthened to 8 or 10 seconds. The Eg has the same length and, as in the human Ecg, we may distinguish at the beginning of the systole the QRS-group, at the end the T-wave. With continued poisoning the duration of the systole increases to about half a minute.

Between the QRS-group and the T-wave the line of the Eg practically coincides with the zero-axis and thus displays a striking want of similarity with the mechanogram. But when we consider what the conditions are, to which the development of an electric and a mechanical force are subjected, we can explain the difference readily. In the curious form of the Eg—the QRS-group at the beginning and the T-summit 30 seconds later at the end of the systole—we may even see a striking confirmation of the view, that a close connection exists between contraction and action-current.

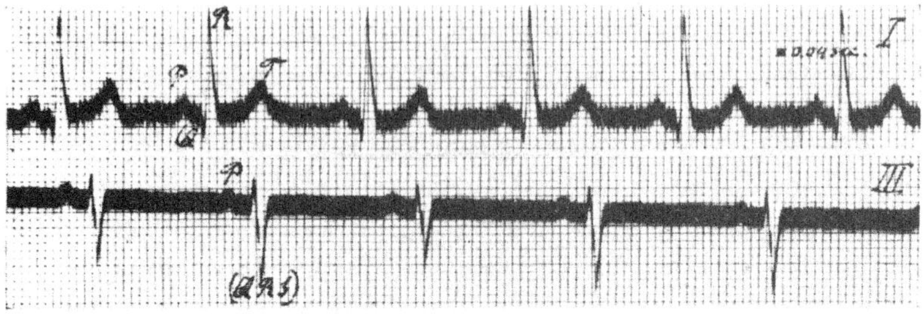

FIG. 13.—Two electrocardiograms of the same person. The upper curve is taken from lead I, the bottom curve from lead III. In the latter curve the *T*-wave practically disappears, so that the duration of the ventricular complex is reduced to 0,1 sec.

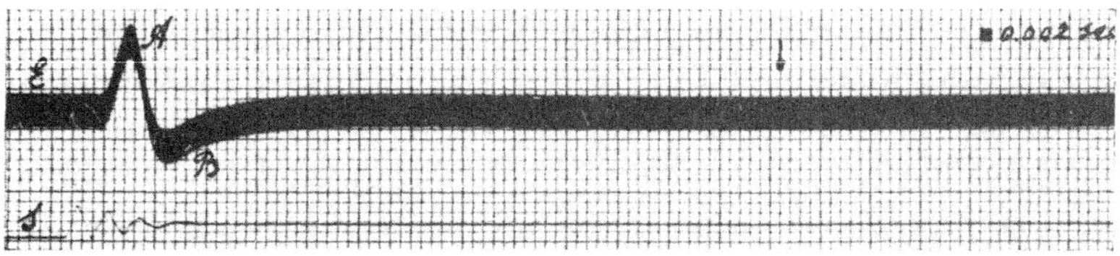

FIG. 14.—Diphasic action current of the gastrocnemius muscle of a frog. *E*, electromyogram; *S*, signal. After the two phases *A* and *B*, there is to be seen an inconspicuous, slow, long continued negative deflection, the top of which is indicated by an arrow. *Battaerd*.

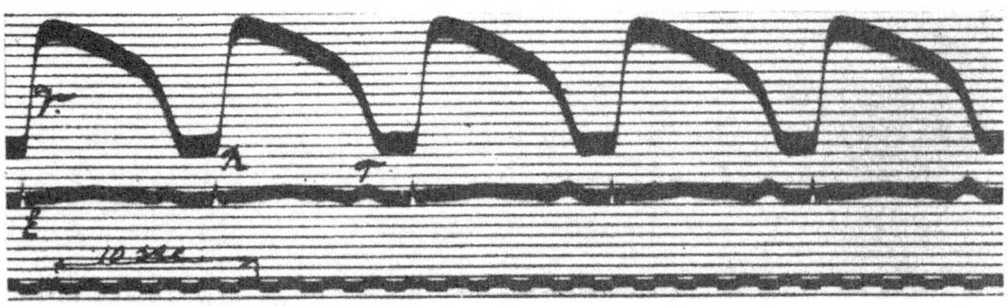

FIG. 15.—Frog's heart poisoned with veratrin. *V*, ventricular mechanogram; *E*, ventricular complex of the electrogram. The duration of the mechano- and of the electrogram is equally lengthened. *v. Lawick v. Pabst.*

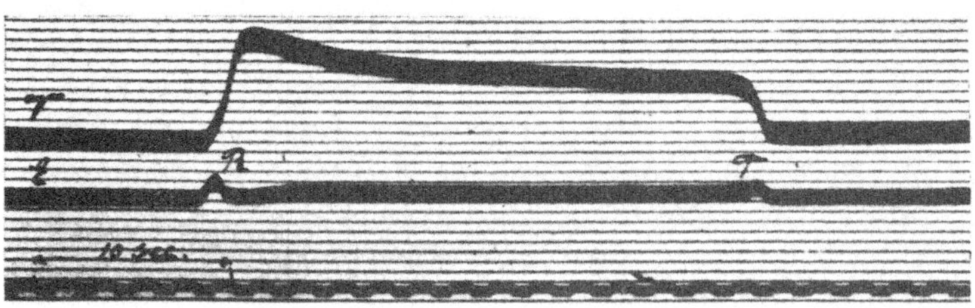

FIG. 16.—Same conditions as in Fig. 15 with continued poisoning. *v. Lawick v. Pabst.*

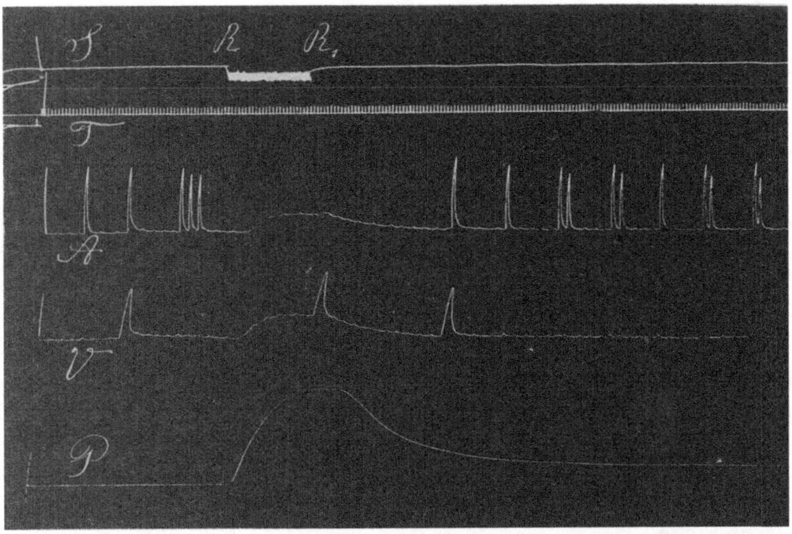

FIG. 17.—Tortoise. *S*, signal; *T*, time-axis, the distance between two vertical lines corresponds to one sec. *A*, mechanogram of the right auricle; *V*, mechanogram of the ventricle; *P*, pneumogram. Between *R* and R_1 the vagus is stimulated. *Rademaker*.

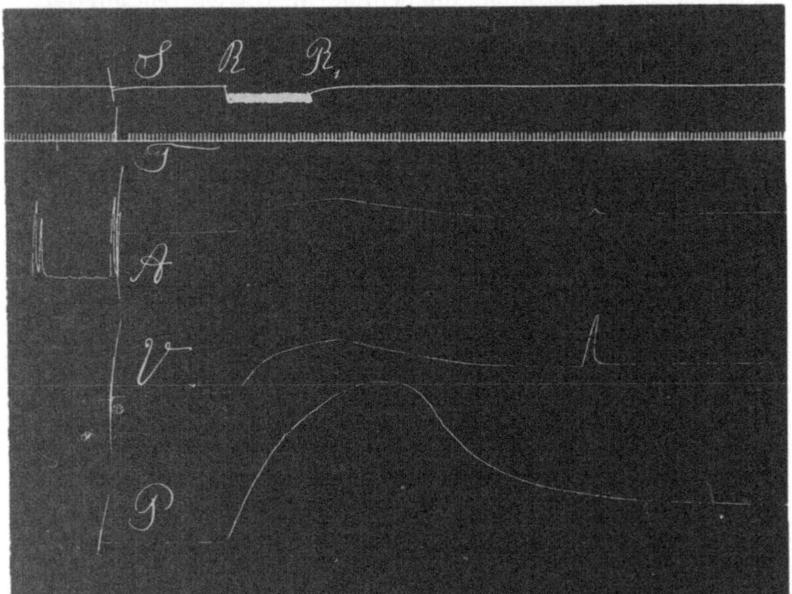

FIG. 18.—Similar conditions as in the previous figure. The heart had come to a standstill. *Rademaker*.

We may now proceed to the discussion of Gaskell's well-known experiments. They were carried out in the following way. The heart of a tortoise is prepared in such a manner that the auricles are separated by a cut from the sinus and brought to a standstill. The apex of the right auricle is drawn up a little and injured. From the injured apex and from the uninjured auricular tissue near its base the demarcation-current is led off to the galvanometer. Care is taken that in separating auricle and sinus the vagus nerve remains intact. Thus with a stimulation of this nerve its effect on the heart might still be expected.

Now what did Gaskell observe? That with a stimulation of the vagus the demarcation-current increased and thus in contrast with any skeletal-muscle, whose nerve is stimulated, showed a positive fluctuation. This experiment, described by *Gaskell* in 1887, has had a great influence and has helped to establish the theory, that the electric current would be the expression in the one case of a wave of excitation corresponding to a katabolic effect, in the other of a wave of inhibition corresponding to an anabolic effect; and that the contraction was to be looked upon as secondary, something independent of the electric current.

A closer examination, however, shows that this conclusion cannot be correct. The cause of the positive fluctuation of the current is to be found in a movement of the auricle. When the peripheral end of the vagus is stimulated, the lungs of the tortoise contract. In Gaskell's preparation the heart rests on the lungs, and when these contract the heart drops backwards with them. The right auricle, which is fastened to a hook by a thread, is thereby somewhat extended, and this extension is the cause of the current-fluctuation.

We shall try by means of a few curves to demonstrate, first, that when the lungs contract on excitation of the vagus the auricle is actually extended; in the second place, this extension of the auricle leads to positive variation of the demarcation-current.

In figure 17 *S* represents the signal; *T* is the time-axis.

The distance between two vertical lines here has the value of one second. A lever is attached to the apex of the right auricle and describes line *A*; a second lever registers the movements of the ventricle *V* and a third those of the lungs *P*. The preparation is no longer fresh, the heart has suffered much, and the auricle and ventricle only beat in an irregular manner. There is, moreover, a block between auricle and ventricle. Between R and R_I the vagus is stimulated during about 25 seconds. The effect on the lungs is seen, and at the same time that on the heart. The contraction of the auricles has been stopped, but owing to the block the ventricles go on beating.

The next figure 18 gives a confirmation of the previous one. In this case we have a preparation comparable to that of Gaskell. The heart has come to a standstill, and when the vagus nerve is now stimulated we see the curves of the auricle, ventricle and lungs ascend simultaneously. The contraction of the lungs in the tortoise is very slow. It begins after a latent period of about 3 to 4 seconds, reaches its maximum in about half a minute and is not finished till after three or four minutes. This exceptional slowness has probably been the cause of the contraction not having been noticed previously.

We now show the curves which prove that an extension of the auricle occasions a positive variation of the demarcation-current.

In figure 19 *L* is the pneumogram, *E* the electrogram of the right auricle, the electro-atriogram. Between R and R_I the peripheral end of the vagus is stimulated. A remarkable correspondence between the contraction of the lung and the electro-atriogram will be seen here. Even small oscillations, displayed by the contraction of the lung, are similarly found in the galvonometric curve. It is true that the similarity is not an absolute one, but we cannot expect that, in comparing two phenomena, the one mechanical and the other electrical. As it is, the similarity is, indeed, sufficiently striking.

In the next figure 20 we have a heart which has been poisoned with muscarin and thus brought to a standstill. The right auricle is again injured, in the same way as in the previous experiment, and the current is also collected from the auricle to the galvanometer in the same manner. Again the corre-

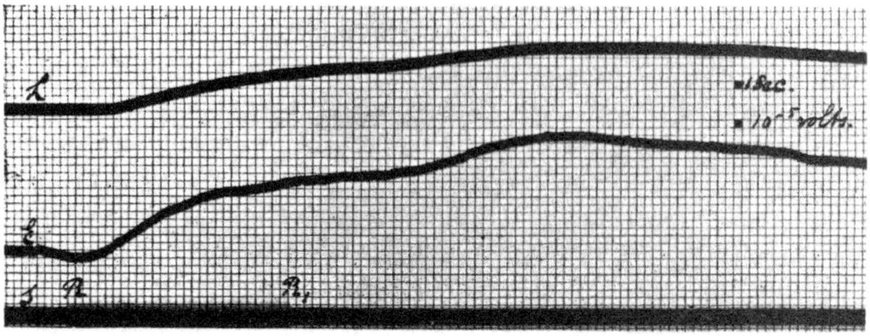

FIG. 19.—Tortoise, *L*, pneumogram; *E*, electrogram of the right auricle. Between *R* and R_1 vagus stimulation. *Rademaker.*

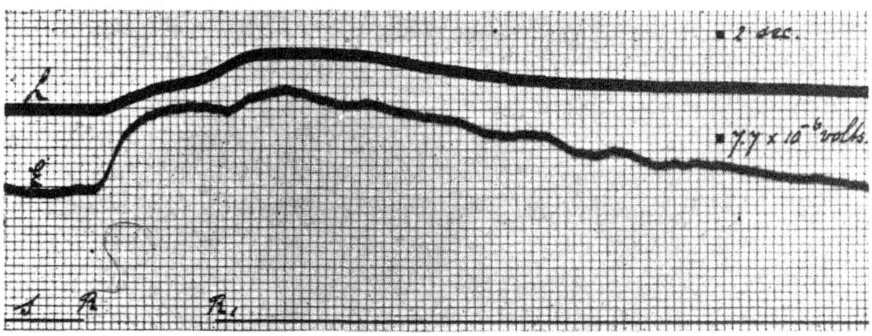

FIG. 20.—Tortoise poisoned with muscarin. Similar conditions as in the previous figure. *Rademaker.*

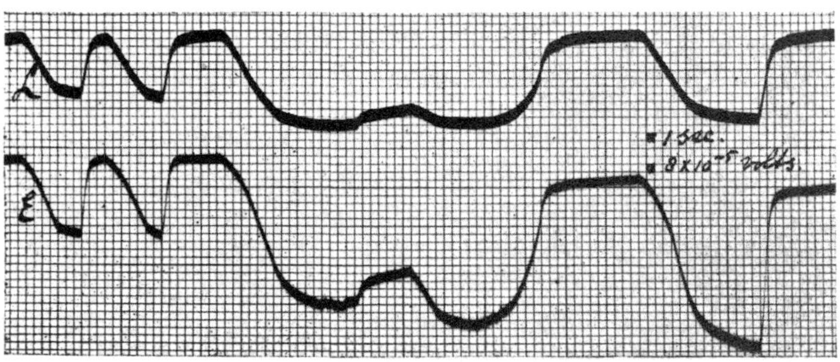

FIG. 21.—Tortoise. *L*, pneumogram; *E*, electro-atriogram. The lungs are alternately inflated and slightly deflated. *Rademaker.*

spondence between pneumogram and the electrical phenomenon is striking.

In the next figure 21 we did not stimulate the vagus, but the lungs were alternately inflated and slightly deflated. By the movement thus produced, the right auricle was necessarily extended more or less and we notice again a correspondence between the variations in the volume of the lungs and the current fluctuations of the right auricle. Purposely the inflating and deflating of the lungs was made to take place irregularly. That all these irregularities are also found in the electro-atriogram may be looked upon as a definite proof that the current fluctuations in the auricle are caused by increase or diminution of the extension of this organ. Gaskell's positive current variation is not a vital process, not an expression of the inhibitory action of the vagus, but a physical process, a physical effect of the extension of the organ.

The curves shown here prove more than the incorrectness of Gaskell's interpretation. They allow the drawing of a positive conclusion. The inhibition of a heart's action by the vagus is a phenomenon studied by all physiologists. There probably is not a physiological laboratory where this vagus-experiment has not been made. The proof is repeated annually in hundreds of courses of medicine or physiology as being equally easily demonstrated as instructive to the audiences. If in an inhibition experiment so clear and easily controlled a *positive* current-variation cannot be demonstrated, we have the right to assume, that neither is the *negative* current fluctuation of a striated muscle caused by the excitation-wave, but is closely connected with the contraction itself.

Finally, we shall discuss the experiments which have made the deepest impression on investigators, and which seemed to be the most conclusive towards proving that the mechanical and electrical phenomena may be separated. They have been described by various experimenters from different countries. It is said that a heart may be brought to a mechanic standstill by injury, removal of indispensable constituents and also by the action of various drugs, while the rhythmic electrical variations continue. Here we have an instance in which the mechano-cardiogram ceases, whereas the electro-cardiogram continues to be recorded undisturbed. A more striking experiment to demonstrate the separability of the two processes can hardly be conceived.

These experiments have reference to the frog's heart; they are easily made, and in the hands of the various investigators have so far yielded corresponding results. There is no denying the fact itself that the marking lever of an ordinary registering apparatus may stop, while the galvanometer quietly continues to record the electro-cardiogram. But the conclusion drawn from this fact, that the mechanical and electrical processes are actually separable, is incorrect. This beautiful and seemingly so conclusive proof is not a proof at all, and the phenomenon only arises through the imperfection of the instruments used and the inadequacy of the methods adopted.

In the first place, attention must be drawn to the vast difference in sensitiveness between the mechanical and the electrical measuring instruments, as universally used. Thus, for instance, the string-galvanometer is many hundred-thousand times more sensitive than the ordinary mechanical registering arrangement. It can register an electric current, the energy of which corresponds to that which is required to lift 1 $mm.^3$ of the heart to a height of 10^{-11} mm. If the weight of a frog's heart is put at 100 mg., we may also say that the energy required to produce a visible deviation of the string corresponds to that of the lifting of one-ten-thousandth part of the heart to a level of one-millionth of a micron. The mechanical recording contrivance does not exist which would approach anything like this sensitiveness. This fact must not be lost sight of when we wish to compare the results.

The second remark which we wish to make has reference to the friction. A mechanical registering apparatus, as a rule, has to overcome the mutual friction of solid parts. Unless the registering is done photographically, the marker travels with its point over the writing surface, neither does the axle of a rotating lever move without friction in its bearings, whereas in the elec-

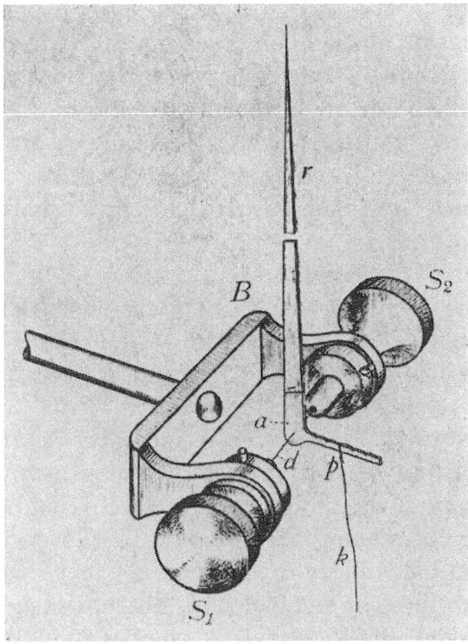

FIG. 22.—String recorder. Vertical motions of the cord *k* produce horizontal ones of the pointer *r*.

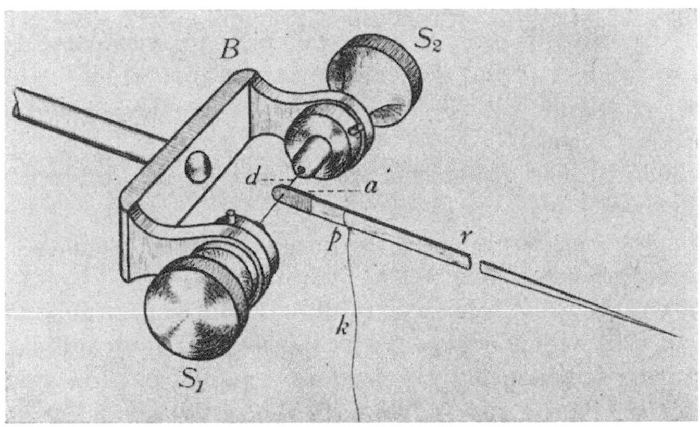

FIG. 23.—Similar apparatus as in Fig. 22. The pointer *r* and the cord *k* move in the same direction.

trical registration there is only some air-friction to be overcome. There is this great difference between the friction of solid parts, on the one hand, and air-friction on the other; the latter approaches zero, as the velocity of motion becomes very small or disappears. On the contrary, solid friction increases as the motion becomes slower and approaches a maximum as the motion reduces to nothing.

In the third place we draw attention to the fact which may lead to a false conclusion and is connected with the heart itself. If a heart is brought to a standstill by poisoning it with digitalis, when it will be in a condition of strong systole, or if it is injured by pouring paraffine over it in order thus to bring it to a mechanical standstill, it remains possible that differences in tension develop in it, which may produce mutual displacement of the separate fibres, but are unable to displace the external surface of the heart and thus impart motion to a lever. Under these circumstances there are isometric contractions in the heart which can produce an electrogram, but not a mechanogram.

When the heart is perfused, the friction of the perfusing solution in the heart will also have to be taken into account. This friction is not sufficiently removed by cutting the two aortic arches or even opening the bulb, especially if the severed parts of the wall should come in contact again and stick together. When the heart is very much weakened, we again meet with a condition that external movements are absent, while in the inside forces are acting which are associated with the development of electric currents.

When all these difficulties are avoided, totally different results are obtained.

For the registration of the mechanogram, we have used a recording arrangement acting without friction. To a tightly drawn metal wire *d* a lever is soldered. The long arm of the lever is a pointer which registers the motions photographically; the short arm is attached by a cord to a point of the heart's ventricle at *k*. At S_1 and S_2 we have the screw heads by means of which the torsion of *d* may be increased or diminished. This metal wire may be considered as perfectly elastic. Each movement of the heart will be thus transmitted without the least chance of friction. We may call this piece of apparatus a "string-recorder" and I may mention that it is very similar to that constructed by Mines.

The recorder of figure 22 registers vertical motions in such a manner that they are changed to horizontal ones. It is, of course, also possible to design the apparatus so that vertical motions remain vertical, as shown in figure 23. We shall now describe a number of records obtained.

In figure 24 are seen the curves obtained when the heart's action is registered in a case of KCl poisoning. The current is taken from the apex and the base of the heart. Previously the apex has been injured, with the object that with each contraction the same regular form of electrocardiogram may be registered. If the heart had been left uninjured, it would have been possible for the contraction-wave to change its direction in the course of the experiment. The form of the Ecg would thereby become variable while the mechanogram remained practically unchanged. Here is another instance of dissimilarity between electrogram and mechanogram, although it does not in the least prove that the two phenomena are not most closely connected. To avoid this we have always injured the apex.

A is the curve of the auricular, *V* that of the ventricular movement, *E* the electrogram of the ventricle.

In the first part of the figure before the beginning of the poisoning we notice large deflections of both mechano- and electrogram, which on the application to the heart of drops of KCl-solution diminish in height, almost proportionally, until both groups of waves in the last part of the figure become so small that they can hardly be perceived.

The opinion prevailed, that by means of the poisonous KCl it was possible to demonstrate the mutual independence of the electro- and mechanogram quite easily. But the curves show that if the experiments are made with sufficient accuracy, both groups of phenomena are about equally susceptible to the action of the poison and remain parallel to the end.

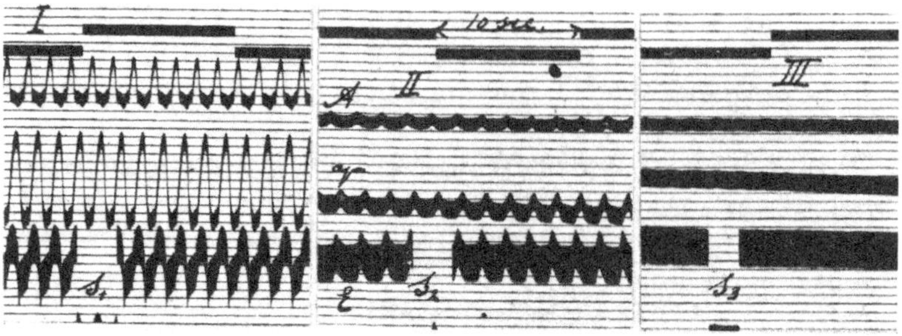

FIG. 24.—Frog. I, before poisoning. II, poisoned by means of a KCl solution. III, poisoning continued. *A*, Mechanogram of the auricle, *V*, mechanogram of ventricle, *E*, ventricular complex of the electrocardiogram. At S_1, S_2, S_3, the sensitiveness of the galvanometer is tested by introducing 10^{-2} volts in the circuit. *Arbeiter.*

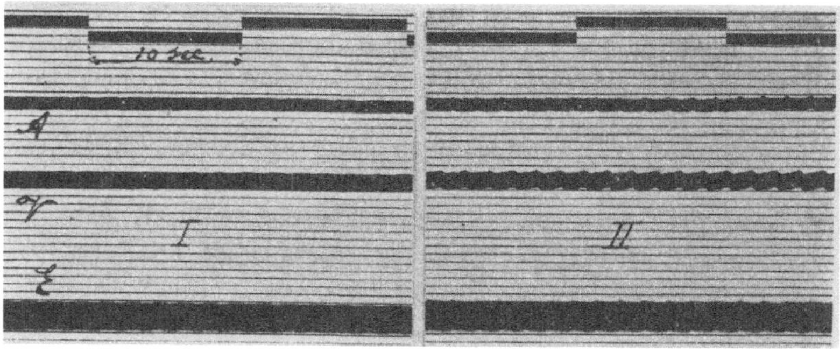

FIG. 25.—Frog's heart. I, after being perfused for 24 hours with a Ca-free Ringer-solution. II, Gradual increase of the mechanical and electrical phenomena on the addition of lime-salt. *A*, mechanogram of the auricle, *V*, of the ventricle, *E*, Ecg. *Arbeiter.*

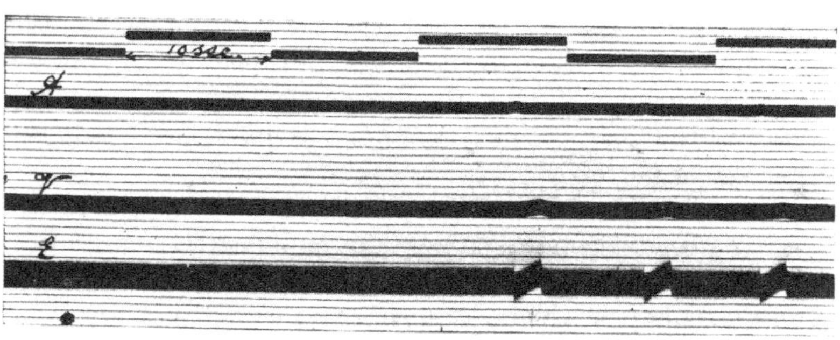

FIG. 26.—Frog's heart. Standstill produced by perfusion with a Ca-free Ringer-solution. Sudden recovery on addition of Ca. Simultaneous reappearance of the mechano- and the electrogram. *Arbeiter.*

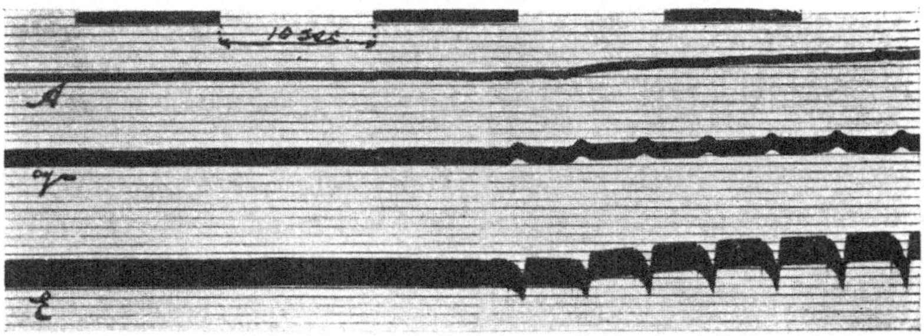

FIG. 27.—Another instance of sudden recovery and simultaneous reappearance of the two groups of phenomena. *Arbeiter.*

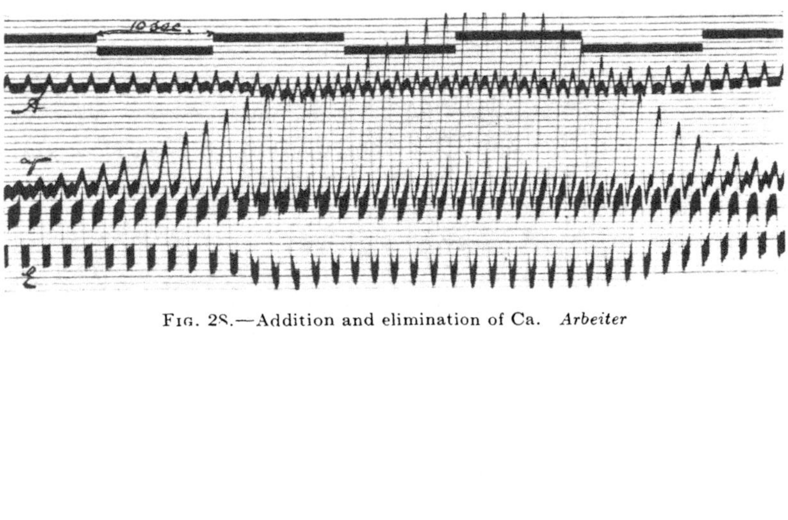

FIG. 28.—Addition and elimination of Ca. *Arbeiter*

On the other hand, it is quite simple to arrange the experiment in such a manner that the mechanogram disappears before the Eg. We have only to make the marker of the mechanical heart-action work with some friction.

Another means of separating the two groups of phenomena consisted in the removal of calcium from the heart. The heart was perfused with a Ringer-solution, from which the calcium had been removed. Soon the heart was then found to come to a mechanical standstill.

Against this we have found that even after being perfused for 24 hours with a Ca-free Ringer-solution the heart does not cease to contract. It is true that after a relatively short time—about half an hour—the power of the heart's contraction is very considerably diminished, and this circumstance has probably induced investigators to assume that the heart has stopped. But if the recording apparatus is sufficiently sensitive, one can even after 24 hours continue to register the regular rhythmic contractions, while the electrical deflections always run parallel to the mechanical action.

In figure 25 a curve is seen in which the mechanical and electrical actions are both very weak, but still distinctly visible, after the heart had been perfused for 24 hours with a solution without a trace of lime salt. On the addition of Ca a slow and gradual return of both groups of phenomena took place, as is shown in the second part of the curve.

Sometimes the heart recovers suddenly, when fresh calcium is added, but always a simultaneous reappearance of the two oscillations will be noticed, comp. figures 26 and 27.

In figure 28 we have a curve in which, after removal of calcium followed by its replacement a diminution of the waves in the mechano- and electrogram can be noticed followed by an increase. The proportionality is not so close as might be expected, but we had omitted in this case to remove the friction in the heart as much as possible. For that purpose one must cut open the apex of the heart completely, in order that the solution may be able to flow off freely. Otherwise, the friction of the liquid which has to flow off through the bulb and the two aortic

XII
The string galvanometer and the measurement of the action currents of the heart, Nobel lecture 1925

Einthoven was awarded the Nobel Prize for "his discovery of the mechanism of the electrocardiogram". Professor Johansson in his statement on behalf of the Nobel Committee,* made it clear that this meant in effect, that Einthoven first discovered the true electrocardiogram (by correction of the capillary electrometer curve and subsequently by constructing the string galvanometer) and thereupon elucidated the mechanism of it. Einthoven's functional appreciation of the conducting system was seen as his most fundamental contribution in this respect, whereas Lewis was said to have shown the importance of the difference in conducting velocity between the specific system and cardiac muscle.

It will be seen from this reprint that Einthoven was deeply convinced of the value of Lewis's contribution to electrocardiography. In fact, as early as 1911 Einthoven wrote a letter to Lewis on June 22rd after receiving the book "The Mechanism of the Heart Beat" (written by Lewis and dedicated to James Mackenzie and Einthoven): " I consider the dedication an honour and also a token of your kindness towards me. An instrument takes its value not so much from the work that it possibly might do, but from the work that it really does. So your discoveries in the field of the pathology of the heart increase the value of the string galvanometer greatly..."

Einthoven's lecture at the Nobel Prize Ceremony constitutes an important review of a lifetime's work. Doubtful or still unsolved questions have mostly been left out. One issue which should have been in doubt, but appeared to be firmly established, was the diagnosis of right and left bundlebranch block. It is curious to see, that the crucial point i.e. that the general pattern of laevogram (with differences such as widening) was associated with *left* ventricular hypertrophy, but also with *right* bundlebranch block, and vice versa, was not questioned by Einthoven at all, but accepted on the basis of the work of Lewis and others (in particular Rothberger). Presumably this was so because the theory of the electrical predominance of one ventricle in the first part of systole under these two circumstances and in ventriculas extrasystoles appeared to fit

* Nobel Ed. Physiology or Medicine (1922-1941). Amsterdam, New York, Barking, Elsevier 1965.

in so well with the experimental findings in the dog and the pathological observations in humans (see ch. 1). Einthoven's observation of a patient in whom extrasystoles could be evoked by tapping on the chest is also interpreted in the light of the theory of laevo- and dextrogram.

WILLEM EINTHOVEN

The string galvanometer and the measurement of the action currents of the heart

Nobel Lecture, December 11, 1925

May I be permitted to communicate something about the string galvanometer, its latest improvements and its use in electrocardiography.

The string galvanometer consists of a thin thread conducting the electric current which is stretched as a string in a magnetic field. The thread, as soon as the current passes through it, is displaced from its position of equilibrium in a direction at right angles to the direction of the lines of magnetic force. The amount of displacement is proportional to the strength of the current passing through the thread, so that this current can be easily and accurately measured.

The less the tension in the thread, the weaker are the currents which are adequate to cause a visible displacement. But, if the current sensitivity is in this way increased, the string movements are at the same time slowed down, whilst in most uses of the instrument, one has to deal with rapid variations in the current. To assess the usefulness of the instrument, we therefore introduce instead of current sensitivity the concept of normal sensitivity and define this as the sensitivity at a certain arbitrarily established, constant duration of the deviation of the string. In more precise form we write

$$G = \frac{u}{T^2\sqrt{A}}$$

in which G is the normal sensitivity and A that strength of current which causes the deviation u . T is the natural frequency of the freely oscillating string.

We assume that the movements of the string are damped down and u is the permanent deviation for a constant current. But T is the frequency which would be present if the damping down were removed.

In the string galvanometer the normal sensitivity is conditioned by the magnification v, the field strength H, the mass M of the string and the characteristics of the material of which the string is made, thus

$$G' = \frac{vH}{\sqrt{mwM}} \times \text{constant}$$

The quality of the material is rendered by mw, if m = the mass and w the resistance of the string per cm of length. If H is expressed in gauss, m and M in grams, and w in ohms, the constant equals 1/320.

The normal sensitivity of a string galvanometer can be made 1000 times greater than that of the most sensitive mirror galvanometer.

In order to increase the normal sensitivity one must select a favourable material for the manufacture of the string, use a high magnification and a strong field, and finally reduce the mass M of the string.

The possible improvement of the material soon reaches a limit and this also applies to the increase of the magnification and of the magnetic field used. A suitable electromagnet with a field of about 20,000 gauss can be constructed without special difficulty; it will however hardly be deemed possible to build a galvanometer with a field ten times bigger than this. The cost would be in any event disproportionately high.

If we now consider the mass M of the string and restrict ourselves to strings of a certain constant length, we then see from the formula that the normal sensitivity is inversely proportional to the diameter of the string. We must therefore make the string as thin as possible, only reaching the limit when it is so thin that the observation and reproduction of it are connected with difficulties.

While in many of the instruments in use for the most diverse purposes the string is 2 or 3 μ thick it is however possible to use strings of 0.1 μ diameter and still thinner ones with good results. The figure below (Fig. 1) shows a thin string which was photographed at a magnification of 1800. Its diameter could not be accurately measured. But there were good grounds to estimate this as 0.04 μ, i.e. about 15 times smaller than the wavelength of yellow light and nevertheless it was possible to obtain a photograph which, although it was not rich in contrasts, was still reasonably satisfactory.

A thin string can be induced to move rapidly and under suitable conditions to achieve almost aperiodic displacement, about 0.1 σ. Under these conditions the string is strongly stretched and its current sensitivity is only small. For most purposes a greater current sensitivity is needed, so that it is necessary to slacken the string. But then one encounters the difficulty of air-damping which in such a thin string is troublesome and inhibits the movement of the string excessively.

Engineer W. F. Einthoven has therefore made a model in which the string lies in a vacuum and this is specially suitable for the use of very thin strings. We obtained with this model with a string about 2 cm long and 0.1–0.2 μ thick and a magnification of the image of the string of 1800 times, a displacement of 1 mm in 0.01 sec for a current of 10^{-11} A. This corresponds to an unparalleled normal sensitivity and one could think that these conditions would be uncommonly suitable for the study of the small variations of current which play so great a role in physiology and medicine.

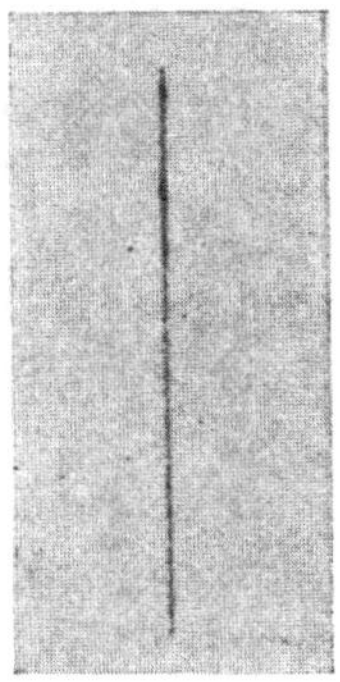

Fig. 1. A string the diameter of which is estimated to be of the order of 0.04μ.

There is however an insurmountable difficulty. The string does not remain still. Molecular movements due to the temperature cause the whole string to remain in continuous movement. These movements could be named Brownian string vibrations. If one puts the mean energy of a molecule at a certain temperature at $\frac{1}{2}\, m\, v^2$, the string movement which corresponds to one degree of freedom at the same temperature has a mean energy of $\frac{1}{6}\, m\, v^2$. In fact, one obtains about this amount if one calculates the mean energy from the mass of the string and the movement actually observed.

In a high vacuum the string oscillates very regularly with its natural frequency; if a little air enters the movements become irregular. It is self-evident that the air cannot damp down the movements of the string because the movement of the air molecules is itself the cause of the movements of the string. If the string is strongly stretched, its natural frequency is high but the amplitude of the oscillations is small. If one reduces the tension of the string

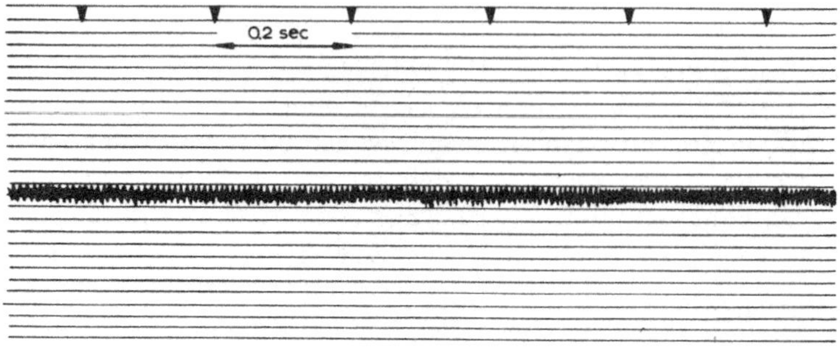

Fig. 2. Brownian string vibrations magnified about 2,000 times. The string is 18 mm long and has a diameter of less than 0.2 μ and a resistance of 250,000 ohm. High vacuum. No field-magnet current. The string-circuit is open.

its natural frequency will be lower, but at the same time the amplitude of the oscillations is greater to such an extent that the mean energy of the string's movement remains unchanged.

If the string is in a strong magnetic field and in a closed electrical circuit the usual string movements will be electromagnetically damped down. They induce currents in the circuit outside the galvanometer and must transmit heat there.

Since one might at first sight perhaps think that the Brownian string vibrations had the same result it will appear that here we have a case of « perpetuum mobile » of the second kind. Then, if the circuit is closed by an external resistance, this would be warmed even if its temperature were warmer than that of the galvanometer.

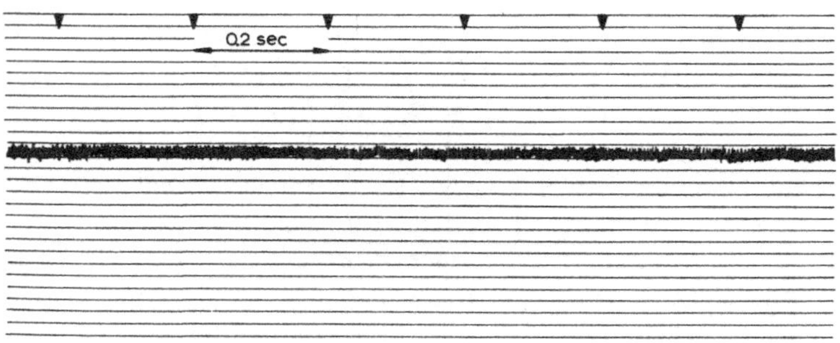

Fig. 3. Air pressure 100 μ Hg. Otherwise as in Fig. 2.

The Brownian string vibrations are made irregular by electromagnetic influences, but in fact they experience no trace of damping. The explanation of the phenomenon is found if one takes into account the thermal movements of the electrons in the circuit. These cause Brownian currents which can neither increase nor reduce the Brownian string vibrations.

We thus see that measurement of weak currents with thin strings is in practice limited. But if one has to deal with stronger currents which can cause a sufficiently large displacement of a strongly stretched string, the thinnest string is the best because one reaches with it the greatest normal sensitivity.

The string galvanometer is within the limits mentioned useful for numerous purposes. For wireless telegraphy a model has been built which has rendered very good service as a receiving apparatus. A short string *in vacuo* is tuned to the frequency of the ether oscillations which are sent from some transmitting station. From the ether oscillations high-frequency alternating currents are obtained by one of the usual methods which one sends through the accurately tuned string. As soon as a signal is sent the string is set in motion and its movements are photographed on a moving strip of paper, so that the dots and dashes can be recorded. Thus one has a recording apparatus which is very sensitive, and its decrement can be made precisely controllable and extraordinarily small.

A string 1 mm long can be so stretched that its natural frequency is 300000 cycles per second which corresponds to a wavelength of 1 km. It is difficult to obtain such rapid oscillations of a material in any other way.

Another technical use of the string galvanometer is the recording of sound

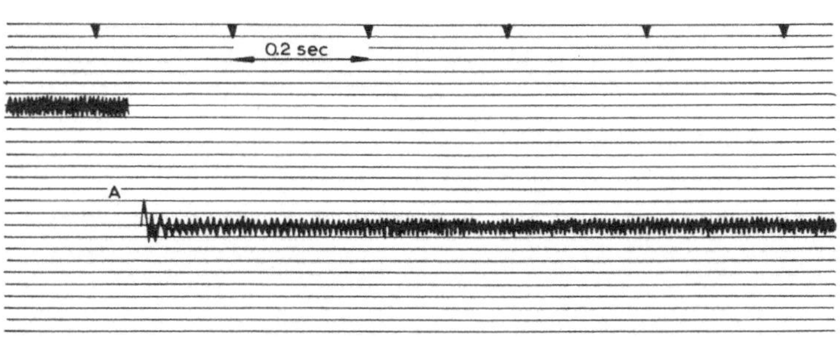

Fig. 4. High vacuum as in Fig. 2. The field-magnet current passes through and the galvanometer circuit is closed. At *A* a constant potential difference is applied to the galvanometer. Otherwise as in the two preceding figures.

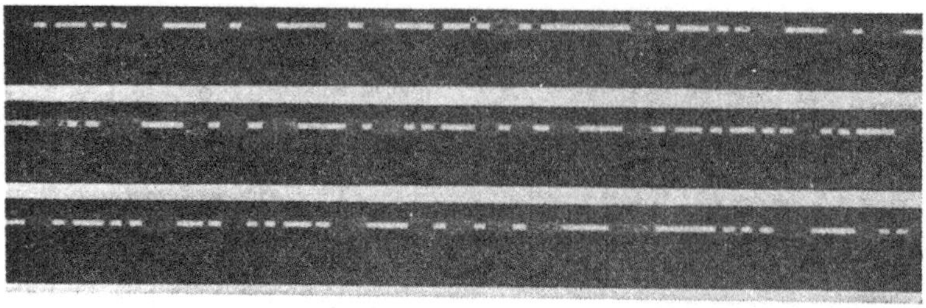

Fig. 5. String-galvanometer recording made in Leiden of wireless signals from Bandoeng, Netherlands Indies. Distance 12,000 km. The string is 6 mm long and is tuned accurately to the incoming waves of $\lambda = 7.5$ km. It thus has a natural frequency of 40,000 whole oscillations per sec. The dots and dashes of the signals are clearly seen in the figure.

waves which can by means of the telephone or microphone set the string in oscillations. One has made full use of the instrument in locating the source of the sound.

In physiology the string galvanometer has been used with success for recording muscle, nerve and skin currents and also those of sense organs.

We mention also the psychogalvanic reflex phenomenon, the heart sounds and the action currents of the heart, and must discuss the latter in further detail.

Just as each muscle when it contracts generates an electric current, so the heart develops electricity at each systole. This was first described by Kölliker and Müller. The English physiologist Augustus D. Waller then showed that the differences in potential which arise in the heart are transmitted to various parts of the body and that with a sensitive measuring instrument, the capillary electrometer, variations in potential in the human heart can be observed. One needs only lead the current from the hands and feet to the measuring instrument in order to see the variations of the current which show the same rhythm as that shown by the heart's action.

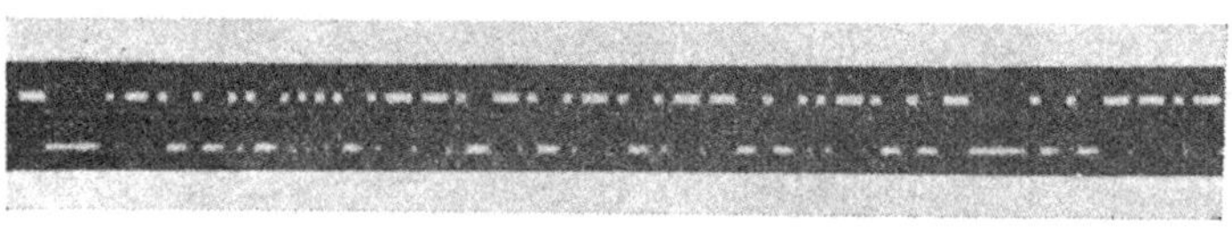

Fig. 6. Reception of wireless signals from an arc transmitter with two galvanometers. The string of one is tuned to the working wavelength and that of the other to the wavelength used when not transmitting signals. Whilst one string oscillates the other remains quiescent and vice versa.

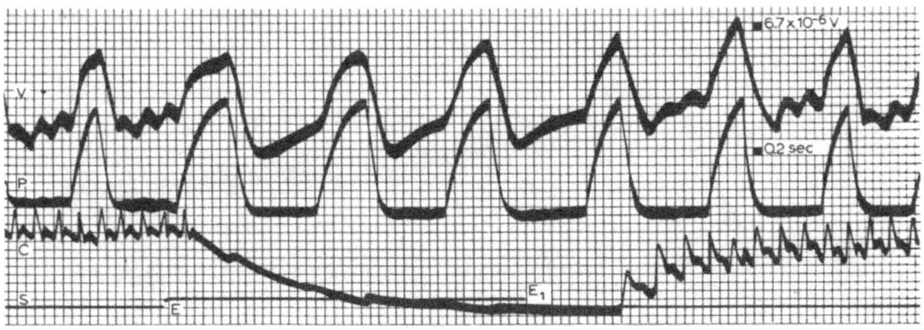

Fig. 7. Vagus currents of the dog. Recording of the currents from the peripheral stump of the left N. vagus. *V*, vagus currents; *P*, pneumogram of the own respiratory movements of the animal; *C*, blood-pressure curve; *S*, signal. Between *E* and E_1 the peripheral stump of the right vagus nerve was stimulated by induction currents. The heart became arrested. The heart waves disappear in the left electrovagogram, whilst the respiratory waves persist.

If one records the displacements in the measuring instrument, one obtains a curve called the electrocardiogram (ECG). But because of the imperfections of the capillary electrometer the directly recorded curve does not give an accurate picture of the actual variations in the potential. In order to obtain a fairly accurate picture one must construct a new curve based upon the properties of the instrument used and the data of the recorded curve and this takes much time. This stood in the way of the practical use of electrocardiography for the investigation of heart diseases, and general interest in the ECG only developed later, after the string galvanometer had made it possible to record easily and quickly the required shape with satisfactory accuracy.

There was a certain satisfaction in learning that the picture constructed by means of the time-consuming measurements and calculations from the data of a capillary-electrometer curve corresponded in shape and measurements

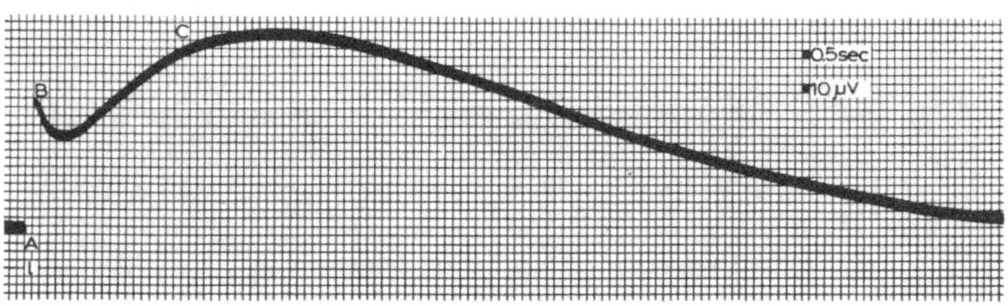

Fig. 8. Retinal currents. Combined reaction of the three substances *A*, *B*, and *C*. Eyes in darkness. At *l* instantaneous illumination with strong light for 0.01 sec.

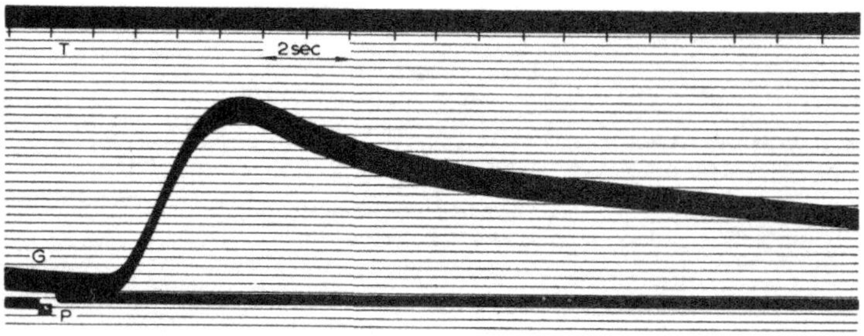

Fig. 9. Psychogalvanic reflex phenomenon. Current lead from the thumbs and fingers of a hand. At *P* acoustic stimulus is applied. The curve *G* gives the resultant change in the resistance of the skin of the person investigated and an upward deflection of one scale division corresponds to a reduction in the resistance of 20 ohm.

with the electrocardiogram directly recorded with the string galvanometer. Because this correspondence signified firstly that the earlier calculations were correct, and secondly that the new galvanometer fulfilled its purpose.

An advantage of electrocardiography over other graphic methods for the study of the heart and pulse is that the ECG can record in absolute units, and the shape of the curve no longer depends on the properties of the instrument used. Provided a string galvanometer is correctly built and is suited to its purpose, i.e. is sensitive and rapid enough, each curve, whenever and wherever in the world it may be recorded, is directly comparable to any other curve.

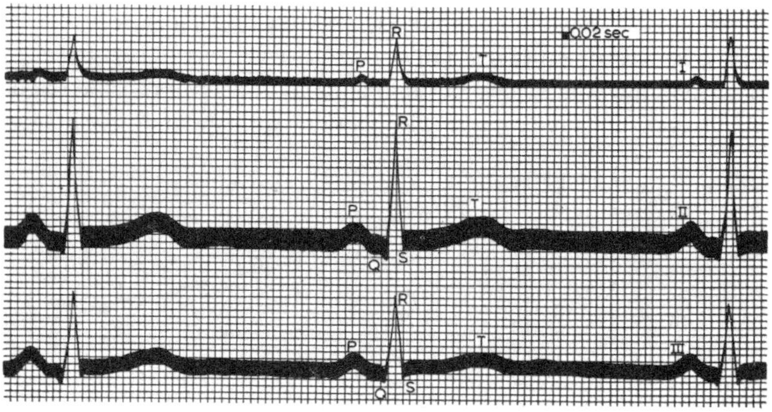

Fig. 10. Normal electrocardiogram taken with three leads simultaneously.

The investigator cannot be satisfied with the fact that he determines the shape of the potential variations at the hands and feet. This measurement is rather the means of bringing to light the functions of the heart. It is therefore desirable to take the ECG by three leads: I from the right and left hand; II from the right hand and the left foot; III from the left hand and left foot. Curves taken by these three leads have a certain relation to each other, i.e. the degree of potential variation in Lead III is equal to the difference in the potential variations recorded at the same time in Leads I and II.

Lead III = Lead II — Lead I

By means of these multiple leads it is possible to measure the direction and manifest magnitude of the potential variations in the heart itself. The technique of electrocardiography has developed so far that it is now possible to record curves with three strings simultaneously. This enables us to control the quality of the instruments and the accuracy of the methods used. For when one can confirm the formula practically by means of the curves, one demonstrates in this way that these curves have been correctly obtained.

What must we regard as the cause which determines a specific shape of the ECG or better: What determines the direction and the degree of the potential difference present in the heart at a given moment?

The process of contraction of the heart is associated, just as is contraction

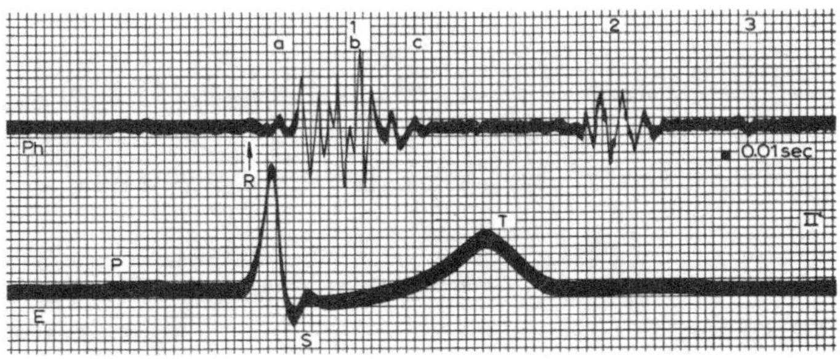

Fig. 11. Heart sounds and electrocardiogram. The sounds are taken from the apex of the heart and are indicated by *1*, *2*, and *3*. The third sound is only weak. In the phonocardiogram of the first sound, one can differentiate between the initial oscillations *a*, the main oscillations *b*, and the subsequent oscillations *c*. The arrow indicates both the beginning of the ventricular complex and that of the systolic heart sound. Both begin simultaneously.

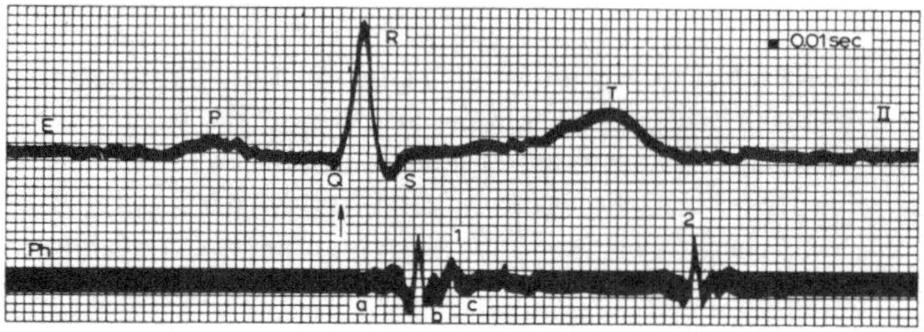

Fig. 12. Similar to Fig. 11. The ventricular complex and the systolic heart sound begin almost simultaneously.

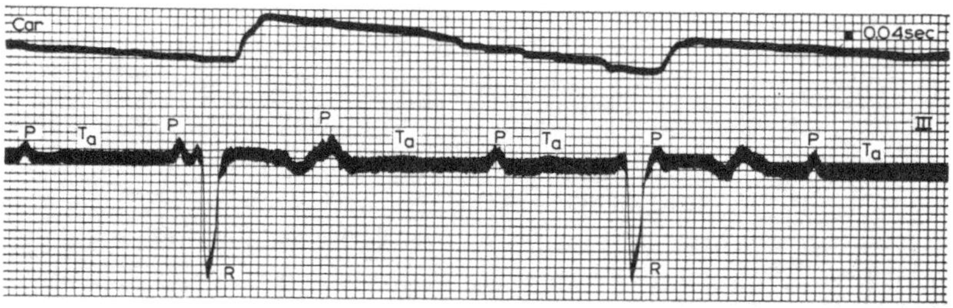

Fig. 13. Stokes-Adams disease with hypertrophy of the left ventricle. A positive T_a-wave.

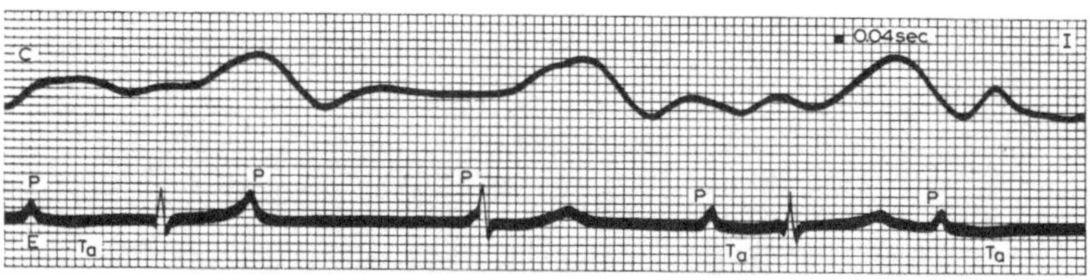

Fig. 14. Stokes-Adams disease. The T_a-wave is negative.

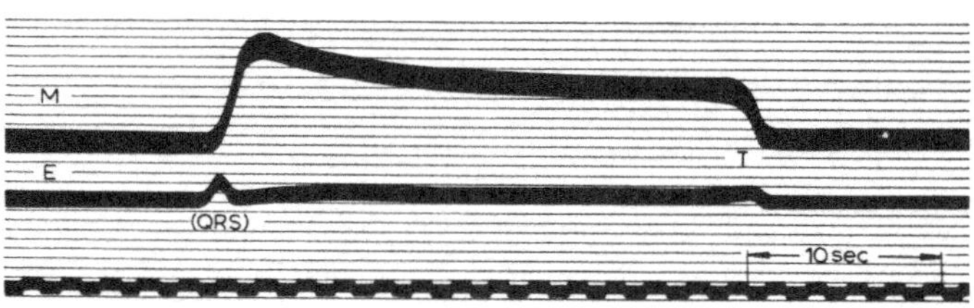

Fig. 15. A frog's heart poisoned with veratrin. *M*, mechanogram; *E*, electrogram of the ventricle. The mechanical systole and the electrogram are slowed to the same degree. They lasted almost half a minute.

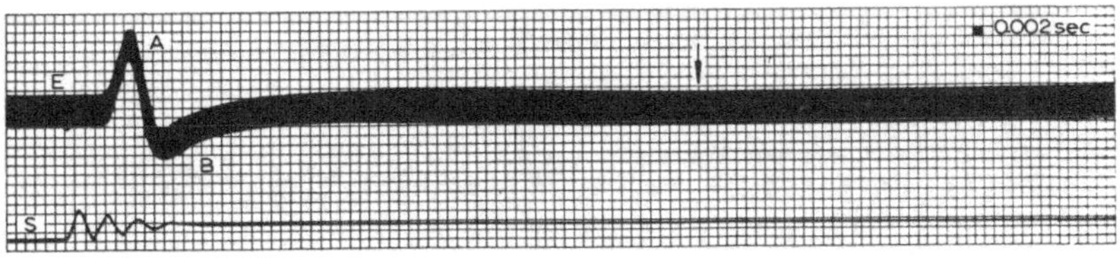

Fig. 16. Diphasic action current of a striated muscle. Stimulation at *S*. After going through the two phases *A* and *B* there is still a late, shallow depression of the curve visible. This is comparable to the *T*-wave of an electrocardiogram.

of a skeletal muscle, with the development of an electrical wave. Still the heart as a whole may not simply be compared with a skeletal muscle. It has a different structure. The skeletal muscle consists of fibres which are often of the same length as the muscle itself. When a contraction wave passes over a skeletal muscle, the locality at which the summit of the wave is found is electronegative with regard to the other parts of the muscle.

The heart muscle, however, consists of microscopically small segments, which are separated from one another by certain septa. So far as the production of electricity is concerned, each segment has to be considered an individuality. When a contraction wave passes over a segment of heart muscle, the point at which the summit of the wave occurs is electronegative towards all other points *in that same segment*. Thus it is for example possible that a contraction wave passing over the heart at a given moment may have its summit

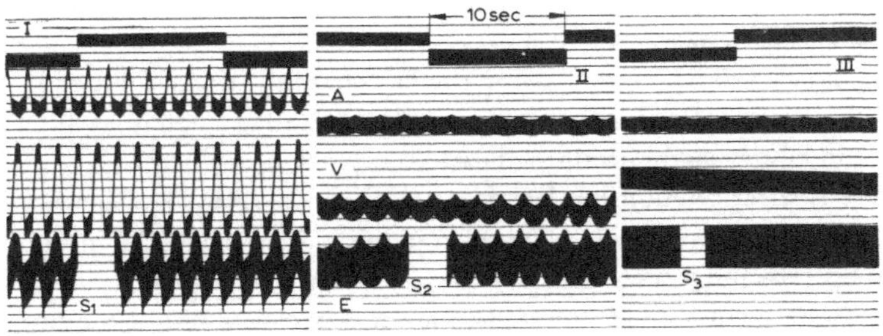

Fig. 17. Frog's heart poisoned with KCl. *I*, before the use of the KCl solution. *II* and *III*, during continued poisoning. *A*, mechanogram of the auricles; *V*, mechanogram of the ventricle; *E*, electrogram of the ventricle; S_1, S_2, S_3, calibration curves. It is evident from the curves that the mechanical and electrical phenomena decrease to the same extent. In *III*, the summits of the ventricular systole, as well as those of the electrogram are just visible.

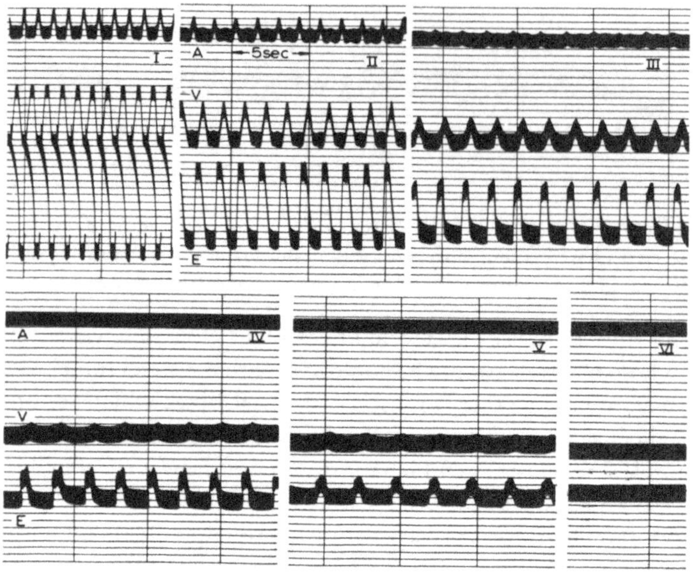

Fig. 18. Similar to Fig. 17, only the poisoning was with chloroform in stead of KCl.

in the base of the heart whilst nevertheless the direction of potential difference measured at the hands and feet indicates a negativity of the apex to the base. For, the direction of the created potential difference is determined not by the position of the wave in the heart, but by the position of the wave *in each individual segment.*

One has also to take into account the fact that the potential difference observed by indirect leads is always the resultant of all the potential differences present in all the segments of the heart.

There is strict relationship between the electrical and the mechanical phenomena of the heart systole. The accurate measurement of the moments at which both begin is beset with difficulties, but in so far as the measurements are made by a suitable technique and an appropriate method they indicate that at the moment at which the electrical current begins the first mechanical results of the contraction are also visible.

Also the duration of the mechanical contraction corresponds in general to the duration of the production of electricity.

And finally there is also a relationship between the force of the contraction and the magnitude of the potential difference produced.

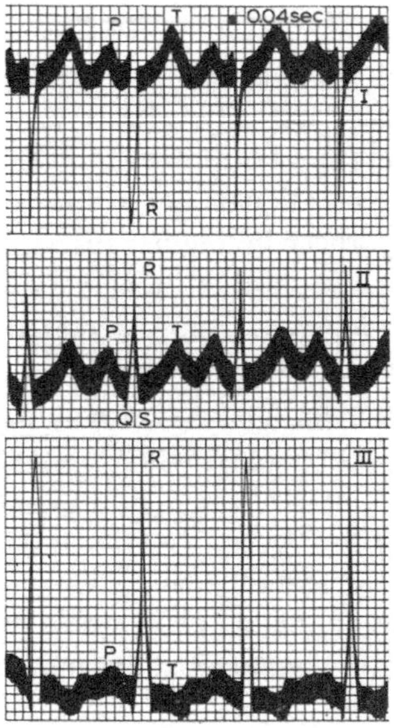

Fig. 19. Preponderance of the right ventricle, negative R_{I}-wave and very high R_{III}-wave. The three curves were taken successively.

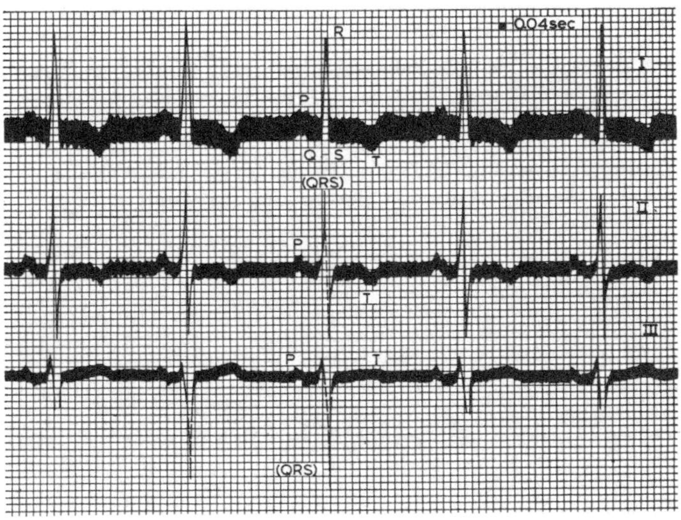

Fig. 20. Preponderance of the left ventricle. Strongly negative R_{III}-deflection. The record was taken simultaneously at the three usual leads.

In pathology and clinical work the ECG has attained great significance because it often facilitates the diagnosis of a disease. This is true for example in cases of unilateral hypertrophy of the heart.

In other cases new light has been thrown on known phenomena. As an example we can mention occasional cases in which a pulse becomes small or disappears in a series of otherwise regular successive pulses all of the same magnitude. Formerly one could think that the cause of this intermittence lies in a heart systole which because it appeared prematurely was so weak that it could not cause a forceful pulse. Now we know that also the premature systoles are of full strength and that the weakening or disappearance of the pulse is due to the fact that in the premature contraction the heart lacks time to fill its chambers with a sufficient amount of blood. A ventricle empty of blood cannot, when it contracts, even if its contraction occurs with full force, send blood into the arteries and thus cannot cause a pulse.

Fig. 21 shows a strong premature extrasystole with absence of the pulse, while some seconds later in the same patient and on the same photographic

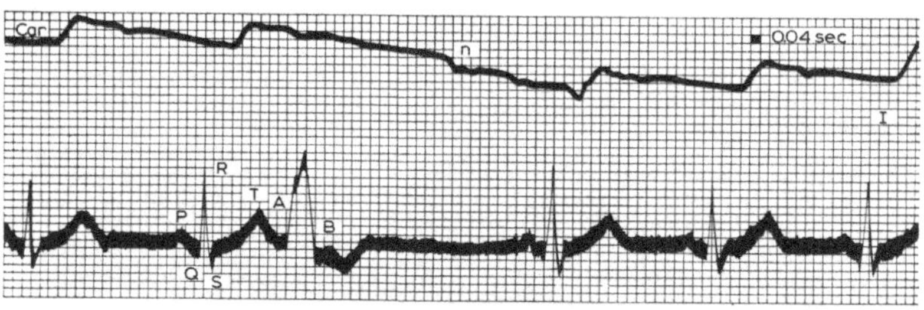

Fig. 21. Extrasystole which because of its premature occurrence caused no pulse. The heart was empty of blood during the extrasystole.

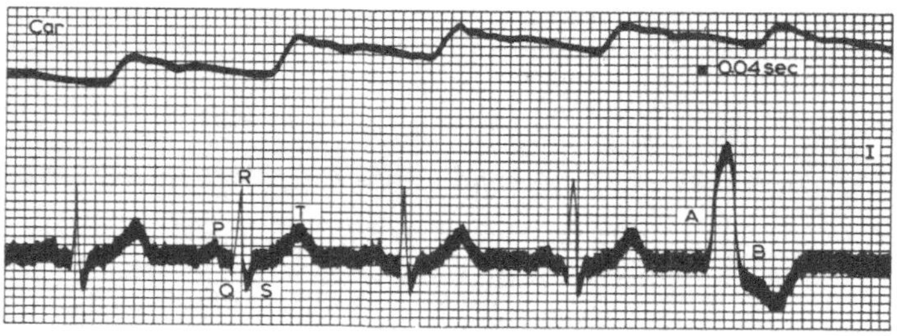

Fig. 22. An extrasystole similar to the one in the preceding figure. Because of its later appearance it caused a strong pulse. The heart had had time to fill with blood.

plate a similar but much less premature extrasystole appears (see Fig. 22). Although in both cases the kind and manner of the heart's contraction was the same, in the second case a forceful pulse was caused. This shows that what was lacking in the first case was not force but blood.

In Fig. 23 we see in succession an extrasystole *with* a pulse and one *without* it. The latter which is very premature is however very similar to the former. The atypical electrocardiograms shown in Figs. 21, 22, and 23 are all laevograms. In the main they are diphasic and in Lead I the first phase is positive as in Figs. 21 and 22; in Leads II and III it is negative as in Fig. 23.

The name laevogram indicates that the curve corresponds to a systole in which the contraction begins in the left side of the heart and passes from this to the right heart. A dextrogram gives the reverse picture.

It has been doubted whether in man a diphasic action current of the heart with downwardly directed phase 1 in Leads II and III corresponds to a laevogram and it has been believed on theoretical grounds that the position may be the reverse. But we have by chance had the opportunity to apply a direct control in man.

There was a hitherto quite healthy man whose sternum had been surgically removed. His heart was covered only by a thin layer of skin. Light tapping on the area of the heart caused an extrasystole. Because the right half of the heart lies in man on the anterior side and thus must be stimulated mechanically by the tapping this must cause a dextrogram. Fig. 24 confirmed this prediction.

It may also be stated that this finding is in full agreement with the theory of the heart muscle segments mentioned above.

In many cases of disease the diagnosis is possible only by electrocardiography. This is especially true of certain diseases of the auricles and of anom-

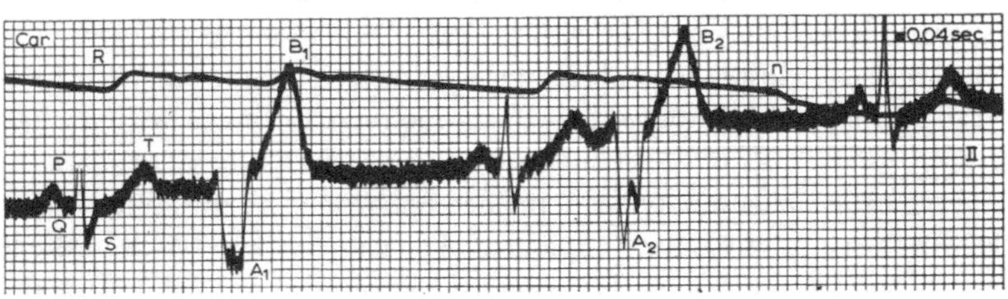

Fig. 23. Two extrasystoles. A_1 B_1 appeared late and caused a fairly strong pulse. A_2 B_2 appeared earlier. Instead of the pulse corresponding to them the record shows at *n* a depression.

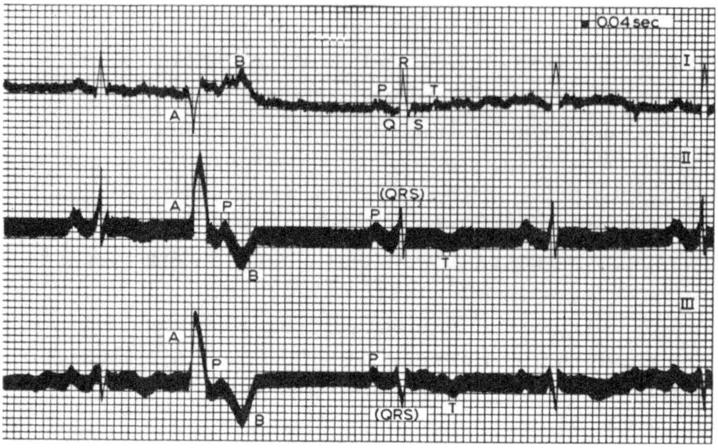

Fig. 24. Man without a sternum. The heart was as good as naked and covered only by a thin layer of skin. A light tapping on the heart area caused an extrasystole. This is a pure dextrogram which is in agreement with the theory that the segments of the heart muscle are electrically to be regarded as being individual entities.

alies in various parts of the conduction system which can nowadays be accurately localized.

I may be permitted to return in a few words to the capillary electrometer. In 1894 we recorded with this instrument an ECG which had a shape markedly diverging from curves up till then recorded, which puzzled us. The oscillations of the mercury meniscus were so slow that the recorded curve must in itself already reproduce *approximately* the variations in potential actually present. Thus a detailed calculation and construction were not carried out.

In the course of 1925 we had the opportunity to investigate the same person who is now 79 years old with the string galvanometer. In Figs. 25 and 26 one sees how closely the capillary electrometer curve taken with Lead I 31 years earlier corresponds to the galvanometric curve taken with the same lead.

The typical heart anomaly has remained unchanged all this long time but what was then a puzzle is now explained. The patient had a block in the left branch of the bundle of His. The ventricles execute abnormal contractions and produce dextrograms. Clinically it is important that a patient can have this anomaly for more than 31 years without experiencing excessive discomfort and this case is for that reason alone well worth mentioning because un-

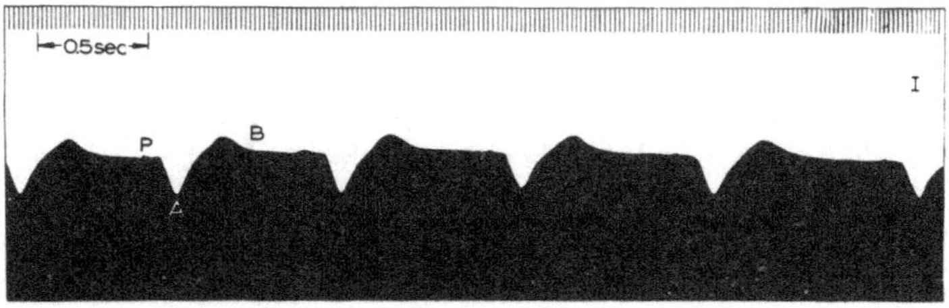

Fig. 25. Record of an electrocardiogram by means of a capillary electrometer taken on June 15, 1894, i.e. before the construction of the string galvanometer. Lead I. Blocking of conduction in the left branch of the bundle of His. Aberrant dextrogram.

til now clinical work on the whole has had at its disposal only experience in electrocardiography of limited duration.

The insight into the true nature of the deficiency has been given to us by later investigators. Among them the English investigator Thomas Lewis, who has played a great part in the development of electrocardiography deserves special mention. It is my conviction that the general interest in ECG would certainly not have risen so high, nowadays, if we had had to do without his work, and I doubt whether without his valuable contributions I should have the privilege of standing before you today.

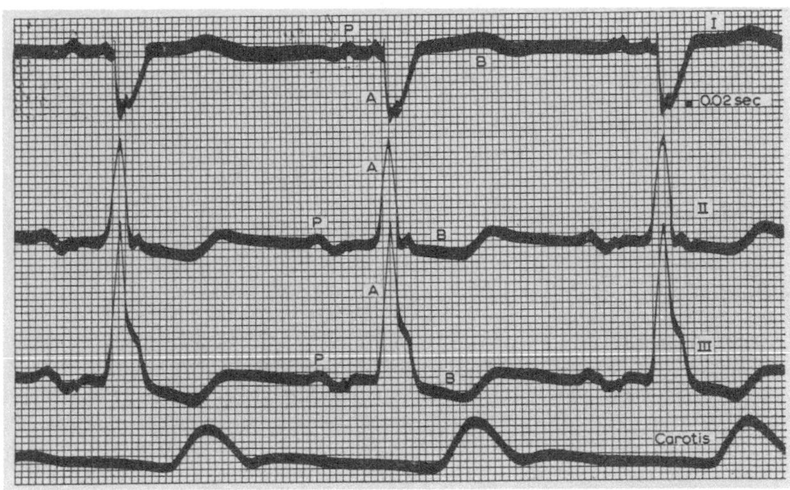

Fig. 26. The same patient as in Fig. 25 but investigated 31 years later with three leads simultaneously. The disease has remained unchanged. One notes the similarity of the curves taken with the capillary electrometer and the galvanometer with Lead I.

But in addition, innumerable other workers in the field of electrocardiography have gained great merit. We cannot now name them all but we conclude with a reference to the happy circumstance that investigators of the whole world have worked together. A new chapter has been opened in the study of heart diseases, not by the work of a single investigator, but by that of many talented men, who have not been influenced in their work by political boundaries and, distributed over the whole surface of the earth, have devoted their powers to an ideal purpose, the advance of knowledge by which, finally, suffering mankind is helped.

GPSR Compliance

The European Union's (EU) General Product Safety Regulation (GPSR) is a set of rules that requires consumer products to be safe and our obligations to ensure this.

If you have any concerns about our products, you can contact us on ProductSafety@springernature.com

In case Publisher is established outside the EU, the EU authorized representative is:

Springer Nature Customer Service Center GmbH
Europaplatz 3
69115 Heidelberg, Germany

Batch number: 10607320

Printed by Printforce, the Netherlands